Case Reports in Cardiology

From the earliest days of medicine to the present, case reports have been a critical aspect of clinical education and knowledge development. In this comprehensive volume, Dr. William C. Roberts, a renowned expert in the field, explores the rich history and ongoing importance of case reports in cardiology.

Through engaging and insightful analysis, the book demonstrates how case reports have provided physicians with crucial insights into rare diseases, complex conditions, and ground-breaking treatments. Drawing on a vast range of sources, from seminal manuscripts to cutting-edge journals, it presents a unique perspective on the role of case reports in medical education and practice of valvular heart disease and analogous cardiac morbidities, including carcinoid heart disease with a rich coverage of heart valve bioprostheses. It underscores how case reports can be used to enhance diagnostic accuracy, identify new treatment options, and promote innovation in the field. In addition, the book provides valuable insights into the process of writing and publishing case reports, including tips for young physicians looking to break into the field.

The book will be an indispensable guide to the history, practice, and ongoing significance of case reports for medical students, physicians, and researchers alike.

KEY FEATURES

- Provides a rich repository of diverse case reports in cardiology published by the editor and his colleagues over 61 years

- Features 65 clinical case studies related to Valvular Heart Disease useful for medical students and practicing cardiologists

- It is a valuable resource for young physicians seeking to establish a foothold in medical research and academics

Case Reports in Cardiology

Series Editor

William C. Roberts, MD

Baylor Heart and Vascular Institute, Baylor University Medical Center, Dallas

Case Reports in Cardiology: Congenital Heart Disease
Edited by Dr. William C. Roberts, MD

Case Reports in Cardiology: Valvular Heart Disease
Edited by Dr. William C. Roberts, MD

Case Reports in Cardiology: Coronary Heart Disease and Hyperlipidemia
Edited by Dr. William C. Roberts, MD

Case Reports in Cardiology: Cardiomyopathy
Edited by Dr. William C. Roberts, MD

Case Reports in Cardiology: Cardiac Neoplasm
Edited by Dr. William C. Roberts, MD

Case Reports in Cardiology: Cardiovascular Diseases with a Focus on Aorta
Edited by Dr. William C. Roberts, MD

For more information on this series, please visit https://www.routledge.com/Case-Reports-in-Cardiology/book-series/CRIC

Case Reports in Cardiology
Valvular Heart Disease

Edited by
William C. Roberts, MD

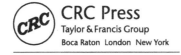

CRC Press
Taylor & Francis Group
Boca Raton London New York

CRC Press is an imprint of the
Taylor & Francis Group, an **Informa** business

Designed cover image: Shutterstock

First edition published 2024
by CRC Press
6000 Broken Sound Parkway NW, Suite 300, Boca Raton, FL 33487–2742

and by CRC Press
4 Park Square, Milton Park, Abingdon, Oxon, OX14 4RN

CRC Press is an imprint of Taylor & Francis Group, LLC

© 2024 selection and editorial matter, William C. Roberts; individual chapters, the contributors

ISBN: 978-1-032-52937-0 (hbk)
ISBN: 978-1-032-52936-3 (pbk)
ISBN: 978-1-003-40928-1 (ebk)

DOI: 10.1201/9781003409281

Typeset in Palatino LT Std
by Apex CoVantage, LLC

William Clifford Roberts, MD [1932–2023]
A Remembrance

As a cardiac surgical associate at the NIH in Bethesda for 2 years, I attended my father's Monday conference regularly. There was a case of a healed traumatic aortic rupture. The fellow discovered that the patient was in a motor vehicle accident "several years before death." To this fellow, WCR said, "Write this case up and have it on my desk by Friday." He added, "It takes about as long to write a brief report as it does to write up the chart. Know the case precisely before going to the library to search the literature." He told the fellow to put the aorta in his pocket to remind him what it looked like. "This is a single task, a single mission." What to search for in the library? "Are there any cases of healed traumatic aneurysm of the descending thoracic aorta." In 30 years, WCR had seen only 1 other, who died 7 days later, not 7 years. This was 1989, of course, before the ubiquitous use of CT scans.

The material for his case reports was this weekly conference in cardiovascular pathology over 6 decades. During these conferences, WCR would personally examine each surgical and autopsy cardiovascular specimen that was submitted—a heart or valve or aorta—and a chart would be created for each patient. He would typically examine each specimen as "an unknown." To him it was a provocative way to conduct the conference. He urged his students and residents and fellows to "remember one thing about each case." To him that was >600 "new things" a year. He believed that studying the case at hand was better than general reading.

In a personal review of his own publications, William Clifford Roberts, MD (WCR) listed 269 case reports out of a total of 1784 publications over a 60-year period, 1961–2022. This sheer number of case reports by one physician in cardiovascular disease is perhaps a record in the field.

As an editor in chief of 2 medical journals, he carefully considered the value of case reports:

> Usually, case reports have only 1 point, and information not pertinent to that point is unnecessary. Indeed, unnecessary words and nonessential details actually prevent clear focus on the patient. Thus, these "Brief Reports" must be brief—no more than 2 or 3 double-spaced typed pages with few references. Reports only 1 page long will be favored over those 3 pages long. Pertinent illustrations may be the dominant element in conveying the message . . . Brief Reports require clear thinking. Each word must count.

In nearly every case report of WCR, there is an illustration or photograph. WCR preferred "drawings not words." He would say, "There is nothing more important than absolutely perfect photographs." In his first 20 years at NIH, he spent every Tuesday and Thursday morning from 9am to noon with a photographer. He believed the subject should occupy "85% of the frame."

WCR graduated from Southern Methodist University (1954) and Emory University School of Medicine (1958), then had 6 years of residency training. For the next 60 years (1964–2023), he focused exclusively on cardiovascular pathology. The first 30 years were spent at NIH in Bethesda and the second 30 years at Baylor University Medical Center in Dallas. He held his weekly conference past 90 years of age.

My younger brother, John David Roberts, observed that WCR was "an intense scholar, but also a loving person. He had both qualities. He was loved for the person, not the accomplishments. One would never know he was a physician in daily interactions. He was satisfied to be unknown. Though in the Public Health Service for 30 years, he never wore the Navy uniform, even when it was recommended at NIH. As a father he required respect, which included "Yes Sir" and "No Sir." Manners were important to him, especially at the table for the evening meal, where each of his children was asked to express what he or she learned that day."

He will be remembered by his family not only for his contribution to the field of medicine, but for his hungry intellect, his indominable work ethic, his high standards, and his loyalty to loved ones.

Charles Stewart Roberts, MD
October 1, 2023

Contents

Preface xiii

About the Editor xv

Introduction xvii

Case 8.   Roberts WC, Rabson AS. Focal Glomerular Lesions in Fungal
           Endocarditis. *Ann Intern Med.* 1962;56(4):610–618 1

Case 14.   Levine RJ, Roberts WC, Morrow AG. Traumatic Aortic
           Regurgitation. *Am J Cardiol.* 1962;10(5):752–763 11

Case 26.   Friedman RM, Roberts WC. Myocardial Embolus—A
           Complication of Mitral Valvulotomy. *N Engl J Med.*
           1965;272(5):251–252 27

Case 32.   Roberts WC, Mason DT, Wright LD Jr. The Nondistensible Right
           Atrium of Carcinoid Disease of the Heart. *Am J Clin Pathol.*
           1965;44(6):627–631 29

Case 35.   Berard CW, Roberts WC, Kahler RL. Pulmonary Arteriovenous
           Fistula and Rheumatic Cardiac Disease. *Am Heart J.*
           1966;71(3):390–392 35

Case 38.   Brawley RK, Roberts WC, Morrow AG. Intestinal Infarction
           Resulting from Nonobstructive Mesenteric Arterial Insufficiency.
           With a Note on Hepatic Hypoglycemia as a Possible Aid in
           Diagnosis. *Arch Surg.* 1966;92(3):374–378 39

Case 56.   Roberts WC, Berard CVV, Braunwald NS. Roentgenogram of the
           Month. *Dis Chest.* 1967;51(4):439–440 46

Case 65.   Carpenter DF, Golden A, Roberts WC. Quadrivalvular
           Rheumatoid Heart Disease Associated with Left Bundle Branch
           Block. *Am J Med.* 1967;43(6):922–929 49

Case 78.   Roberts WC, Kehoe JA, Carpenter DF, Golden A. Cardiac Valvular
           Lesions in Rheumatoid Arthritis. *Arch Intern Med.* 1968;122(2):141–146 . . . 59

Case 89.   Glancy DL, Massumi RA, Roberts WC. Fatal Acute Rheumatic
           Fever in Childhood Despite Corticosteroid Therapy. A Note
           on the Spectrum of Childhood Rheumatic Fever. *Am Heart J.*
           1969;77(4):534–537 67

Case 97.   Ewy GA, Lotz M, Geraghty M, Marcus FI, Roberts WC. Clinical
           Pathologic Conference. *Am Heart J.* 1969;78(2):259–265 72

Case 114. Roberts WC, Levinson GE, Morrow AG. Lethal Ball Variance
           in the Starr-Edwards Prosthetic *Mitral* Valve. *Arch Intern Med.*
           1970;126(3):517–521 80

Case 156. Shepherd RL, Glancy DL, Stinson EB, Roberts WC. Hemodynamic
           Confirmation of Obstruction to Left Ventricular Inflow by
           a Caged-Ball Prosthetic Mitral Valve. Case Report. *J Thorac
           Cardiovasc Surg.* 1973;65(2):252–254 85

Case 182. Roberts WC, Hollingsworth JF, Bulkley BH, Jaffe RB, Epstein
           SE, Stinson EB. Combined Mitral and Aortic Regurgitation in

*Note: Cases are numbered based on their number in WCR's CV.

Ankylosing Spondylitis. Angiographic and Anatomic Features. *Am J Med.* 1974;56(2):237–243 88

Case 231. Hammer WJ, Hearne MJ, Roberts WC. Cocking of a Poppet-Disc Prosthesis in the Aortic Position. A Cause of Intermittent Aortic Regurgitation. *J Thorac Cardiovasc Surg.* 1976;71(2):259–261 96

Case 243. McReynolds RA, Ali N, Cuadra M, Roberts WC. Combined Acute Rheumatic Fever and Congenitally Bicuspid Aortic Valve: A Hitherto Unconfirmed Combination. *Chest.* 1976;70(1):98–100 99

Case 267. Arnett EN, Kastl DG, Garvin AJ, Roberts WC. Clinical Pathologic Conference: A Conversation on Prosthetic Valve Endocarditis. *Am Heart J.* 1977;93(4):511–517 104

Case 274. Jones AA, Otis JB, Fletcher GF, Roberts WC. A Hitherto Undescribed Cause of Prosthetic Mitral Valve Obstruction. *J Thorac Cardiovasc Surg.* 1977;74(1):116–117 114

Case 301. Breyer RH, Arnett EN, Spray TL, Roberts WC. Prosthetic-Valve Endocarditis Due to *Listeria Monocytogenes. Am J Clin Pathol.* 1978;69(2):186–187 116

Case 369. Waller BF, Reis RL, McIntosh CL, Epstein SE, Roberts WC. Marfan Cardiovascular Disease Without the Marfan Syndrome. Fusiform Ascending Aortic Aneurysm with Aortic and Mitral Valve Regurgitation. *Chest.* 1980;77(4):533–540 119

Case 402. Davis WA, Isner JM, Bracey AW, Roberts WC, Garagusi VF. Disseminated *Petriellidium Boydii* and Pacemaker Endocarditis. *Am J Med.* 1980;69(6):929–932 130

Case 413. Ishihara T, Ferrans VJ, Jones M, Cabin HS, Roberts WC. Calcific Deposits Developing in a Bovine Pericardial Bioprosthetic Valve 3 Days After Implantation. *Circulation.* 1981;63(3):718–723 136

Case 458. Borkon AM, McIntosh CL, Jones M, Roberts WC, Morrow AG. Inward Stent-Post Bending of a Porcine Bioprosthesis in the Mitral Position: Cause of Bioprosthetic Dysfunction. *J Thorac Cardiovasc Surg.* 1982;83(1):105–107 144

Case 491. McManus BM, Katz NM, Blackbourne BD, Gottdiener JS, Wallace RB, Roberts WC. Acquired Cor Triatriatum (Left Ventricular False Aneurysm). Complication of Active Infective Endocarditis of the Aortic Valve with Ring Abscess Treated by Valve Replacement. *Am Heart J.* 1982;104(2 Pt 1):312–314 148

Case 497. Waller BF, Kishel JC, Roberts WC. Severe Aortic Regurgitation from Systemic Hypertension. *Chest.* 1982;82(3):365–368 152

Case 523. Roberts WC, Arnett EN, Aisner SC, Techlenberg P. Aortic Valve Stenosis and Left Ventricular Apical Aneurysm and/or Rupture. Real or Potential Complications of Persistent Left Ventricular Systolic Hypertension After Acute Myocardial Infarction. *Am Heart J.* 1983;105(3):513–514 158

Case 531. Ferrans VJ, McManus B, Roberts WC. Cholesteryl Ester Crystals in A Porcine Aortic Valvular Bioprosthesis Implanted for Eight Years. *Chest.* 1983;83(4):698–701. 160

Case 543. Silver MA, Orenburg PR, Roberts WC. Severe Mitral Regurgitation Immediately After Mitral Valve Replacement with a Parietal Pericardial Bovine Bioprosthesis. *Am J Cardiol.* 1983;52(1):218–219 166

Case 633. Lester WM, Roberts WC. Fatal Bioprosthetic Regurgitation *Immediately After* Mitral and Tricuspid Valve Replacements with Ionescu-Shiley Bioprostheses. *Am J Cardiol.* 1985;55(5):590–592. 168

Case 724. Barbour DJ, McIntosh CL, Roberts WC. Extensive Calcification of a Bioprosthesis in the Tricuspid Valve Position and Minimal Calcification of a Simultaneously Implanted Bioprosthesis in the Mitral Valve Position. *Am J Cardiol.* 1987;59(1):179–180. 171

Case 788. Potkin BN, McIntosh CL, Cannon RO III, Roberts WC. Bioprostheses in Tricuspid and Mitral Valve Positions for 100 Months with Heavier Calcific Deposits on the Left-Sided Valve Followed by New Bioprostheses in Both Positions for 95 Months with Heavier Calcific Deposits on the Right-Sided Valve. *Am J Cardiol.* 1988;61(11):947–949 173

Case 806. Mann JM, Roberts WC. "Quadricuspidization" of a Previously Three-Cuspid Aortic Valve. *Am Heart J.* 1988;116(3):889–890 177

Case 811. Kalan JM, McIntosh CL, Bonow RO, Roberts WC. Development of Severe Stenosis in a Previously Purely Regurgitant, Congenitally Bicuspid Aortic Valve. *Am J Cardiol.* 1988;62(13):988–989. 179

Case 840. Dollar AL, Pierre-Louis M-L, McIntosh CL, Roberts WC. Extensive Multifocal Myocardial Infarcts from Cloth Emboli After Replacement of Mitral and Aortic Valves with Cloth-Covered, Caged-Ball Prostheses. *Am J Cardiol.* 1989;64(5):410–412 . . . 182

Case 876. Roberts CS, Roberts WC. Huge, Unattached Left Atrial Thrombus in Mitral Stenosis. *Clin Cardiol.* 1990;13(4):295–297 186

Case 898. Kragel AH, Lapa JA, Roberts WC. Cardiovascular Findings in Alkaptonuric Ochronosis. *Am Heart J.* 1990;120(6 Pt 1):1460–1463 190

Case 903. Roberts WC, Dollar AL. Extreme Obstruction to Left Ventricular Outflow by a Bioprosthesis in the Mitral Valve Position. *Am Heart J.* 1991;121(2 Pt 1):607–608 194

Case 919. Klues HG, Statler LS, Wallace RB, Roberts WC. Massive Calcification of a Porcine Bioprosthesis in the Aortic Valve Position and the Role of Calcium Supplements. *Am Heart J.* 1991;121(6 Pt 1):1829–1831 197

Case 1167. Lander SR, Taylor JE, Roberts WC. Congenitally Bicuspid Stenotic Aortic Valves in Octogenarians. *Am J Geriatr Cardiol.* 1999;8(6):304–306 200

Case 1306. Grayburn PA, Hamman BL, Roberts WC. Severe Late (16 Years) Dysfunction of a Bioprosthesis in the Mitral Valve Position Without Dysfunction of a Bioprosthesis in the Aortic Valve Position. *Proc Bayl Univ Med Cent.* 2004;17(2):214 203

Case 1335. Farooq H, Grayburn P, Roberts WC. Severe Regurgitation Immediately After Replacement of a Dysfunctional Bioprosthesis in the Mitral Valve Position. *Am J Cardiol.* 2005;95(5):703–704 205

CONTENTS

Case 1357. Theleman KP, Grayburn PA, Roberts WC. Mitral "Annular" Calcium Forming a Complete Circle "O" Causing Mitral Stenosis in Association with a Stenotic Congenitally Bicuspid Aortic Valve and Severe Coronary Artery Disease. *Am J Geriatr Cardiol.* 2006;15(1):58–61 208

Case 1359. Sims JB, Roberts BJ, Roberts WC, Hebeler RF Jr, Grayburn PA. The Heaviest Known Operatively-Excised Aortic Valve. *Am J Cardiol.* 2006;97(4):588–589 212

Case 1361. Peterman MA, Donsky MS, Matter GJ, Roberts WC. A Starr-Edwards Model 6120 Mechanical Prosthesis in the Mitral Valve Position for 38 Years. *Am J Cardiol.* 2006;97(5):756–758 215

Case 1374. Roberts WC, Grayburn PA. Sudden Onset of "Cardiac" Symptoms, (?) Mild or Severe Aortic Valve Stenosis Involving a Congenitally Bicuspid Aortic Valve, and Nearly Normal Coronary Arteries in an Octogenarian. *Am J Geriatr Cardiol.* 2006;15(3):185–187 . . . 219

Case 1390. Roberts WC, Ko JM, Matter GJ. Isolated Aortic Valve Replacement Without Coronary Bypass for Aortic Valve Stenosis Involving a Congenitally Bicuspid Aortic Valve in a Nonagenarian. *Am J Geriatr Cardiol.* 2006;15(6):389–391 223

Case 1423. Roberts WC, Ko JM, Schussler JM. Sudden Collapse in Aortic Stenosis. *Am J Geriatr Cardiol.* 2007;16(5):319–320 226

Case 1445. Gibbs WN, Hamman BL, Roberts WC, Schussler JM. Diagnosis of Congenital Unicuspid Aortic Valve by 64-Slice Cardiac Computed Tomography. *Proc Bayl Univ Med Cent.* 2008;21(2):139 229

Case 1502. Roberts WC, Velasco CE, Ko JM, Matter GJ. Comparison of the Quantity of Calcific Deposits in Bovine Pericardial Bioprostheses in the Mitral and Aortic Valve Positions in the Same Patient Late After Double-Valve Replacement. *J Thorac Cardiovasc Surg.* 2009;138(6):1448–1450 231

Case 1506. Roberts WC, Ko JM, Schumacher JR, Henry AC III. Combined Mitral and Aortic Stenosis of Rheumatic Origin with Double-Valve Replacement in an Octogenarian. *Int J Cardiol.* 2010;140(1):e1–e3 235

Case 1531. Roberts WC, Varughese CA, Ko JM, Grayburn PA, Hebeler RF Jr, Burton EC. Carcinoid Heart Disease Without the Carcinoid Syndrome but with Quadrivalvular Regurgitation and Unsuccessful Operative Intervention. *Am J Cardiol.* 2011;107(5):788–792 240

Case 1559. Head SJ, Ko J, Singh R, Roberts WC, Mack MJ. 43.3-Year Durability of a Smeloff-Cutter Ball-Caged Mitral Valve. *Ann Thorac Surg.* 2011;91(2):606–608 248

Case 1589. Roberts WC, Zafar S, Ko JM, Carry MM, Hebeler RF. Combined Congenitally Bicuspid Aortic Valve and Mitral Valve Prolapse Causing Pure Regurgitation. *Proc Bayl Univ Med Cent.* 2013;26(1):30–32 252

Case 1611. Sarmast S, Schussler JM, Ko JM, Roberts WC. Infective Endocarditis Superimposed on a Massively Calcified Severely Stenotic Congenitally Bicuspid Aortic Valve. *Proc Bayl Univ Med Cent.* 2014;27(1):37–38 256

Case 1636. Roberts CC, Parmar RJ, Grayburn PA, Patankar GR, Ko JM, Hamman BL, Roberts WC. Clues to Diagnosing Carcinoid Heart Disease as the Cause of Isolated Right-Sided Heart Failure. *Am J Cardiol.* 2014;114(10):1623–1626 259

Case 1723. Fathima S, Hall SA, Grayburn PA, Roberts WC. The Mitral Valve 16 Months After Operative Insertion of the Alfieri Stitch. *Am J Cardiol.* 2019;123(4):695–696. 266

Case 1727. Thakkar SJ, Grayburn PA, Hall SA, Roberts WC. Orthotopic Heart Transplantation for Ankylosing Spondylitis Masquerading as Nonischemic Cardiomyopathy. *Am J Cardiol.* 2019;123(10):1732–1735 . . 270

Case 1729. Roberts WC, Grayburn PA, Lander SR, Meyer DM, Hall SA. Effect of Progressive Left Ventricular Dilatation on Degree of Mitral Regurgitation Secondary to Mitral Valve Prolapse. *Am J Cardiol.* 2019;123(11):1887–1888 276

Case 1733. Roberts WC, Lee AY, Lander SR, Roberts CS, Hamman BL. Libman-Sacks Endocarditis Involving a Bioprosthesis in the Aortic Valve Position in Systemic Lupus Erythematosus. *Am J Cardiol.* 2019;124(2):316–318 279

Case 1735. Chalkley RA, Kim CW, Choi JW, Roberts WC, Schussler JM. Smeloff-Cutter Mechanical Prosthesis in the Aortic Position for 49 Years. *Am J Cardiol.* 2019;124(3):457–459 284

Case 1740. Roberts WC, Siddiquiz S, Rafael-Yarihuaman AE, Roberts CS. Management of Adults with Normally Functioning Congenitally Bicuspid Aortic Valves and Dilated Ascending Aortas. *Am J Cardiol.* 2020;125(1):157–160 288

Case 1753. Ather N, Roberts WC. Cardiovascular Ochronosis. *Cardiovasc Pathol.* 2020;48:107219 295

Case 1760. Roberts WC, Kapoor D, Main ML. Virtually All Complications of Active Infective Endocarditis Occurring in a Single Patient. *Am J Cardiol.* 2020;137:127–129 305

Case 1763. Sovic WR, Ngo Q, Patlolla S, Guileyardo JM, Roberts WC. Isolated Mitral Valve Endocarditis with Ring Abscess and Pericarditis in End-Stage Renal Disease. *Proc Bayl Univ Med Cent.* 2021; 34: 403–404 309

Case 1780. Makhdumi M, Meyer DM, Roberts WC. Malignancy-Associated Non-Bacterial Thrombotic Endocarditis Causing Aortic Regurgitation and Leading to Aortic Valve Replacement. *Am J Cardiol.* 2021;154:120–122 312

Index 317

Preface

When these case reports (numbering 272) were sent to the publisher my intention was that all would be published in one or two volumes. The publisher, however, convinced me that the collection of case reports would be too large if they were all published together, and that decision resulted into dividing the collection into six smaller books arranged by subject. I find case reports useful and often they are the first publication of many authors. William Osler published many case reports in the later decades of the 19th century. Today, the JACC has a journal devoted solely to case reports. The doctor-patient relationship is one on one. Most journals today publish case reports, but their name is usually disguised as something else.

William C. Roberts, MD

About the Editor

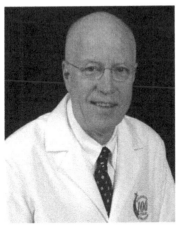

William C. Roberts, MD, was born in Atlanta, Georgia, on September 11, 1932. He graduated from Southern Methodist University (1954) and Emory University School of Medicine (1958). He did his training in internal medicine at the Boston City Hospital and at The Johns Hopkins Hospital. He had a 1-year fellowship in cardiology at the National Heart, Lung and Blood Institute. He did his training in anatomic pathology at the National Institutes of Health (1959-1962). From July 1964 to March 1993, he was Chief of Pathology in the National Heart, Lung, and Blood Institute, National Institutes of Health, Bethesda, Maryland. He has written 1784 articles. Additionally, he has edited 31 books and lectured in more than 2200 cities around the world.

From December 1992 through December 2018, Dr. Roberts was program director of the Williamsburg Conference on Heart Disease held every December in Williamsburg, Virginia. The American College of Cardiology Foundation sponsored this conference for 30 years. Since March 1993, Dr. Roberts had been the executive director of the Baylor Heart and Vascular Institute at Baylor University Medical Center in Dallas, Texas. He served as the editor in chief of the *Baylor University Medical Center Proceedings* from 1994 to 2022 (29 years) and the editor in chief of *The American Journal of Cardiology* from June 1982 until July 2022 (40 years).

He received many honors, including the 1978 Gifted Teacher Award from The American College of Cardiology; the 1983 College Medalist Award of the American College of Chest Physicians; the Public Health Service Commendation Medal in 1979; the 1984 Richard and Hilda Rosenthal Foundation Award from the Council of Cardiology of the American Heart Association; an honorary Doctor of Science degree from Far Eastern University, Manila, Philippines in 1995; the designation of *Master* from The American College of Cardiology in 2004; the Lifetime Achievement Award of The American College of Cardiology in 2016; and the Lifetime Achievement Award for D's CEO's Excellence in Healthcare Awards in 2021.

Sadly, Dr. William C. Roberts passed away in June 2023 at the age of 90, just as this book series went into production.

Introduction

Case reports have had a long history. Many diseases have been reported initially as a case report. The first publication of many authors, including the present author, was a case report. William Osler's curriculum vitae (CV) is loaded with individual case studies on a variety of conditions. Paul Dudley White's CV, particularly his early publications, is loaded with individual case reports. Indeed, he indicated that he tried to write a case report on a variety of cardiovascular conditions to familiarize himself quickly with them.

The physician-patient relationship is a one-on-one encounter. Although randomized clinical trials are favored today, often it is difficult to fit a single patient into these types of studies due to the heterogeneous nature of the populations. Some patients or circumstances cannot be described except in the case-report format. An example might be case #342 included in volume 6, which described a man who was shot; the bullet coursed through the right atrium and then through the right ventricular outflow tract, preventing flow to the left side of the heart. Autopsy disclosed the left atrial appendage to have protruded through the mitral orifice, suggesting that the left ventricle had a negative pressure during ventricular diastole, something confirmed physiologically in a subsequent publication. We recently received a manuscript describing a young boy who was thrown from his vehicle and landed on a rattlesnake who bit him on his leg that was the site of a compound fracture suffered during the accident. The case-report format is the only mechanism to report such events.

Many disease entities have been described initially as case reports: Ochronosis by Rudolph Virchow (1821–1920), sickle-cell anemia by James B. Herrick (1861–1954), and the Pickwickian syndrome (obesity-hyperventilation syndrome) by Charles Sydney Burwell (1893–1967) are just a few examples. Multiple first operations were described initially in the case report format, as well as the first effective anesthetic drug.

Another benefit of case reports is that they provide the opportunity for young physicians to break into the medical publishing arena. They can be used to describe a new facet of a disease or provide a fuller description of an entity described previously. New journals often begin by publishing case reports. (See the early issues of the *Mayo Clinic Proceedings* or the *Cleveland Clinic Medical Quarterly* or the *Baylor University Medical Center Proceedings*.)

Some authors, editors, and readers minimize the usefulness of case reports to medical education. We recently received a case report from an important and established investigator who indicated that he was really not in favor of publishing case reports but that his was "special" and deserved rapid acceptance and publication. This type of comment is fairly frequent.

In more modern times, several collections of case reports have been published. *The New England Journal of Medicine* calls them "Images in Clinical Medicine" or "Case Records of the Massachusetts General Hospital"; *The Lancet* calls them "Clinical Picture"; *Circulation* calls them "Cardiovascular Images" or "Cases and Traces" or "ECG Challenge"; *JAMA Cardiology* calls them "JAMA Cardiology Clinical Challenge"; and *The American Journal of Medicine* calls them "Diagnostic Dilemma" or "Images in Dermatology" or "Images in Radiology" or "ECG Image of the Month," to name a few examples. *The Journal of the American College of Cardiology* has an entire journal devoted to case reports (*JACC Case Reports*).

The present collection of case reports, of course, is not the first. An early collection of case studies was by Ambroise Pare called *Oeuvres* in 1628 (in French) and compiled and edited by Wallace B. Hamby and titled *The Case Reports and Autopsy Records of Ambroise Pare* (in English) in 1960. These short descriptions of patients are fascinating and enjoyable reading. Richard C. Cabot, who started the clinicopathologic conferences at the Massachusetts General Hospital, published *Case Teaching in Medicine—A Series of Graduated Exercises in the Differential Diagnosis, Prognosis and Treatment of Actual Cases of Disease* in 1906. Cabot described 78 patients, most of whom went to autopsy and some to surgery. The collection included patients with a variety of conditions. Cabot's 1906 book led to "The Case History Series": *Case Histories in Pediatrics* by John Lovett Morse; *Surgical Problems* by James G. Mumford in 1911 (100 cases); and *Case Histories in Neurology* by E. W. Taylor in 1911.

In more modern times, several collections of case reports have been published. The most popular are under the general heading of *Clinicopathologic Conferences of The Massachusetts General Hospital:* the collection of cases, published individual books, are variously titled *Selected Medical Cases; Surgical; Bone and Joint; Neurologic;* and *Cardiac.* The latter by Benjamin Castleman and Roman W. De Sanctis presents 50 cases of various cardiovascular diseases studied both clinically and at necropsy. (The gross photos of the hearts cannot be recommended.)

Finally, case reports are fun reading (particularly Ambroise Pare's *Selections*). They are a "break" from the data-heavy multicenter placebo-controlled trials and metaanalyses.

When these 272 case reports were sent to the publisher, my intention was that all would be published in one or two volumes. The publisher, however, convinced me that the collection of case reports would be too large if they were all published together, and that decision resulted into dividing the collection into six smaller books arranged by subject:

1. Congenital Heart Disease
2. Valvular Heart Disease
3. Coronary Heart Disease and Hyperlipidemia
4. Cardiomyopathy
5. Cardiac Neoplasm
6. Cardiovascular Diseases with a Focus on Aorta

The case reports were written by me and colleagues over a 61-year period (1961 to 2022). All 272 describe a single patient with a cardiovascular disease, nearly all of whom were studied both clinically and morphologically, i.e., at autopsy or after cardiac transplantation or after another cardiovascular operation. Thus, the collection is unique. Each report is numbered as it appears in my CV, which includes as of August 15, 2022, a total of 1784 publications (Table 1). Some were book chapters, published interviews of prominent physicians, or published symposia in which I participated, but most (952) were patient-centered studies.

William C. Roberts, MD
May 5, 2022

Disclaimer:

All case reports are reprinted exactly as first published.

Table 1: Number and types of articles published by William C. Roberts, MD, 1961–2022

Article type		N
1. Patient-centered studies		952
a. Single patient	269	
b. Multipatient	666	
c. Nonpatient	17	
2. From-the-editor columns		342
a. AJC (1982–2022)	234	
b. BUMC (1994–2021)	108	
3. Other editorials, mini reviews, forewords, historical pieces (all journals)		67
4. Chapters in books		143
5. Interviews		197
a. AJC	77	
b. BUMC	96	
c. Visiting professors	24	
6. Published symposia ("AJC editor's roundtable")		43
7. AJC in month (25 years earlier) (May 1983–August 1988)		40
Total		**1784**

AJC indicates *American Journal of Cardiology;*
BUMC, *Baylor University Medical Center Proceedings.*

Note: Additional publications were added after this table was compiled, including additional case studies, with a new total of 272.

Case 8   Focal Glomerular Lesions in Fungal Endocarditis

William C. Roberts, M.D., and Alan S. Rabson, M.D.
Bethesda, Maryland

FOCAL AREAS of necrosis and sclerosis have frequently been seen in the renal glomeruli of autopsied patients with subacute endocarditis due to bacteria. These glomerular lesions have been called "focal embolic (endocarditic) glomerulonephritis," with the implication that they were the result of multiple small emboli, which were dislodged from cardiac vegetations and landed in the glomerular capillaries. Allen[1] summarized the reasons for rejecting the embolic theory of the pathogenesis of these lesions and agreed with Longcope[2] who considered these lesions to be of an allergic nature. Since fungal infections in man are commonly associated with manifestations of hypersensitivity to the organisms, the presence of focal glomerular lesions in some patients with endocarditis caused by fungi might be expected. Focal glomerular lesions have been mentioned in four[3-6] of the 44 autopsy-proven cases of endocarditis caused by the higher fungi (*Eumycetes*) reported in the literature,[3,7,8] and all four have been in patients with endocarditis caused by organisms of the Candida species. Nine[3,8] of these 44 patients with fungal endocarditis were studied clinically and at autopsy at the Clinical Center of the National Institutes of Health, and one of the nine showed the typical renal lesion of "focal embolic glomerulonephritis." The latter patient is the subject of this communication.

CASE REPORT

A 26-year-old Puerto Rican man (C.C. No. 02–78–74), who was a narcotic addict, was transferred to the Clinical Center (National Institute of Allergy and Infectious Diseases) from a federal penitentiary hospital two months prior to death. He gave no history of rheumatic heart disease. He was in good health until 11 months before death, when he experienced acute left upper quadrant abdominal pain, and was believed to have a splenic infarct. Shortly after this episode he had the onset of fever which persisted until his death. A heart murmur and splenomegaly also were noted, and three blood cultures were positive for *Candida parapsilosis*. Hemolytic *Staphylococcus aureus*, coagulase negative, grew in one of the blood cultures. The patient was treated with penicillin, streptomycin, and neoantimosan (Fuadin) without clinical response. Five months before death, anemia and thrombocytopenia were noted. His urine showed hematuria, pyuria, albuminuria, and cylindruria.

On admission to the Clinical Center, his temperature was 38.6°C; heart rate, 132/min; respiratory rate, 30/min; and blood pressure, 100/60 mm Hg. He was chronically ill, thin, and pale. Petechiae were present in the lower conjunctival sac and over the right buttock. The heart was not enlarged. A loud,

Received August 14, 1961; accepted for publication November 22, 1961.

From the Pathologic Anatomy Department, Clinical Center, National Institutes of Health, Bethesda, Maryland.

Requests for reprints should be addressed to William C. Roberts, M.D., Pathologic Anatomy Department, Clinical Center, National Institutes of Health, Bethesda 14, Maryland.

high-pitched, blowing systolic murmur was heard over the precordium. The liver and spleen were markedly enlarged and tender. There was clubbing of the fingers bilaterally.

During the hospital course, the hemoglobin ranged from 6.9 to 8.9 g/100 ml; platelet count, from 44,000 to 120,000/mm^3; and leukocyte count, from 2,400 to 4,300/ mm^3. The leukocyte differential count showed more than 50% lymphocytes on all determinations. The erythrocyte sedimentation rate (Westergren method) was 104 to 140 mm/hr; blood urea nitrogen was 36 to 63 mg/100 ml; uric add, 6.7 to 9 mg/100 ml; creatinine, 2.6 to 3.5 mg/100 ml; calcium, 8.4 to 9.2 mg/100 ml; alkaline phosphatase, 20 to 53 King-Armstrong units; albumin, 1.6 to 2.1, and globulin, 5.5 to 6.5 g/100 ml; bromsulphalein retention in the blood, 6 to 16% at 45 min; cephalin flocculation test, 3 to 4+; and thymol turbidity, 13 to 20 units. Multiple urinalyses revealed the presence of innumerable erythrocytes and leukocytes with persistent 1 to 3+ albumin, and "occasional" to a "moderate number" of granular casts. Serial Addis counts disclosed persistently abnormal values for erythrocytes, leukocytes, and casts. Nine urine cultures were positive for *Klebsiella* and hemolytic *Staphylococcus albus*, coagulase negative, hemolytic *Staphylococcus aureus*, coagulase positive, or both, but colony counts were less than 50,000 bacteria/ml of urine, except once when the count was greater than 1 million/ml of urine. The phenolsulfonphthalein test showed 12% excretion at the end of two hours, and the Fishberg concentration test showed maximal concentration to be only 1.010. Thirty-one blood cultures and one bone marrow culture were positive for *Candida parapsilosis*. None of the blood cultures were positive for bacteria.

Two days after admission to the Clinical Center, the patient had clinical and electrocardiographic evidence of a massive anterior wall myocardial infarct. His last two months of life were characterized by a progressive downhill course with congestive heart failure, marked personality changes, slurring of speech, ptosis of the left upper lid, increasing weakness, and enlargement of the liver and spleen. The day prior to death he had an extension of the previous myocardial infarct, and he exhibited ventricular fibrillation at death the following day. During the last two months of life, he was treated with amphotericin B via a nasogastric tube and an experimental antifungal drug (RO–2), without apparent benefit.

AUTOPSY FINDINGS

Necropsy was started 15 hours after death. See Figures 1A–1D. Effusions were present in the abdominal cavity (925 milliliters), pleural spaces (420 and 150 milliliters), and pericardial sac (70 milliliters). The heart weighed 400 grams. The right and left atria, tricuspid and mitral valves, right ventricle, and pulmonic valve were unremarkable. There was aneurysmal dilatation of an infarct, 5 by 3.5 by 0.2 centimeters, in the anterior wall of the left ventricle. The left anterior descending coronary artery was totally occluded just proximal to the myocardial infarct. A soft, friable, greyish vegetation was present on the ventricular aspect of each of the three cusps of the aortic valve (Figures 1A and 1B). The largest vegetation measured 2 centimeters in longest diameter.

The kidneys (Figure 2A) were enlarged; the left weighed 190 grams, and the right, 180 grams. The surface of each kidney was glistening, greyish purple, and smooth, except for two focal indentations in the right kidney. No petechiae were noted on the surfaces. On section, the corticomedullary junctions were well delineated. The ureters were widely patent. The large renal arteries and veins were free of atheromata and of emboli.

The spleen weighed 1,000 grams and contained several infarcts. The liver weighed 3,650 grams and, on section, had a nutmeg appearance. There was marked generalized lymphadenopathy. The left internal iliac and left femoral arteries were

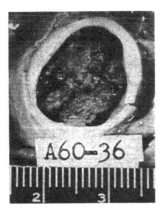

Figure 1A Aortic valve viewed from above. The large vegetations almost totally occlude the aortic valve orifice.

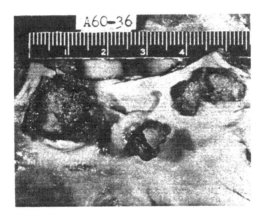

Figure 1B Aortic valve opened. Note the presence of a vegetation on the ventricular aspect of each of the cusps of the aortic valve.

occluded by soft yellow emboli. Cultures were taken of the aortic valve vegetation, spleen, liver, hilar lymph node, and left femoral artery and all grew *C. parapsilosis*.

Microscopically, Candida organisms were identified in the aortic valve vegetations, left anterior descending coronary artery, myocardial infarct, left femoral artery, and brain. The vegetations consisted of eosinophilic and basophilic debris, fibrous tissue, and large colonies of Candida organisms (Figures 1C and 1D). The left anterior descending coronary artery was totally occluded except for a small organizing channel which contained Candida organisms. Sections of the myocardial infarct disclosed that the myocardial fibers were largely replaced by fibrous tissue, which contained macrophages, lymphocytes, plasma cells, fibroblasts, Langhans type giant cells, and a few Candida organisms.

In the sections from the kidneys, there were focal areas of fibrinoid necrosis and fibrosis in numerous glomeruli (Figures 2B–2D). Some of the glomeruli were completely hyalinized. Approximately 90% of the glomeruli were involved in some manner by the fibrinous and fibrous processes. No abnormalities were noted in the uninvolved glomeruli or in the uninvolved portions of the affected glomeruli. The diseased portions of the glomeruli were frequently adherent to Bowman's capsule.

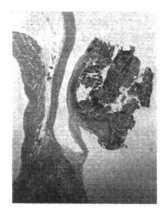

Figure 1C Photomicrograph of section through the largest vegetation illustrated in Figure 1B. The darker areas in the vegetation represent collections of Candida organisms. Note that the sinus of Valsalva is free of vegetation. Gomori's methenamine silver stain, × 10.

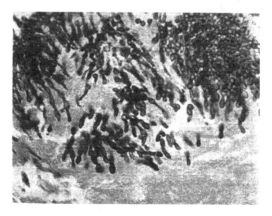

Figure 1D Photomicrograph (high power) of candida organisms present in vegetation shown in Figure 1C. Gomori's methenamine silver, × 495.

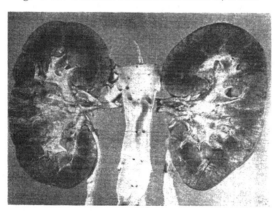

Figure 2A Surface of cut section of each kidney, showing marked congestion.

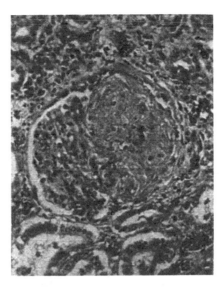

Figure 2B Photomicrograph of kidney showing focal glomerular lesion which is adherent to Bowman's capsule. Hematoxylin and eosin stain, × 310.

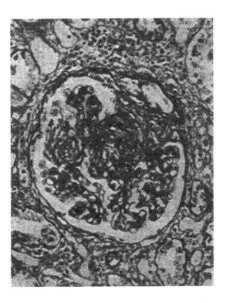

Figure 2C Photomicrograph of renal glomerulus demonstrating "focal embolic glomerulonephritis." Some malpighian tufts are hyalinized; other tufts are normal. Periodic acid-Schiff stain, × 310.

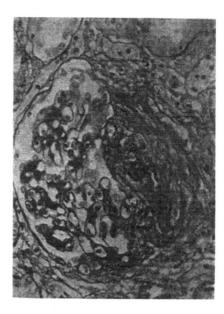

Figure 2D Photomicrograph of glomerulus. Periodic acid-Schiff stain, × 415.

There was no cellular proliferation in the glomerular tufts. Proliferation of the epithelium of Bowman's capsule, however, to form epithelial crescents, occasionally was seen. The basement membrane of involved glomeruli was usually thickened. In some places, it was thickened in the absence of involvement of the glomerular tufts. Heidenhain's azan modification of Mallory's connective tissue stain disclosed that most of the focal glomerular lesions were of the "healed fibrous" type as described by Bell.[9,10] The "fresh hyalin" lesion of Bell was seen only occasionally, and then frequently was associated with a "healed fibrous" lesion in the same glomerulus. Red blood cells were present to a limited extent in Bowman's space and commonly were seen in the lumen of the tubules. The tubules immediately adjacent to some of the more severely involved glomeruli were atrophic. Prussian blue stain revealed the presence of iron pigment in numerous tubular cells, and in the lumina of some tubules. Hyaline and granular casts also were present in the lumina of many tubules. The interstitial tissue contained many focal collections of lymphocytes and plasma cells. No fungi or bacteria were identified in the sections from the kidneys.

COMMENT

"Focal embolic glomerulonephritis" at one time was considered to be associated only with subacute streptococcal endocarditis.[11,12] Subsequently, it was seen in endocarditis produced by a number of other bacteria.[13] Furthermore, "focal embolic glomerulonephritis" has been reported in septicemia without endocarditis,[9,14] in rheumatic endocarditis,[9] in acute bacterial endocarditis—that is, of less than six weeks' duration—,[9] and in systemic lupus erythematosus.[15,16] The use of the renal biopsy has disclosed the presence of focal glomerular lesions in a group of patients who heretofore would not have been suspected of having this disorder. Bates, Jennings, and Earle[17] found focal glomerular lesions on renal biopsy in four of ten patients with proteinuria, hematuria, and pharyngitis, without bacterial or immunological evidence of a recent hemolytic streptococcal infection. Heptinstall and Joekes[16] reported "focal glomerulonephritis" in 13 of 100 patients from whom renal biopsies were obtained because of some urinary abnormality (usually proteinuria and hematuria). Four of the patients were believed to have systemic lupus erythematosus or polyarteritis nodosa, three appeared to have Schönlein-Henoch purpura, and the remainder would have been diagnosed clinically as having Ellis type II glomerulonephritis had the renal biopsies not been done.

The cause of "focal embolic glomerulonephritis" has not been definitely determined. Löhlein,[18] Baehr,[11,12] Fahr,[14] and Bell[9] ascribed the glomerular lesions to the embolization of minute fragments from the vegetations on the heart valves. However, there are several reasons, which Allen[1] has summarized, to doubt this concept. First, bacteria rarely are seen in the involved glomeruli. Second, focal glomerular lesions are rarely found in acute endocarditis, which has even more friable vegetations than does the subacute variety. Third, focal glomerular lesions are seen, although rarely, in the presence of bacteremia alone, without endocarditis, and in certain collagen diseases. In addition, "focal embolic glomerulonephritis" has been seen with endocarditis that involved only valves on the right side of the heart.[19] Fourth, it is difficult to accept the idea that hundreds of approximately equal-sized minute emboli are dislodged from a vegetation and seed only one organ, the kidneys, practically to the exclusion of others. Fifth, "focal embolic glomerulonephritis" cannot be produced experimentally by injecting solid particles into the blood stream of an animal. Thus, since these focal glomerular lesions do not appear to result from the implantation of minute emboli in the glomerular capillaries, since they occur in the absence of endocarditis, as well as in its presence, and since there usually is no inflammatory response in the glomeruli, the terms "embolic," "endo-carditic," and "-nephritic" should be discarded. We favor, as does Fishberg,[13] simply the descriptive term, "focal glomerular lesions." (As pointed out by Heptinstall and Joekes,[16] the glomerular lesions are local as well as focal. The "local" refers to the condition in which only a part of an individual glomerulus is involved by the lesion and the "focal," to the condition in which some glomeruli are involved and others are uninvolved, the latter being normal.)

Since the embolic mechanism seems untenable, the immuno-allergic theory has found much favor. Originally suggested by Longcope[2] and advanced later by Allen,[1] this idea ascribes the glomerular lesion to sensitization of the glomerular capillaries, to the bacteria themselves, or to the products of the bacteria present in the blood. This hypothesis is consistent with the occurrence of "focal embolic glomerulonephritis" in occasional cases of acute bacterial endocarditis, in bacteremias without endocarditis, and in isolated right-sided endocarditis. Since it is known that Candida organisms are good antigens, the immuno-allergic theory also is consistent with the occurrence of "focal embolic glomerulonephritis" in Candida endocarditis. Drake[20] has shown that 45% of normal human sera agglutinate C. albicans, and that approximately 40 or 50% of adults show a positive skin test to vaccine of C. albicans. It seems reasonable to believe that the same mechanisms which produce "focal embolic glomerulonephritis" in bacterial endocarditis also may play a role in the focal glomerulonephritis associated with Candida endocarditis.

Of the 44 cases reported of endocarditis caused by the higher fungi and proven at autopsy, 23 were due to Candida species.[3,21,22] The endocarditis in each of the four patients with well-documented "focal embolic glomerulonephritis" was caused by organisms of the Candida species. No focal glomerular lesions have been reported in patients with endocarditis due to Coccidioides immitis, Cryptococcus neoformans, Blastomyces dermatitidis, Histoplasma capsulatum, Aspergillus, or Mucor, although several of these fungi appear to be good antigens. "Focal embolic glomerulonephritis" has been mentioned in the protocols of three other patients[22-24] who died of endocarditis due to fungi, probably of Candida species, but these cases are omitted from this report because of inadequate diagnostic information. None of the four patients with "focal embolic glomerulonephritis" listed in Table 1 had an associated bacterial endocarditis. The patient reported by Kushner and Szanto,[21] with "focal embolic glomerulonephritis" associated with fungal endocarditis, also had bacteria in the cardiac vegetations and is therefore excluded from this report. The incidence of "focal embolic glomerulonephritis" associated with fungal endocarditis may be less than 10%, whereas the incidence of focal glomerulonephritis associated with subacute bacterial endocarditis is in the order of 50 to 90%.[9–11] There was no mention of organs other than the heart in several reports of patients with fungal endocarditis; consequently, the former percentage is probably low. Diffuse glomerulonephritis is uncommon in bacterial endocarditis and has not been mentioned in any reports of patients with fungal endocarditis.

Table 1 summarizes the renal findings in the documented cases of "focal embolic glomerulonephritis" associated with fungal endocarditis. Examination of the urinary sediment is of little help in distinguishing "focal embolic glomerulonephritis" from diffuse glomerulonephritis. Although the hematuria associated with focal glomerular lesions is classically microscopic and transient, massive, though intermittent, hematuria does occur (patient 2, Table 1). Leukocytes were described in the urinary sediment of two patients, but pyelonephritis was present histologically in all four patients (Table 1) at autopsy. Bacteria rarely are present in the glomeruli of patients with focal glomerular lesions associated with subacute endocarditis due to bacteria. In contrast, fungi were seen in the kidneys in two of the four patients with "focal embolic glomerulonephritis" associated

Table 1: Patients with focal glomerular lesions (focal embolic glomerulonephritis) in fungal endocarditis

Patients	1	2	3	4
Author	Pasternack	Neil-Kohlmeier	Neil-Kohlmeier	Present Author
Year	1942	1953	1953	1962
Age (years), sex	45 M	41 M	60 F	26 M
Length of illness (months)	1¼	3	2	11
Location of endocarditis (heart valve)	Aortic	Aortic Mitral	Aortic Mitral	Aortic
Organism causing endocarditis	C. parapsilosis	C. albicans	C. guilliermondi	C. parapsilosis
Renal function				
Specific gravity		1.018	1.027	1.010
Pyuria		0	+	+
Hematuria		+	0	+
Cylindruria		+	+	+
Uremia		+		+
Renal morphology				
Pyelonephritis	+	+	+	+
Infarcts	+	0	0	0
Size	↑	Normal	Normal	↑
"Flea-bitten" surface (petechiae)	0	+	0	0
No. of glomeruli involved	"Occasional"	"Severe"	"Slight"	90%

with endocarditis due to fungi. The fungi were present in the glomeruli as well as in the lumina of the tubules and in the interstitial tissues. In each of the two patients with *C. tropicalis* without endocarditis reported by Richart and Dammin,[25] Candida organisms were present in the glomeruli, as well as intratubularly and interstitially. In addition, in one of their patients, there was "partial destruction of the glomerular tuft without inflammatory response." The latter finding may represent an example of "focal embolic glomerulonephritis" associated with candidiasis without endocarditis.

Uremia was present in two of the four patients with focal glomerular lesions associated with fungal endocarditis (Table 1). Uremia on the basis of "focal embolic glomerulonephritis" associated with subacute bacterial endocarditis has been considered a rarity. Indeed, Libman is quoted by Fishberg[13] as saying that in 800 cases of subacute bacterial endocarditis he never had seen uremia due to focal glomerular lesions. Boyarsky, Burnett, and Barker,[26] however, found reports in the literature of 16 patients with "focal embolic glomerulonephritis" that produced uremia, and they added one of their own. Baehr[11] felt that renal function was rarely altered in the presence of focal glomerular lesions because the uninvolved portions of the damaged glomeruli remained normal, leaving enough healthy glomerular tissue to maintain normal glomerular functions.

SUMMARY

"Focal embolic glomerulonephritis" may occur in patients with endocarditis due to organisms other than bacteria, and indeed may occur occasionally in patients without endocarditis. A young man is presented who had endocarditis due to a fungus (*Candida parapsilosis*) and whose kidneys at autopsy showed the classical lesion of "focal embolic glomerulonephritis." It is mentioned that "focal embolic glomerulonephritis" probably occurs, proportionally, less commonly in fungal than in bacterial endocarditis. This lesion has been described in only four of 44 autopsied patients who died of fungal endocarditis, and in each of the four the endocarditis was caused by organisms of the Candida species. The term "focal embolic glomerulonephritis" is considered unsatisfactory, since the process appears not to be "embolic," and there rarely is an inflammatory response in the glomeruli. The descriptive term "focal glomerular lesions" is preferred.

ACKNOWLEDGMENT

The authors wish to thank Doctors Arthur Allen and Paul Kimmelsteil for reviewing the histological sections from the kidneys, and Doctors Louis B. Thomas and Ross C. MacCardle for reviewing the manuscript.

SUMMARIO IN INTERLINGUA

"Focal glomerulonephritis embolic" pote occurrer in patientes con endocarditis causate per organismos altere que bacterios; de facto, illo pote occurrer in patientes qui ha nulle endocarditis del toto. Es presentate le caso de un juvene homine qui habeva endocarditis causate per un fungo (*Candida parapsilosis*) e in qui le renes revelava al necropsia le lesion classic de "focal glomerulonephritis embolic." Es mentionate que "focal glomerulonephritis embolic" occurre probabilemente in un plus basse procentage del casos in endocarditis fungal que in endocarditis bacterial. Iste lesion esseva notate in solmente quatro de 44 necropsiate patientes morte ab endocarditis fungal, e in omne ille quatro casos le endocarditis esseva causate per organismos del specie Candida. Le termino "focal glomerulonephritis embolic" es considerate como non satisfactori in vista del facto que le processo non pare esser embolic e que il occurre rarmente un responsa inflammatori in le glomerulos. Le termino descriptive "focal lesiones glomerular" es preferite.

REFERENCES

1. ALLEN, A. C.: *The Kidney, Medical and Surgical Diseases*. Grune & Stratton, Inc., New York, 1951, pp. 164–170.
2. LONCCOPE, W. T.: The susceptibility of man to foreign proteins. *Amer. J. Med. Sci.* 152: 625, 1916.
3. ANDRIOLE, V. T., KRAVETZ, H. M., ROBERTS, W. C., UTZ, J. P.: Candida endocarditis: Clinical and pathological studies. *Amer. J. Med.* 32: 251, 1962.
4. PASTERNACK, J. G.: Subacute monilia endocarditis: New clinical and pathological entity. *Amer. J. Clin. Path.* 12: 496, 1942.
5. NIEL, K.: Zur Klinik der Candidainfektionen. *Klin. Med. (Wien)* 8: 49, 1953.
6. KOHLMEIER, W.: Zur Kenntnis der Candidainfektionen. *Klin. Med. (Wien)* 8: 54, 1953.
7. COOPER, T., MORROW, A. G., ROBERTS, W. C., HERMAN, L. G.: Postoperative endocarditis due to Candida: Clinical observations and the experimental production of the lesion. *Surgery* 50: 341, 1961.
8. MERCHANT, R. K., LOURIA, D. B., GEISLER, P. H., EDGCOMB, J. H., UTZ, J. P.: Fungal endocarditis: Review of the literature and report of three cases. *Ann. Intern. Med.* 48: 242, 1958.
9. BELL, E. T.: Glomerular lesions associated with endocarditis. *Amer. J. Path.* 8: 639, 1932.
10. BELL, E. T.: *Renal Diseases*, Lea & Febiger, Philadelphia, 1950, pp. 165–169.
11. BAEHR, G.: Glomerular lesions of subacute bacterial endocarditis. *Amer. J. Med. Sci.* 144: 327, 1912.
12. BAEHR, G.: Glomerular lesions of subacute bacterial endocarditis. *J. Exp. Med.* 15: 330, 1912.
13. FISHBERG, A. M.: *Hypertension and Nephritis*, 5th ed., Lea & Febiger, Philadelphia, 1954, pp. 665–671.
14. FAHR, T.: In *Handbuch der Speziellen pathologischen Anatomie und Histologie*, vol. 6, pt. 1, ed. by HENKE, F., and LUBARSCH, O. Springer, Berlin, 1925, pp. 355–362.
15. KLEMPERER, P., POLLACK, A. D., BAEHR, G.: Pathology of disseminated lupus erythematosus. *Arch. Path.* 32: 569, 1941.
16. HEPTINSTALL, R. H., JOEKES, A. M.: Focal glomerulonephritis. *Quart. J. Med.* (new series) 28: 329, 1959.
17. BATES, R. C., JENNINGS, R. B., EARLE, D. P.: Acute nephritis unrelated to group A hemolytic streptococcus infection: Report of ten cases. *Amer. J. Med.* 23: 510, 1957.
18. LÖHLEIN, M.: Ueber hämorrhagische Nierenaffektionen bei; chronischer ulzeröser Endokarditis. (Embolische nichteiterige Herdnephritis.) *Med. Klin.* 6: 375, 1910.
19. BAIN, R. C., EDWARDS, J. E., SCHEIFLEY, C. H., GERACI, J. E.: Right-sided bacterial endocarditis and endarteritis. *Amer. J. Med.* 24: 98, 1958.
20. DRAKE, C. H.: Quoted by Dubos, R. J. In *Bacterial and Mycotic Infections of Man*, 2nd ed., J. B. Lippincott Company, Philadelphia, 1952, p. 664.
21. KUSHNER, D. S., SZANTO, P. B.: Heart failure, fever, and splenomegaly in a morphine addict. *J. A. M. A.* 166: 2162, 1958.
22. CASSELS, D., STEINER, P.: Mycotic endocarditis: Report of a case with necropsy: review of the literature. *Amer. J. Dis. Child.* 67: 128, 1944.
23. CAPLAN, H.: Monilia (Candida) endocarditis following treatment with antibiotics. *Lancet* 2: 957, 1955.
24. NICOLAIDES, N. J.: Fungal endocarditis complicating staphylococcal endocarditis. *Med. J. Aust.* 1: 793, 1957.
25. RICHART, R., DAMMIN, G. J.: Candida tropicalis as a pathogen for man. *New Engl. J. Med.* 263: 474, 1960.
26. BOYARSKY, S., BURNETT, J. M., BARKER, W. H.: Renal failure in embolic glomerulonephritis as a complication of subacute bacterial endocarditis. *Bull. Johns Hopkins Hosp.* 84: 207, 1949.

Case 14 Traumatic Aortic Regurgitation

Robert J. Levine, M.D., William C. Roberts, M.D. and Andrew G. Morrow, M.D.
Bethesda, Maryland

NONPENETRATING TRAUMA to the chest often results in injury to the heart,[1,2] which may vary in severity from rapidly fatal cardiac rupture to asymptomatic lesions detectable only by serial electrocardiograms or serum enzyme determinations. It is not generally appreciated that as many as 38 per cent of patients sustaining chest injuries may also show evidence of cardiac damage.[3]

A patient herein described had a variety of manifestations of trauma to the heart. These included pericardial effusion, myocardial contusion, complete heart block and rupture of the aortic valve. For several reasons the diagnosis was elusive at first. The chest trauma, which the patient considered too trivial to mention, was followed after several symptom-free days by the gradual onset of disability associated with atypical auscultatory findings. Of the several cardiac lesions in this patient, we have considered the ruptured aortic valve in greatest detail because it is potentially amenable to a definitive corrective procedure. In addition, the clinical and pathologic findings in previously reported patients with aortic regurgitation due to nonpenetrating chest trauma are summarized.

CASE REPORT

W. R., a 35 year old prize fighter, was in excellent health until May 1960, when a box weighing over 500 pounds slid from the back of a truck and knocked him to the ground, causing sudden violent compression of his chest. He was stunned momentarily and had difficulty catching his breath but recovered spontaneously within ten minutes without residual discomfort. He regarded this trauma as trivial. Two or three days later he developed night sweats, progressively increasing fatigability and, after one week, dyspnea with exertion. Two weeks following the injury he began to have spontaneous episodes of nausea, vomiting and dizziness. After three days of such attacks he lost consciousness during a particularly severe bout of vomiting. He was brought to a hospital near his home where he was found to have a pulse rate of 30 per minute and a blood pressure of 90/50 mm Hg. There were physical signs of complete heart block, but no murmurs or cardiomegaly were evident. The electrocardiogram (Figure 1A) showed complete heart block with a ventricular rate of 29 but no evidence of left ventricular ischemia or hypertrophy. Laboratory studies gave normal values; these included hematocrit, white blood cell count with differential, erythrocyte sedimentation rate, urinalysis, serologic test for syphilis, serum glutamic oxalacetic transaminase, C-reactive protein, multiple blood cultures, blood urea nitrogen, fasting blood sugar, cholesterol and electrolytes. Chest roentgenogram and gastrointestinal x-ray series showed no abnormalities. On the third hospital day there was a rise in the sedimentation rate which persisted for about three weeks. The patient remained afebrile during six weeks of observation, and there was no significant alteration in the white blood count or the serum transaminase.

From the Clinics of Experimental Therapeutics and Surgery, National Heart Institute and Department of Pathologic Anatomy, The Clinical Center, National Institutes of Health, Bethesda, Maryland.

DOI: 10.1201/9781003409281-2

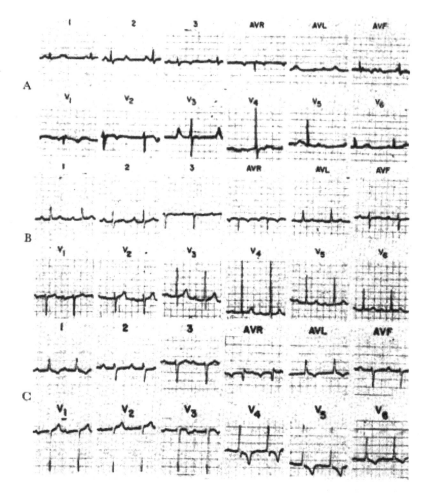

Figure 1 Serial electrocardiograms. A, May 20, 1960, two weeks after injury. Complete heart block is present. B, July 14, 1960, seven weeks later. There is a prolonged P-R interval and a shift of the electrical axis to the left. C, October 11, 1960, five months after injury. First degree heart block persists. There is now evidence of left ventricular hypertrophy and ischemia and further shift of the electrical axis to the left.

The heart rate responded to sympathomimetic amines, and the cardiac rhythm in the electrocardiogram gradually returned to first degree heart block within two weeks. By this time he had developed a pericardial friction rub and an apical systolic murmur. The heart sounds became quite distant, and this finding was interpreted as being due to pericardial effusion. A blowing diastolic murmur was later heard along the left sternal border. Because he was thought to have myocarditis, treatment with prednisone, 20 mg. daily, was given for about three months without apparent benefit.

In August 1960 he was readmitted to his local hospital because of persistent cough and dyspnea on exertion. At this time the pulse rate was 76 per minute and the blood pressure 110/60 mm. Hg. The heart was not clinically enlarged. A grade 2, blowing, diastolic decrescendo murmur was best heard at the left sternal border, and there was a grade 2 systolic murmur at the apex of the heart. The electrocardiogram now showed left axis deviation and persistent prolongation of the P-R interval (Figure 1B). Again several blood cultures were negative and the sedimentation rate was elevated. Digitalis was added to his treatment because of evidence of left ventricular failure.

Physical Examination: On October 10, 1960, the patient was admitted to the National Heart Institute. The blood pressure was 110/60 mm. Hg, the pulse rate 100 per minute, and he was in no distress. The lungs were clear. There was a prominent left ventricular lift. The heart sounds were faint and regular. A short, rough, early systolic murmur which appeared to originate in the aortic area was heard over the entire precordium. A grade 3 early diastolic blowing murmur was heard best along the left sternal border. At the apex, in late diastole, this murmur assumed a rumbling quality (Austin Flint murmur). Near the apex was a high-pitched systolic rub heard with inspiration (pleuropericardial rub). Neither hepatomegaly nor peripheral edema was present. Numerous hematologic, bacteriologic and chemical studies were normal, with the following exceptions: The BUN was 27 mg. per 100 ml., and the sedimentation rate was 23 mm. per hour.

Roentgenographic study of the chest (Figure 2) with barium swallow showed moderate cardiomegaly with left ventricular predominance. The ascending aorta bulged to the right, having the appearance of aneurysmal dilation. No intracardiac calcification was observed. The *electrocardiogram* showed a P-R interval of 0.34 second with evidence of left ventricular hypertrophy and ischemia and left axis deviation (Figure 1C).

During the patient's hospital stay a marked variation in his blood pressure was recorded with systolic readings as high as 140 mm. Hg and diastolic values ranging from 0 to 60 mm. Hg. After several weeks of observation, when questioned specifically about the occurrence of chest trauma, he mentioned for the first time to a physician the injury described previously.

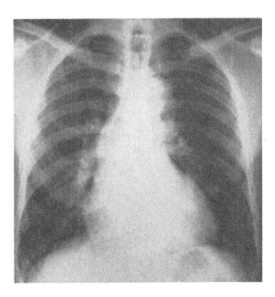

Figure 2 Chest roentgenogram (PA projection). There is generalized cardiomegaly with left ventricular predominance and striking dilation of the ascending aorta.

Cardiac catheterization was performed in November 1960. Right-sided pressures were normal with the exception of a pulmonary artery pressure of 42/25 mm. Hg (mean pressure 32). There was no evidence of an intracardiac shunt. Left heart catheterization by the transseptal technic demonstrated a mean left atrial pressure of 26 mm. Hg. The left ventricular systolic pressure was 100 mm. Hg, and the end-diastolic pressure in the ventricle was 50 mm. Hg. The brachial artery pressure was 110/50 mm. Hg. The cardiac output, determined by dye dilution technic, was 3.1 liters per minute.

Retrograde aortography showed gross aortic regurgitation. Indicator dye injected into the aorta at the level of the eleventh thoracic vertebra was detected by sampling within the left ventricle.[4]

Surgical Findings: On the basis of the findings noted above, the diagnosis of traumatic rupture of the aortic valve seemed established, and an operation for its correction was undertaken. Through a longitudinal incision in the ascending aorta, the valve was exposed during complete cardiopulmonary bypass and hypothermic cardiac arrest. It appeared that the left anterior leaflet had been avulsed from its attachment at the commissure between it and the posterior leaflet (Figure 3). The leaflet was re-attached and the commissure plicated with two mattress sutures reinforced with Teflon® felt, as shown in Figure 4. Following the repair, however, efforts to restore ventricular action were unsuccessful.

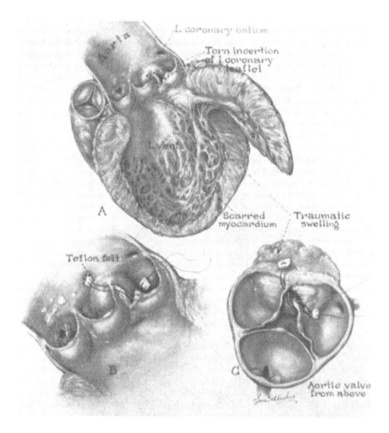

Figure 3 Appearance of the aortic valve lesion and method of surgical repair employed.

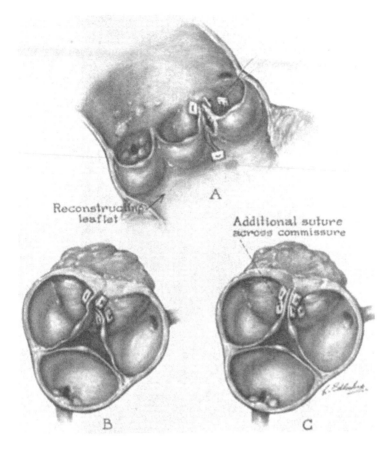

Reconstructing leaflet

A

Additional suture across commissure

B

C

Figure 4   Following re-attachment of the valve leaflet, another similar suture was placed across the newly reconstructed commissure.

The intact, fresh heart was placed in the Davila pulse duplicator[5] in order to study the function of the aortic valve. At a rate of 70 to 80 per minute, the aortic valve, both with the surgical repair intact and following the removal of the sutures, was incompetent. It was observed, however, that the more rapid the heart rate, the more competent was the reconstructed aortic valve. Indeed, when the heart rate was approximately 130 per minute, the orifice of the surgically repaired aortic valve closed well during ventricular diastole (Figure 5). After the sutures were removed, the valve was grossly incompetent at all rates (Figure 6).

PATHOLOGIC FINDINGS

Gross Findings

The heart was enlarged and weighed 600 gm. The right atrium and ventricle were hypertrophied and moderately dilated. A valvular-competent patent foramen ovale was present. The tricuspid and pulmonic valves were normal. The left atrium was also moderately dilated and hypertrophied, and its endocardium, particularly that portion between the anterior mitral leaflet and the foraman ovale, was thickened.

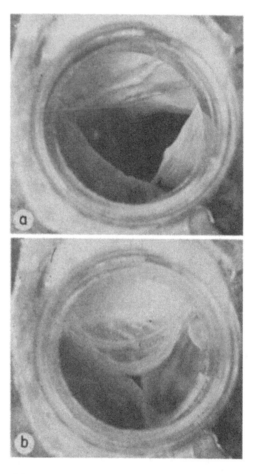

Figure 5 Views of the aortic valve as it functioned on the Davila pulse duplicator. The surgical repair is intact. The heart rate was approximately 130 per minute. a, maximal opening of aortic valve during ventricular systole. b, maximal closure of aortic valve during ventricular diastole.

The anterior leaflet of the mitral valve was thickened, but the posterior leaflet and the mitral chordae tendineae were normal. The left ventricle was hypertrophied and dilated. Its wall measured 1.7 cm. in greatest thickness, and 0.8 cm. at its thinnest point, the apex. A fibrous scar, measuring 3 by 1 by 1 cm., was present in the anterolateral wall of the left ventricle (Figure 7). Several smaller fibrous scars also were noted in the adjacent anterolateral papillary muscle.

The aortic valve "ring" measured 8 cm. in circumference; the pulmonic valve ring, 7 cm. Within the aortic valve there was a localized, smooth-surfaced, firm "bulge," measuring 2.5 by 2.5 by 1.5 cm., which was located directly behind the commissural attachments of the posterior and left anterior aortic cusps and which protruded equally into the dilated left anterior and posterior sinuses of Valsalva (Figure 8). In the space produced by the separation of the left anterior and posterior (noncoronary) cusps, and overlying the mid-portion of the bulge, there was a depressed area, measuring 0.2 by 0.3 cm., which was covered by necrotic material. The commissural

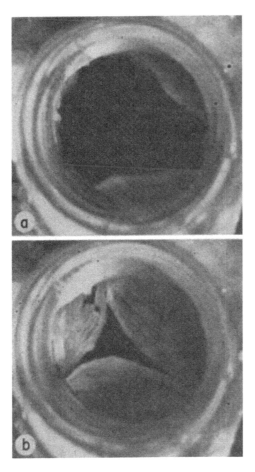

Figure 6 Views of aortic valve functioning on the Davila pulse duplicator following the removal of the sutures reattaching the leaflet. The heart rate was 70 to 80/min. a, maximal opening of the aortic valve during ventricular systole. b, maximal closure of the aortic valve during ventricular diastole.

attachment of the left anterior aortic cusp was torn free and displaced downward toward the left ventricle. The portions of the aortic leaflets adjacent to the protruding nodule were thickened, particularly in their margins; otherwise, these leaflets were delicate and pliable. On section through the nodule or bulge, it was found to lie between the intimal surface of the aortic sinus and the epicardial surface of the left atrium (Figure 9A). The ostium of the left coronary artery was displaced upward, arising above the commissural attachments (Figure 8). The ostium of the right coronary artery was normally located. The distribution of each coronary artery was normal. The right one showed a mild degree of atherosclerosis. A few atheromata were present in the ascending aorta, particularly about the ostium of the right coronary artery. Approximately one centimeter distal to the aortic valve, the ascending aorta became extremely thin and fragile, but at no point was its wall interrupted or broken.

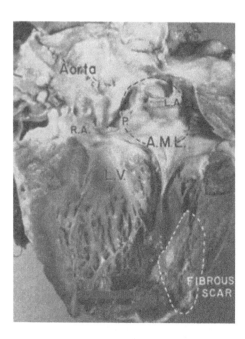

Figure 7 The left ventricle, aortic valve and aorta are opened. The "bulge" at the aortic valve is enclosed in the black-lined circle. A fibrous scar, which probably represents an old contusion, is enclosed in the white-lined circle. L.V. = left ventricle; A.M.L. = anterior mitral leaflet; R.A. = right anterior cusp; P = posterior cusp; L.A. = left anterior cusp of the aortic valve. Both the left ventricle and aortic valve are dilated. The surgical incision is apparent in the ascending aorta.

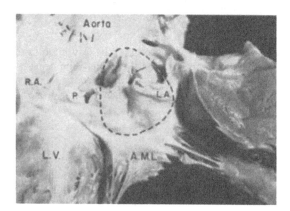

Figure 8 A close-up view of the aortic valve "bulge." It is continuous with the anterior mitral leaflet (A.M.L.) and lies behind the left anterior (L.A.) and posterior (P) cusps of the aortic valve. The commissural attachment of the left anterior cusp has been torn. The area of necrosis in the bulge is identified by the arrow. The ostium of the left coronary artery is displaced upward. The ostium of the right coronary artery, which is normally located, is hidden behind the right anterior (R.A.) cusp of the aortic valve. The tear in the posterior (P) aortic cusp was produced by the prosector and is an artifact.

Microscopic Findings

Aorta and Aortic Valve: Histologically the nodule consisted predominantly of fibrocollagenous tissue (Figure 9B). Within the extremely thick fibrous wall of the sinus of Valsalva an area of necrosis was present, and just proximal to the base of the aortic cusp a large abscess was noted (Figure 10). The central portion of the abscess contained many necrotic cells surrounded by a thin irregular band of epithelioid cells. Around this was a large collection of plasma cells, lymphocytes, fibroblasts and a striking number of eosinophils. Fibrocollagenous tissue, which contained dilated veins, thick-walled arteries, extravasated red blood cells, and occasional foci of plasma cells and lymphocytes surrounded these latter cells.

The area of necrosis within the sinus of Valsalva, in contrast to the abscess, was open to blood traversing the aortic valve (Figure 10). The necrotic material was surrounded by numerous lymphocytes, plasma cells and fibroblasts, but not by eosinophils. The adventitia of the entire ascending aorta consisted of thick fibrous tissue which also contained focal collections of lymphocytes and plasma cells, and many thick-walled arteries, the lumina of some being almost completely occluded. The inflammatory cells in the adventitia were irregularly distributed and not located in the regions of the vasa vasorum. There was virtual absence of elastic fibers in the media of the aorta behind the torn aortic cusp extending approximately

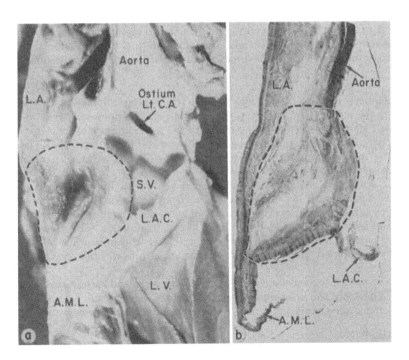

Figure 9 a, view following longitudinal section of the "bulge," anterior mitral leaflet (A.M.L.), left atrium (L.A.) and ascending aorta. The bulge is outlined by the black-dashed circle. The dark portion within the bulge is hemorrhagic material. The anterior portion of the bulge consists of the wall of the aorta behind the left anterior cusp (L.A.C.) of the aortic valve. The sinus of Valsalva (S.V.) is indicated. b, photomicrograph of the cut-surface illustrated in a. The bulge again is circled. There is extreme thickening of the wall of the aorta, particularly its most proximal part. Elastic tissue stain, original magnification ×4.5.

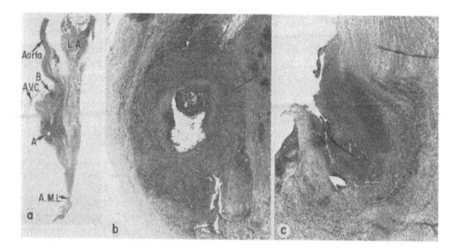

Figure 10 *a*, photomicrograph of longitudinal section through the center of the "bulge." The anterior mitral leaflet (A.M.L.), aortic valve cusp (A.V.G.), aorta, and left atrium (L.A.) are illustrated. A designates the subendocardial abscess which is illustrated in *b*. B represents the focus of necrosis illustrated in *c*. The bulge extends from arrow A to arrow B. Hematoxylin and eosin stain, original magnification ×1.8. *b*, abscess shown in *a*. Hematoxylin and eosin stain, original magnification ×18. *c*, area of necrosis shown in *a*. Hematoxylin and eosin stain, original magnification ×28.

one centimeter distal to the sinus of Valsalva. The configuration of the elastic fibers distal to the aortic valve, however, was normal. No mucopolysacharride material (Rinehart stain) was present in the media of the ascending aorta. Special stains of the sections of the aortic bulge for bacteria (Brown and Brenn), spirochetes (Steiner) and fungi (periodic acid-Schiff and methenamine silver) showed no organisms, and no hemosiderin deposits were seen with the iron stain.

Left Ventricle: Histologic study of the left ventricular fibrous scar (Figure 11) revealed a marked diffuse replacement of myocardial fibers by thick fibrous tissue which was free of inflammatory cells and of hemosiderin deposits (iron stain). The right and left coronary arteries were widely patent, although each showed a mild amount of intimal thickening. The myocardial fibers throughout the left ventricle were hypertrophied. The endocardium of the left atrium was thickened by fibrous proliferation.

There was acute congestion of the lungs, liver, spleen and kidneys. Sections from the vertebrae, hip and knee joints showed no evidence of arthritis. Sections from the bowel, endocrine glands and central nervous system were not remarkable.

DISCUSSION

Gore[6] suggests that many instances of heart disease are incorrectly attributed to trauma or strain, particularly when compensation or disability insurance is involved. He emphasizes the difficulty of being certain of a diagnosis of traumatic heart disease, sometimes even at autopsy. There is, however, no cause for doubt that the cardiac problem in this patient resulted from the traumatic event he described. He was in superb condition, running five miles daily, until his accident. No abnormalities had been detected at the physical examinations which had preceded each of his boxing matches. Shortly following the injury his health began to deteriorate rapidly. It did not occur to him that his injury could have

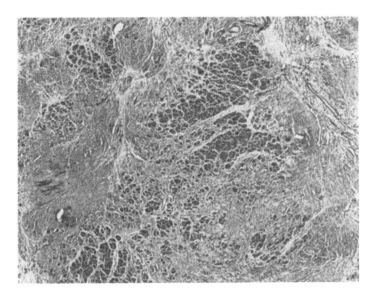

Figure 11 Photomicrograph of section taken from the fibrous scar illustrated in Figure 5 showing severe fibrosis without inflammatory reaction. The darker portions represent myocardial fibers stranded in the fibrous tissue. The coronary artery proximal to this area of fibrosis was widely patent.

contributed to his illness. The clinical and postmortem studies described above disclosed no other cause of heart disease.

This patient had a pericardial effusion and extensive contusion of the myocardium. These are the most common cardiac lesions following blunt chest trauma.[2,7,8] Myocardial contusion may be so mild that it is without symptoms and can be detected only by special studies,[3] or it may be sufficiently severe to result in immediate or delayed cardiac rupture. Myocardial infarction due to coronary arterial occlusion may be closely imitated by contusion.[9] Contusion commonly involves the anterior wall of the left ventricle and the interventricular septum. Involvement of the septum and the conductive tissue may result in atrioventricular conduction defects. Complete heart block is usually transient, as in the patient described herein, but may be permanent.[10]

Rupture of the aortic valve, though unusual, is the valvular lesion most frequently observed in patients surviving nonpenetrating cardiac injury.[2] Howard[11] cites experimental evidence that tears in the cusps of the aortic valve may be produced in dogs and in human cadavers by blunt trauma to the chest or by suddenly increasing the pressure in the aorta.

Previously Reported Cases: Including the patient described herein, the autopsy findings in 52 patients with aortic valvular regurgitation resulting from trauma or muscular strain have been recorded. Of these, 44 were reviewed by Howard[11] in 1928. The clinical and anatomic features in the 8 patients[12-18] described since that date are listed in Table 1. In Howard's 44 proved cases, 14 developed aortic regurgitation as a result of chest trauma and 30 as a result of muscular strain. Ninety-eight per cent were men. The age range in the traumatic group was from 19 to 85, with a mean of 45.6 years; in the strain group, from 20 to 60 with a mean of 37.2 years. Symptoms suggestive of pre-existing valvular disease were mentioned in 2 patients in his strain group, and in 5 in the traumatic group. A history of syphilis was recorded only

21

Table 1: Reported cases of aortic insufficiency due to trauma or muscular strain clinical and pathologic features in the 8 autopsies performed since 1928

Author & Year	Age at Accident Sex	Length of Illness from Accident to Death	Associated Cardio-vascular Disease	Immediate Sign and/or Symptom(s)	Later Signs and Symptoms	Associated Injuries	Blood Pressure (mm. Hg)	Site of Tear	Aortic Valve Cusps Affected	State of Aortic Valve Cusps	State of Aorta	Heart Size (gm.)	Coronary Arteries
1. Kissane Koons Fidler[12] (1936)	22 M	14 mo.	0	Crushing chest pain Dyspnea	CHF syncope	Multiple fractures, lacerations, contusions	110/20	Cusps	All 3	"Torn, frag-mented"		? normal	Normal
2. Beneke[13] (1942)	21 F	9 days	0	0	Fever CHF	0		Cusps Ventricular septum	Posterior R anterior	Normal	Normal	Normal	Normal
3. Bushong[14] (Case 1) (1947)	50 M	2⅓ mo.	0	Chest pain Dyspnea	CHF	0	175/55	Point of attachment of 2 cusp commissures	R anterior Posterior	Normal Separation of commis-sures		650	"Slight" athero-sclerosis
4. Kissane Koons Clark[15] (Case 2) (1948)	58 M	27 mo.	Syphilis	Purring noise in chest Sternal soreness Palpitations Dyspnea	Chest pain CHF	0	220/0	Point of attachment of 2 cusp commissures	L anterior Posterior	Two posterior cusps, fibrous; anterior, normal	Occasional atheromata	"Enormously enlarged"	
5. Proudfit McCormack[16] (1956)	56 M	? 39 mo.	Hypertension Cerebral infarct	0	CHF Gradual lowering of blood pressure	0	150/50	Point of attachment of one cusp Fenestrations in 2 cusps	R anterior L anterior	Normal	Normal except for occasional atheromata	930	Moderate athero-sclerosis

Author & Year	Age at Accident Sex	Length of Illness from Accident to Death	Associated Cardio-vascular Disease	Immediate Sign and/or Symptom(s)	Later Signs and Symptoms	Associated Injuries	Blood Pressure (mm. Hg)	Site of Tear	Aortic Valve Cusps Affected	State of Aortic Valve Cusps	State of Aorta	Heart Size (gm.)	Coronary Arteries
6. Dimond Larsen Johnson Kittle[17] 1957	32 M	? 5 years †	Marfan's syndrome	Chest pain	CHF	Multiple fractures, brain concussion	160/0	Ascending aorta Fenestrations in 2 cusps	L anterior Posterior	Sagging of the commissures with downward displacement of the cusps	Aneurysmal dilatation and medial cystic necrosis, asc. aorta	810	"Stenosis" of ostia by calcareous deposits in aorta
7. Ramage Morgan[18] (1957)	34 M	7 years	0	Cooing noise in chest	CHF Night sweats Fatigability Syncope Arrhythmia	Sprained wrist	160/30	Cusp itself	R anterior	Calcareous, fibrotic, thickened, deformed	Small aneurysm, ascending aorta	630	
8. Present authors (1961)	35 M	7 mo. ‡	0	0	CHF	0	140–110/ 60–0	Point of attachment of one cusp	L anterior	Normal	Thin, fragile occasional atheromata Localized bulge in sinus of Valsalva	600	Minimal athero-sclerosis

* CHF = congestive heart failure.

† Hufnagel valve inserted 4 months before death.

‡ Died during surgical repair of the aortic valve. R = right, L = left.

once and "rheumatism, chorea and tonsillitis" 5 times in the strain group. Neither syphilis nor rheumatic fever was mentioned in any of the 14 traumatic cases. The time interval between the accident and death varied widely, averaging 18 months in the strain group and 40 months in the traumatic group. The most common site of rupture in Howard's series was the aorta, near the base of the aortic valve (22 patients), followed by the rupture of the cusp itself (11 patients), and lastly by the detachment of the cusp from the aortic wall (10 patients). When the rupture affected the cusp itself, most commonly only one cusp was involved. There were only two instances in which all three cusps were torn. The aortic valve cusps were normal in 13 (30%) and fibrous, atheromatous or calcareous in 23 instances. None of the cusps were congenitally deformed.

The aortic regurgitation in the present patient resulted, at least initially, from a partial detachment of one aortic valve cusp from the wall of the aorta. At the time of the detachment there also was probably a tearing of the aorta immediately beneath the commissural attachment. The sequence of events thereafter was probably the following: Erythrocytes, inflammatory cells and fibroblasts entered the wall of the aorta and the adjacent adventitial tissues in the area bounded by the external surfaces of the proximal anterior mitral leaflet and the ascending aorta on one side, and left atrium on the other (Figure 9). The tear in the aorta healed by scarring, and this fibrous proliferation produced severe thickening of the part of the aorta that bordered the sinus of Valsalva. Loose fibrous tissue clumps of chronic inflammatory cells, and scattered erythrocytes remained in the potential space thus created. The bulge thus came into being and further increased the amount of aortic regurgitation. The pathogenesis ot the sterile abscess and of the focus of necrosis (Figure 10) must remain a matter of speculation. The epithelioid cells which surrounded the focus of necrosis have not been noted previously in patients with aortic regurgitation due to trauma or muscular strain, although they have been described in patients with rheumatoid arthritis.[19] The present patient had no clinical signs nor symptoms of arthritis, and sections of two joints at autopsy were normal.

A bulge has been described in one other patient with aortic regurgitation due to muscular strain. This patient, reported by Beneke,[13] was a 21 year old woman who became febrile and in whom a basal diastolic murmur appeared nine days following the spontaneous delivery of a premature fetus. She died shortly after, and at autopsy there was a "walnut-sized nodule" in the subendocardium of the ventricular septum immediately beneath the aortic valve. Two of the aortic valve cusps were torn away at their bases from the wall of the aorta, and this tear was continuous with the nodule, which proved to be a hematoma. The hematoma had dissected through the ventricular septum, and, indeed, was apparent from the right ventricular aspect. Except for the tears, the aortic valve and aorta were normal. There was no evidence of infection at autopsy. This patient is the only recorded one in whom aortic regurgitation presumably resulted from the muscular strain exerted during parturition.

Clinical Features of Traumatic Aortic Regurgitation: The onset of symptoms of traumatic aortic valvular rupture usually follows the causative injury immediately. The most common symptom is agonizing pain in the chest often followed by faintness or syncope. There have been cases, however, in which the onset of symptoms was delayed, sometimes as long as several years. After a variable interval the usual symptoms of aortic regurgitation ensue. About half of the patients complain of a chest sound which is audible, not only to themselves, but to others.

At physical examination there are the usual signs of aortic regurgitation. Although the pulse pressure is usually wide, elevated systolic pressure is not common early in the course of the disease. A rough systolic murmur is often heard and is attributable to vibrations caused by rapid blood flow over the torn cusp. The diastolic murmur commonly has a musical quality and has been compared to such sounds as that of a sea gull, the cooing of a dove, the croaking of a frog, the spinning of a top, or whistling, whining or humming sounds.

Several clinical features that were atypical of traumatic aortic regurgitation were noted in the present patient. The onset of symptoms was delayed by several days, and then the syncope appeared to be caused by the complete heart block rather than by valvular disease. At no time was chest pain prominent, nor was the patient aware of any sound in his chest. The diastolic murmur sounded much like most murmurs of aortic regurgitation and had no musical quality.

Surgical treatment for traumatic aortic regurgitation was apparently first attempted in 1954 by Hufnagel,[20] who successfully inserted a plastic valve in the descending aorta. Fourteen months later the patient continued to do well. A similar operation in a patient with Marian's syndrome was reported by Dimond et al.[17] This patient had no apparent relief from the operation and died a short time later. Spurny and Hara[21] attempted to repair a torn aortic cusp by direct suture but were unable to resuscitate the heart at the end of the procedure. The present patient, had he survived surgery, probably would have derived limited benefit from the operation because of the residual deformity produced by the large aortic valve nodule. It is not possible, however, to determine preoperatively the exact anatomic derangement that will be encountered at operation. Since it represents the only therapeutic approach that potentially offers lasting benefit, operative intervention would seem to be indicated in most patients with traumatic aortic regurgitation.

SUMMARY

A patient is reported who sustained myocardial contusion with complete heart block, pericardial effusion and rupture of the aortic valve following blunt chest trauma. An attempt at direct surgical repair of the valvular lesion was unsuccessful. The diagnostic difficulties presented by traumatic heart disease are discussed, and the previous reports of patients with traumatic aortic regurgitation are summarized.

ACKNOWLEDGMENT

The authors are grateful to Dr. Walter Hasbrouck, who referred this patient to the National Heart Institute.

REFERENCES

1. FRIEDBERG, C. K. Diseases of the Heart, 2nd ed. W. B. Saunders Co, Philadelphia, 1956, p. 1057.
2. PARMLEY, L. F., MANION, W. C. and MATTINGLY, T. W. Nonpenetrating traumatic injury of the heart. *Circulation*, 28: 371, 1958.
3. WATSON, J. H. and BARTHOLOMAE, W. M. Cardiac injury due to nonpenetrating chest trauma. *Ann. Int. Med.*, 57: 871, 1960.
4. BRAUNWALD, E. and MORROW, A. G. A method for the detection and estimation of aortic regurgitant flow in man. *Circulation*, 17: 505, 1958.
5. DAVILA, J. C., TROUT, R. G., SUNNER, J. E. and GLOVER, R. P. A simple mechanical pulse duplicator for cinematography of cardiac valves in action. *Ann. Surg.*, 143: 544, 1956.
6. GORE, I. The question of traumatic heart disease. *Ann. Int. Med.*, 33: 865, 1950.
7. BRIGHT, E. F. and BECK, C. S. Nonperietrating wounds of the heart. *Am. Heart J.*, 10: 293, 1935.
8. BECK, C. S. Contusions of the heart. *J A.M.A.*, 109: 104, 1935.
9. BORODKIN, H. D. and MASSEY, F. C. Myocardial trauma produced by nonpenetrating chest injury. *Am. Heart J.*, 53: 795, 1957.

10. COFFEN, T. H., RUSH, H. P. and MILLER, R. F. Traumatic complete heart block of eighteen years' duration. *Northwest Med.*, 40: 195, 1941.

11. HOWARD, C. P. Aortic insufficiency due to rupture by strain of a normal aortic valve. *Canad. M.A.J.*, 19: 12, 1928.

12. KISSANE, R. W., KOONS, R. A. and FIDLER, R. S. Traumatic rupture of a normal aortic valve. *Am. Heart J.*, 12: 231, 1936.

13. BENEKE, R. Ein Fall spontaner Aortenklappen-Ruptur mit Hämatom im Gebìet des Septum Fibrosum Ventr. als Begleiterscheinung Einer Vorzeitigen Geburt. *Ztschr. Geburtsh. u. Gynak.*, 124:1, 1942.

14. BUSHONG, B. B. Traumatic rupture of the aortic valve: report of two cases, one a proved and the other a probable example of this condition. *Ann. Int. Med.*, 26: 125, 1947.

15. KISSANE, R. W., KOONS, R. A. and CLARK, T. E. Traumatic rupture of the aortic valve. *Am. J. Med.*, 4: 606, 1948.

16. PROUDFIT, W. L. and MCCORMACK, L. J. Rupture of the aortic valve. *Circulation*, 13: 750, 1956.

17. DIMOND, E. G., LARSEN, W. E., JOHNSON, W. B. and KITTLE, C. F. Posttraumatic aortic insufficiency occurring in Marfan's syndrome with attempted repair with a plastic valve. *New England J. Med.*, 256: 8, 1957.

18. RAMAGE, J. H. and MORGAN, J. B. Traumatic aortic incompetence. *Scottish M.*, 2: 299, 1957.

19. BAGGENSTOSS, A. H. and ROSENBERG, E. F. Cardiac lesions associated with chronic infectious arthritis. *Arch. Int. Med.*, 67: 241, 1941.

20. LEONARD, J. J., HARVEY, W. P. and HUFNAGEL, C. A. Rupture of the aortic valve. *New England J. Med.*, 252: 208, 1955.

21. SPURNY, O. M. and HARA, M. Rupture of the aortic valve due to strain. *Am. J. Cardiol.*, 8: 125, 1961.

Case 26 Myocardial Embolus

A Complication of Mitral Valvulotomy*

Robert M. Friedman, M.D.,[†] and William C. Roberts, M.D.[‡]
Bethesda, Maryland

SYSTEMIC arterial embolization is a recognized complication of mitral-valve surgery. These emboli generally consist of fibrin material, which had been dislodged from a clot in the left atrium at the time of commissurotomy. Less commonly, calcium is dislodged from the mitral valve during the procedure and forms the embolus. Rarely, other material may be embolized, as in a forty-four-year-old woman who underwent a second mitral commissurotomy for recurrent stenosis. At operation, finger fracture of the mitral valve was attempted, but believed inadequate, and the valve was further widened by a Tubbs dilator inserted from the left ventricle. Massive mitral regurgitation resulted (V waves in the left atrium rising to 50 mm. of mercury, and the mean pressure rising to 30 mm. from a preoperative valve of 22 mm. of mercury), and on return to the recovery room the patient's pupils were dilated and nonreactive to light. She never regained consciousness and died twelve hours after operation in acute pulmonary edema and shock. Before operation the

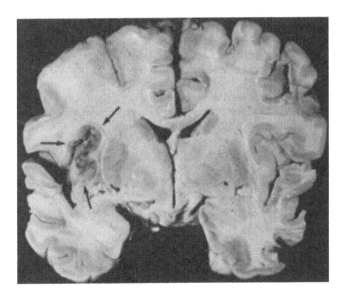

Figure 1   Coronal Section of the Brain, Showing a Fresh Cerebral Infarct (Arrows).

* From the Department of Pathologic Anatomy, Clinical Center, National Institutes of Health.
† Senior investigator, Laboratory of Pathology, National Cancer Institute.
‡ Chief, Laboratory of Pathology, Clinic of Surgery, National Heart Institute.

DOI: 10.1201/9781003409281-3

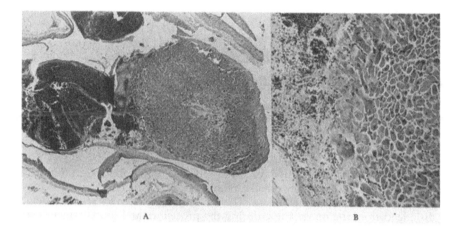

Figure 2 Photomicrographs of the Myocardial Embolus in the Cerebral Artery (Hematoxylin and Eosin Stains). The fragment of myocardium (A), attached to a fibrin clot, lies within the lumen of a longitudinally-cut cerebral vessel (original magnification ×25). The close-up of the myocardial embolus (B) shows the myocardial fibers to be hypertrophied (original magnification ×125).

patient had normal sinus rhythm, an end-diastolic mitral-valve gradient of 20 mm. of mercury and severe pulmonary hypertension (pulmonary arterial pressure of 100 systolic, 40 diastolic). At autopsy the anterolateral mitral commissure was found to have been opened from the free margin to the mitral annulus, and also the anterolateral papillary muscle had been split. No clot was present in the left atrium or ventricle. A fresh infarct was seen in the brain (Figure 1), and histologically a large fragment of myocardium was found in a cerebral artery leading to the area of encephalomalacia (Figure 2).

To our knowledge, myocardial emboli have not previously been reported. The embolus in the present case is believed to have been detached from the anterolateral papillary muscle during the mitral commissurotomy.

Case 32 The Nondistensible Right Atrium of Carcinoid Disease of the Heart

William C. Roberts, M.D., Dean T. Mason, M.D., and Louis D. Wright, Jr., M.D.

Approximately half of the patients with the carcinoid syndrome have carcinoid heart disease.[1] The endocardial fibrous lesions, which are pathognomonic of this disease, almost always involve the tricuspid and pulmonic valves, and whenever the deposits on the tricuspid valve are extensive, similar lesions are generally also present on the endocardium of the right atrium. The chief hemodynamic consequence of diffuse fibrosis of the tricuspid valve in patients with the carcinoid syndrome is tricuspid regurgitation, although some degree of stenosis is almost always present as well. The endocardial fibrous plaques in the right atrium, when diffuse, may prevent this chamber from expanding during ventricular systole as would be expected with tricuspid regurgitation, and thus the right atrial pressure during ventricular contraction may be excessively elevated. This was the case in 2 patients with carcinoid heart disease who underwent cardiac catheterization and finally came to autopsy. Few reports have appeared describing the cardiac morphology in patients with carcinoid heart disease who have undergone catheterization. This paper describes the clinical, hemodynamic, and pathologic features of these 2 patients and calls particular attention to their right atrial pressure pulses.

REPORT OF CASES

Each of the 2 patients had elevated values of urinary 5-hydroxyindoleacetic acid (range 265 to 580 mg. per 24 hr.), and at autopsy the carcinoid primary in each was in the ileum and the only metastases in each were to the liver and regional lymph nodes. One patient (K. W., 01-04-45) was a 59-year-old man who died 6 years after the onset of diarrhea and facial flushing. He had cardiac catheterization 4 years before he died, and the right atrial a-wave pressure was elevated to 24 and the v-wave to 34 mm. Hg (Figure 1). The second patient (C. G., 05-49-35) was a 32-year-old woman who died 9 years after the onset of diarrhea and facial flushing. At catheterization (Figures 2 and 3), performed 8 months before death, the right atrial a-wave pressure was 18, v-wave 23, and mean pressure 15 mm. Hg. The right ventricular pressure was 45/13, and the pulmonary arterial pressure, 20/8 mm. Hg. Cardiac output (dye dilution method) was 4.95 liters per min., and the cardiac index was 3.25 liters per min. per M^2 B.S.A. The arterial hemoglobin oxygen saturation was 92.5 per cent.

On examination, each of the patients was emaciated and demonstrated hepatomegaly, ascites, leg edema, and greatly distended neck veins. A blowing systolic murmur, which increased in intensity during inspiration, was present

Laboratory of Pathology, Clinic of Surgery, the Cardiology Branch, National Heart Institute, and the Pathologic Anatomy Department, Clinical Center, National Institutes of Health, Bethesda, Maryland

Received, June 1, 1965.

DOI: 10.1201/9781003409281-4

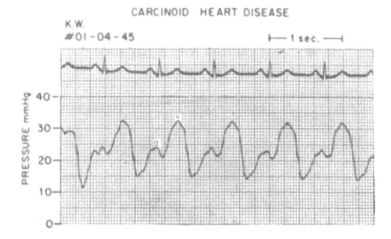

Figure 1 Right atrial pressure tracing in patient K. W. showing marked elevation of peaks of the v- and a-waves.

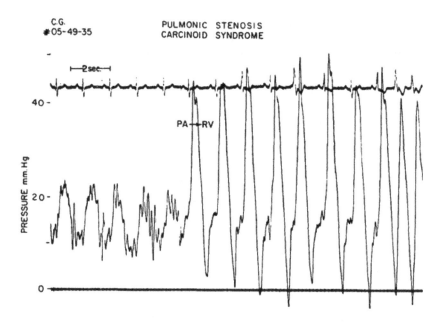

Figure 2 Pullback pressure tracing from the pulmonary artery *(PA)* into the right ventricle *(RV)*, demonstrating the systolic pressure gradient.

over the lower left sternal border, and a harsh systolic murmur was present over the upper left sternal border in each patient. Electrocardiograms (Figure 4) in both patients revealed low voltage and right axis deviation. In addition, right ventricular hypertrophy was present in one (C. G.)

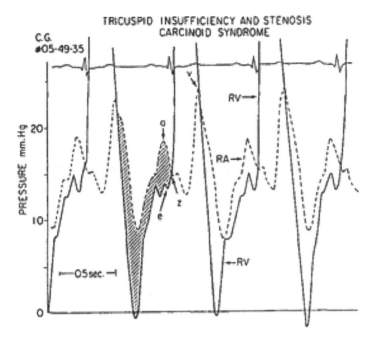

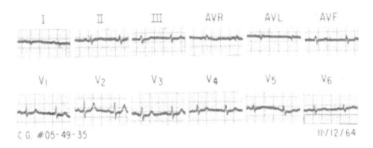

Figure 3 Simultaneously recorded right atrial *(RM)* and right ventricular *(RV)* pressures showing the tall right atrial v-waves with rapid descent, elevated right atrial mean pressure, increased right ventricular end-diastolic pressure (e), and small diastolic pressure gradient *(dashed area)*. Z = z-point, *a* = a-point.

Figure 4 Electrocardiogram in Patient C. G. Low voltage was present in each of the 2 patients described herein and is the most frequent electrocardiographic abnormality found in patients with carcinoid heart disease.[1]

At autopsy, both patients had extensive endocardial fibrosis involving the tricuspid and pulmonic valves and right atrium (Figures 5 to 7). The heart of K. W. weighed 350 Gm., and that of C. G., 250 Gm.

COMMENT AND CONCLUSIONS
The valvular and mural lesions in carcinoid heart disease are specific and characterized by the deposition of an unusual type of fibrous tissue on the

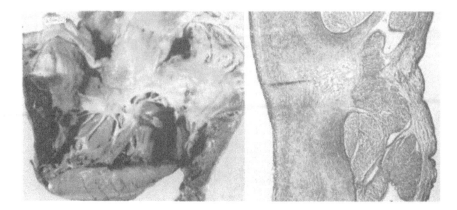

Figure 5 The heart of Patient K. W. *Left,* the right atrium, tricuspid valve, and right ventricle are opened. There is marked carcinoid-type endocardial fibrosis involving the tricuspid valve leaflets and the right atrial wall. The tricuspid valve is incompetent. *Right,* photomicrograph of section of right atrium showing severe thickening of its wall by the deposition of fibrous tissue on the endocardium. The endocardial surface is toward the left, the epicardial surface is on the right. The thickness of the superimposed fibrous tissue at times is greater than that of the right atrial wall. Elastic tissue stain. Reduced 30 per cent from × 40.

endocardial surface. The deposits, which are devoid of elastic fibrils, are located almost entirely on the under or ventricular surface of the tricuspid valve leaflets and on the arterial surface of the pulmonic valve cusps. The underlying valve leaflets and ventricular walls are not involved by this fibrous process and are clearly separated from it by the normal endocardial elastic membrane. The fibrous plaques frequently bind the posterior and septal leaflets of the tricuspid valve to the underlying right ventricular wall, and the result is a fixed regurgitant and slightly stenotic orifice. Tricuspid regurgitation is the most frequent clinical cardiac lesion resulting from this type of fibrosis. When the tricuspid valve is involved, this fibrosing process almost always involves the right atrial endocardium, as well. From study of the extensive right atrial deposits at autopsy in the 2 patients presented, it would seem that the wall of this chamber in these instances is relatively inelastic and consequently not able to distend or to contract normally. This reduction in right atrial elasticity or distensibility as a result of the thick endocardial fibrous deposits probably significantly altered the hemodynamic findings in the right atrial pulse. Thus, there was in each of these 2 patients a greater elevation of the right atrial pressures than would have been expected from the sizes of the tricuspid valve orifices observed at autopsy. It is suggested that even mild tricuspid carcinoid disease may produce significant elevation of right atrial pressures, whereas an equal degree of rheumatic tricuspid disease would not cause right atrial hypertension.

Acknowledgment. Dr. Albert Sjoerdsma, Chief, Experimental Therapeutics Branch, National Heart Institute, gave permission to report these 2 patients and reviewed the manuscript.

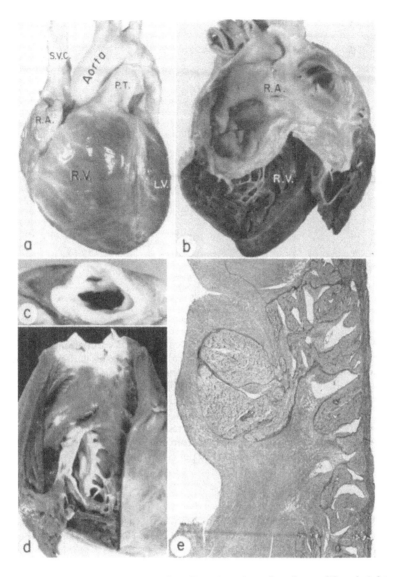

Figure 6 The heart of Patient C. G. *a*. Exterior view showing a dilated right ventricle (*R.V.*) and right atrium (*R.A.*). The apex of the heart is formed by the right ventricle. *S.V.C.* = superior vena cava. *P.T.* = pulmonary trunk. *b*. Opened right atrium, tricuspid valve, and right ventricle. There is marked fibrous thickening of the tricuspid-valve leaflets with fusion of their commissures, and diffuse carcinoid-type fibrosis of the dilated right atrium and superior vena cava. *c*. Unopened, immobile pulmonic valve. *d*. Opened right ventricle and pulmonic valve disclosing marked carcinoid-type fibrosis of both tricuspid and pulmonic valve leaflets producing stenotic and regurgitant orifices. *e*. Photomicrograph of section of right atrial wall which is severely thickened by the deposition of the fibrous tissue which is devoid of elastic fibrils. Elastic tissue stain. × 19.

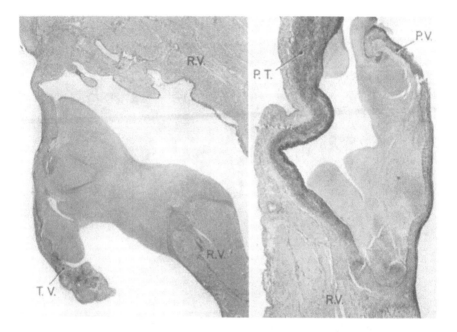

Figure 7 Photomicrographs of right-sided cardiac valves in patient C. G. *Left*, tricuspid valve *(T.V.)*. The superimposed atypical fibrous tissue is deposited only on the undersurface of the leaflet, binding it to the underlying right ventricular *(R.V.)* wall. *Right*, pulmonic valve *(P.V.)*. The cusp itself is normal and sharply outlined by its black-staining elastic membrane, but the superimposed fibrous tissue is adherent to its entire arterial surface and fills much of the sinus. A small deposit also is present on the pulmonic trunk *(P.T.)*. The surface of the pulmonic valve cusp which has the initial contact with blood ejected from the right ventricle is free of fibrous deposits. Elastic tissue stains. Reduced 20 per cent from × 15.

REFERENCE

1. Roberts, W. C., and Sjoerdsma, A.: The cardiac disease associated with the carcinoid syndrome (carcinoid heart disease), *Am J Med* **36**:5–34, 1964.

Case 35 Pulmonary Arteriovenous Fistula and Rheumatic Cardiac Disease

Costan W. Berard, M.D*, William C. Roberts, M.D.** and Richard L. Kahler, M.D.***
Bethesda, MD

The occurrence of peripheral cyanosis (normal arterial oxygen saturation) in patients with severe acquired cardiac valvular disease is not uncommon. However, the occurrence of central cyanosis (reduced arterial oxygen saturation) in these patients is distinctly unusual and suggests the presence of a right-to-left (venoarterial) shunt or extreme pulmonary disease. A patient with severe rheumatic valvular disease was noted to have generalized cyanosis and was found to have a pulmonary arteriovenous fistula. A review of published reports of pulmonary A-V fistulas revealed only 2 other patients with coexistent cardiac valvular disease,[1,2] and consequently prompted this report.

CASE REPORT

M.P. (#05-45-49), a 50-year-old white woman who had had acute rheumatic fever during late childhood, was told during her twenties that she had a "heart murmur." She was asymptomatic until age 47, when exertional dyspnea appeared. Thereafter, symptoms of cardiac decompensation rapidly progressed despite digitalization and diuretic therapy, and, in the 6 months before admission, she became markedly incapacitated, bedridden, and cachectic (35 kilograms).

On admission, she was dyspneic and tachypneic (42 per minute) while sitting up in bed. Her lips and nail beds were cyanotic but there was no digital clubbing or cutaneous or mucosal telangiectasia. The blood pressure was 100/70 mm. Hg, and the heart was enlarged. A Grade 3/6 pansystolic blowing murmur and a Grade 3/6 diastolic rumble were audible over the cardiac apex. A grade 4/6 high-pitched decrescendo diastolic blowing murmur was heard at the lower left sternal border. No murmur was heard over the back. The liver was enlarged, but there was no peripheral edema.

The hematocrit was 46 per cent, and the hemoglobin was 14.3 Gm. per cent. Chest roentgenograms (Figure 1) showed a mass, 6-by-3 cm. in size, in the left lower lung field, cardiomegaly, and calcium in the region of the mitral valve. The electrocardiogram revealed atrial fibrillation, right axis deviation, and right ventricular hypertrophy. Femoral arterial hemoglobin oxygen saturation was 76 per cent while the patient was breathing room air, and rose to 84 per cent after the patient breathed 100 per cent oxygen for 10 minutes. Before cardiac catheterization studies and angiocardiography could be performed, the patient developed acute pneumonia and died.

From the Department of Pathologic Anatomy, National Cancer Institute, the Laboratory of Pathology, Clinic of Surgery, and the Cardiology Branch, National Heart Institute, National Institutes of Health, Bethesda, Md.

Received for publication April 22, 1965.

* Department of Pathologic Anatomy, National Cancer Institute.
** Laboratory of Pathology, Clinic of Surgery, National Heart Institute.
*** Cardiology Branch, National Heart Institute.

DOI: 10.1201/9781003409281-5

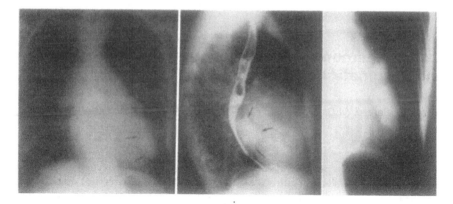

Figure 1 Chest roentgenograms. Posteroanterior view *(left)*, lateral view *(middle)*, and anteroposterior tomogram *(right)*. The pulmonary A-V fistula is designated by the arrows.

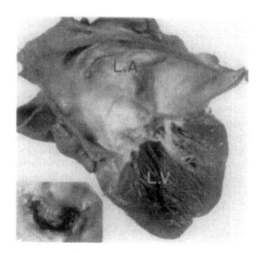

Figure 2 Photograph of the left atrium *(L.A.)*, mitral valve, and the left ventricle *(L.V.)*. The insert shows the unopened diseased mitral valve as seen from the left atrium.

At autopsy (A64–127), the mitral valve was rigid and calcified, and showed evidence of being both insufficient and stenotic (Figure 2). The aortic valve leaflets were thickened and slightly retracted. The left atrial appendage contained old and recent thrombus. In the lingular portion of the left upper lobe, immediately posterolateral to the heart, there was a saccular pulmonary A-V fistula (Figures 3 and 4). Histologic sections of the lungs showed no changes indicative of hypertensive pulmonary vascular disease.

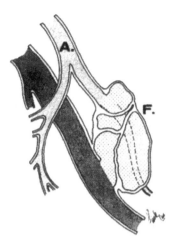

Figure 3 Diagram of the pulmonary A-V fistula. *A:* Pulmonary artery. *V:* Pulmonary vein. *F:* Pulmonary A-V fistula. The diameter of the pulmonary vein is greater than that of the pulmonary artery.

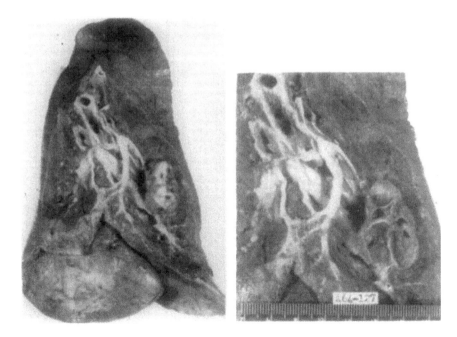

Figure 4 Photograph of the pulmonary A-V fistula in the lingular portion of the left upper lobe. *Left:* The fistula is shown before removal of its medial wall. *Right:* Close-up view showing the quadrilocular fistula.

DISCUSSION

The majority of patients with pulmonary A-V fistula have central cyanosis, digital clubbing, polycythemia, and a localized continuous murmur over the chest.[3] The present patient, however, like 2 previously reported patients with coexistent cardiac valvular disease and pulmonary A-V fistula[1,2] did not have clubbed digits, polycythemia, or a thoracic murmur which could be definitely attributed to a shunt through the fistula. Although occasionally an individual with a pulmonary A-V fistula has no detectable thoracic murmur,[2] it is more likely that in the present patient a murmur was produced by the shunt but was masked by the cardiac murmurs.

REFERENCES

1. Gagnon, E. D., Johnson, R., Siniard, L. C., and Page, A.: Two cases of pulmonary arteriovenous aneurysm with associated rheumatic aortic stenosis in one of them, *Canad MAJ* **79**:906, 1958.
2. Steinberg, L: Pulmonary arteriovenous fistulas of the medial basal segment of the right lower lobe: A note on absence of vascular bruits, *Dis Chest* **33**:86, 1958.
3. Moyer, J. H., Glantz, G., and Brest, A. N.: Pulmonary arteriovenous fistulas, *Am J Med* **32**:417, 1962.

Case 38 Intestinal Infarction Resulting from Nonobstructive Mesenteric Arterial Insufficiency

With a Note on Hepatic Hypoglycemia as a Possible Aid in Diagnosis

Robert K. Brawley, MD; William C. Roberts, MD; and Andrew G. Morrow, MD
Bethesda, MD

GASTROINTESTINAL hemorrhage and necrosis may result from intestinal ischemia secondary to inadequate cardiac output and increased splanchnic vascular resistance.* A variety of conditions, including severe congestive heart failure, acute myocardial infarction, shock, cardiac arrhythmias, and extensive operative procedures, may precipitate intestinal ischemia. The clinical manifestations which accompany this process are determined by the degree of mesenteric vascular insufficiency and range from transient abdominal angina, nausea, and diarrhea to signs of a perforated viscus. The abdominal symptoms and signs resulting from intestinal ischemia are, however, often obscured by the presence of serious disturbances of the nervous and cardiovascular systems. Detailed descriptions of patients who have developed severe abdominal pain secondary to nonobstructive mesenteric arterial insufficiency are unusual. This report describes the clinical, operative, and pathologic findings in such a patient, who had rheumatic mitral stenosis and congestive heart failure.

REPORT OF CASE

Clinical Summary.—A 41-year-old woman, who had acute rheumatic fever at age nine, had been found to have a precordial murmur during her first pregnancy at age 25. At age 32 she was treated with digitalis because of increasing exertional dyspnea, fatigue, and orthopnea. At age 37 (1960) a diagnosis of mitral stenosis was made, and a closed mitral commissurotomy was performed. At operation the valve was found to be heavily calcified, markedly stenotic, and a mild regurgitant jet was also palpable. The patient improved only transiently after this procedure and a year later again developed severe cardiac decompensation, despite digitalis and diuretic therapy. Thereafter, she was hospitalized on numerous occasions, and in December 1963 was admitted to the National Heart Institute. She was dyspneic, afebrile, and in atrial fibrillation with a ventricular response of 110 beats per minute. The blood pressure was 110/80 mm Hg. The trunk, arms, and legs were covered with a maculopapular rash. The jugular veins were distended, and the heart enlarged. A grade 3/6 blowing pansystolic murmur and a grade 2/6 rumbling diastolic murmur were audible at the cardiac apex. The liver was enlarged and tender; the legs and sacrum were edematous. The hematocrit value was 50%; white blood cell count (WBC), 8,300/cu

Submitted for publication Dec 7, 1965.

From the Clinic of Surgery, National Heart Institute, National Institutes of Health, Bethesda.

Reprint requests to National Heart Institute, National Institutes of Health, Bethesda, Md 20014 (Dr. Morrow).

* References 1–10, 18, 19.

DOI: 10.1201/9781003409281-6

mm with a normal differential; whole blood urea nitrogen (BUN), 14 mg/100 ml; and fasting blood sugar, 106 mg/100 ml.

During the first two hospital days the patient was treated with bed rest, sodium restriction, and diuretics; her condition improved and she lost 4 kg in weight. On the third hospital day, however, intermittent bigeminal rhythm was noted, and her rash became urticarial and pruritic. Digitoxin, chlorothiazide, and penicillin were discontinued, and on the sixth hospital day prednisolone was given because of progressive worsening of the rash. On the morning of the eighth day, while walking, the patient developed severe midepigastric pain, a sensation of fullness in the right upper quadrant, and nausea. On examination the abdomen was soft, bowel sounds were present, and there was moderate tenderness in the midepigastrium and right upper quadrant. The heart rate was 120 beats per minute and the blood pressure was 150/90 mm Hg. The WBC was 15,000/cu mm, and roentgenograms of the abdomen were unremarkable. Electrocardiograms (ECG) and roentgenograms of the chest were unchanged in comparison to those obtained at the time of admission. The abdominal pain abated, but 12 hours later the systolic blood pressure was 80 mm Hg. At this time the serum sodium was 138 mEq/liter; potassium, 6.7 mEq/liter; chloride, 82 mEq/liter; carbon dioxide content, 12 mEq/liter; blood sugar, 35 mg/100 ml; serum amylase, 136 Somogyi units; and BUN, 30 mg/100 ml. Repeat blood sugar was 27 mg/100 ml; repeat serum potassium was 7.5 mEq/liter; and the arterial blood had a pH of 7.27, Po_2, 71 mm Hg, and PCO_2, 27 mm Hg. Intravenous fluids containing glucose (25 gm), sodium bicarbonate (7.5 gm) and metaraminol (in amounts sufficient to maintain the systolic blood pressure at 90 mm Hg), digitoxin, and nasal oxygen were administered, and within one hour the abdominal pain had subsided and the patient improved. Two hours later the blood sugar was 135 mg/100 cc, and the BUN was 41 mg/100 ml. The serum potassium was 6.1 mEq/liter; sodium, 132 mEq/liter; chloride, 79 mEq/liter; and carbon dioxide, 12 mEq/liter.

During the next six hours the abdominal pain gradually returned, associated with generalized abdominal tenderness with rebound and rigidity and absent bowel sounds. A stool contained occult blood. Dilated loops of small bowel, with air-fluid levels, were seen on roentgenograms. The blood pressure, which had been about 100 mm Hg systolic during the previous six hours, without the administration of vasopressors, suddenly dropped to 50 mm Hg systolic, and the patient became disoriented and irrational. Intravenous metaraminol, antibiotics, prednisolone, and plasma were given, and an exploratory laparotomy was performed. The peritoneal cavity contained approximately 500 ml of turbid, brown fluid with a fecal odor. The serosal surfaces of the stomach, duodenum, and proximal 10 cm of the jejunum appeared normal. The small bowel distal to this point, however, was dilated and cyanotic, and in some areas appeared to be necrotic. The ascending and transverse colon were gray but appeared viable; the descending colon, from the splenic flexure to the pelvic brim, was black. The superior and inferior mesenteric arteries were nonpulsatile and severely constricted, but no localized obstruction could be detected at any point. Cardiac arrest occurred at the conclusion of the operation, and resuscitation was unsuccessful.

Pathologic Findings.—At autopsy, the stomach and duodenum were normal, but the mucosa of the jejunum, ileum, and colon varied from black to red in color (Figure 1). The serosa of the entire small and large intestine was smooth and glistening, but of dark color. No thrombi or emboli were found in any of the mesenteric vessels, and the mesenteric arteries contained no atheromata. Numerous histologic sections of small and large intestine were examined; some areas were normal while others showed distinct pathologic changes. The most frequent lesion observed was hemorrhagic necrosis of the mucosa (Figure 2). In some areas of the bowel this was the only abnormal finding. At other sites, however, the muscularis

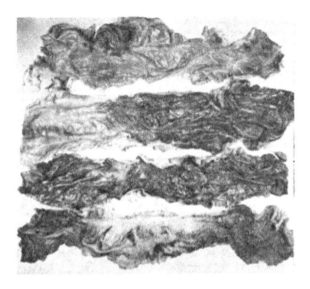

Figure 1 Gross appearance of intestine. Distribution of lesions was irregular and segments of involved mucosa were hemorrhagic.

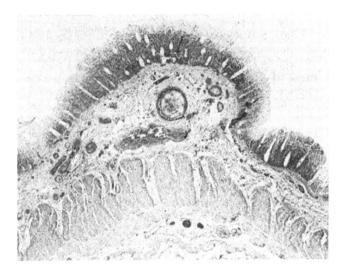

Figure 2 Section of intestine disclosing hemorrhagic necrosis of mucosa and severe dilatation of submucosal blood vessels. Although not apparent in this photomicrograph, there was focal degeneration and necrosis of the smooth muscle of the muscular layer (hematoxylin and eosin, × 25).

mucosae and muscularis externa were also necrotic. In addition, the submucosa was edematous, contained acute inflammatory cells, and its vessels, particularly the veins, were markedly distended by erythrocytes. Variations between these two lesions commonly were seen. The serosa in all sections was intact and free of inflammatory cells, and no mucosal ulcerations were present. Sections of the liver,

41

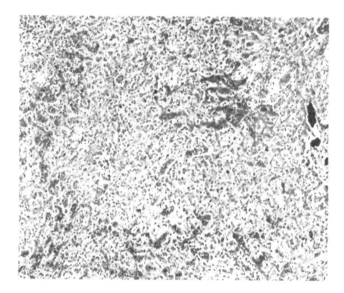

Figure 3 Section of liver disclosing massive necrosis of hepatic lobules. Hepatic architecture was barely discernible (hematoxylin and eosin, × 84).

which weighed 1,700 gm, disclosed massive centrolobular congestion and necrosis, and occasionally infarction of entire lobules (Figure 3). Sections of the kidneys were unremarkable, except for a few old small cortical infarcts.

The heart revealed typical rheumatic mitral valve disease, and the valve orifice was both stenotic and regurgitant (Figure 4). An organized thrombus filled the left atrial appendage. The right ventricle, tricuspid valve ring, and right atrium were dilated, but the tricuspid leaflets and chordae were normal. There was hemorrhagic infarction of the lower lobe of the left lung, and the pulmonary artery to this lobe was completely occluded by a fibrin clot.

COMMENT

Several reviews have emphasized the difficult diagnostic problem posed in the clinical differentiation of nonobstructive and obstructive mesenteric arterial insufficiency.[1-6] The majority of patients with either of these lesions have underlying cardiac disease, and then manifest signs and symptoms related to the abdomen. Abdominal pain, tenderness and distention, nausea and vomiting, bloody diarrhea, and leukocytosis may occur with both conditions. Although abdominal and cardiac manifestations are similar in both obstructive and nonobstructive mesenteric arterial insufficiency, evidences of ischemia in other organ systems is an important diagnostic finding favoring the presence of the nonobstructive lesion. The basic physiologic abnormality in nonobstructive mesenteric arterial insufficiency is an inadequate cardiac output, and the intestine is but one of several areas which receive an insufficient supply of blood. When the cardiac output is abnormally low, the distribution of arterial flow is also abnormal and, by means of selective vasoconstriction, oxygenated blood is shunted to the more vital body areas, such as the heart and brain, and away from the peripheral and splanchnic vascular beds.[7-9] Intestinal ischemia of the nonobstructive type is, therefore, often associated with evidences of decreased perfusion of other body regions, and manifestations of central nervous system, renal, and hepatic ischemia favor this diagnosis. The present

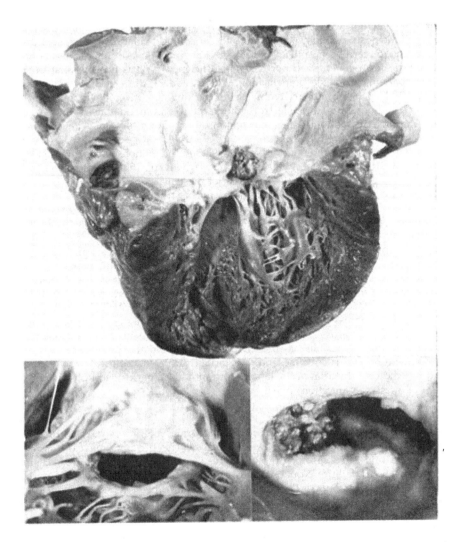

Figure 4　Heart. *Top,* Opened left atrium, mitral valve, and left ventricle. Organized thrombus was present in left atrial appendage. Mitral valve leaflets and chordae tendineae were fibrotic, shortened, and focally calcified. *Bottom,* Mitral valve orifice as seen from left ventricle *(left)* and from left atrium *(right)*. Valve was both stenotic and incompetent.

patient, for example, had evidence of inadequate blood flow to the kidneys (oliguria, azotemia) and liver (hypoglycemia), as well as to the bowel (abdominal pain), before clinical signs of intestinal necrosis appeared. Hypoglycemia has been reported in one other patient with severe cardiac decompensation and nonobstructive mesenteric arterial insufficiency, and may be an important indicator of ischemia of the liver.[10] Hypoglycemia in the present patient appears to have resulted from hepatic ischemia, since necrosis of entire hepatic lobules was found at autopsy.[11,12] In addition, the patient described had severe metabolic acidosis, an abnormality which is also more likely to occur in nonobstructive mesenteric arterial insufficiency than in association with an isolated obstruction of the superior mesenteric artery. Metabolic acidosis, due to tissue hypoxia and anaerobic oxidation, is a consequence of inadequate cardiac output of any cause, and in patients with cardiac failure often indicates a generalized perfusion insufficiency.[13-15] It is possible that in the present patient cardiac decompensation, with a sudden fall in cardiac output, was precipitated by the pulmonary embolus, but the embolus was not evident from the physical, radiographic, and electrocardiographic examinations performed soon after the onset of abdominal pain. Digitalis intoxication also may have been a precipitating factor in this patient.

The diagnostic differentiation of obstructive and nonobstructive mesenteric arterial insufficiency is of vital importance when specific treatment becomes necessary. Organic obstruction of the superior mesenteric artery, or one of its major branches, by an embolus or thrombus necessitates early operative intervention and restoration of a patent aterial lumen before intestinal necrosis occurs.[5,16,17] In contrast, laparotomy prior to bowel infarction is contraindicated in patients with arterial insufficiency secondary to an inadequate cardiac output, since further reduction in cardiac output and intestinal perfusion may result from anesthesia and operative manipulation of the intestine. Optimal therapy in patients with nonobstructive mesenteric arterial insufficiency must be directed to measures which will increase systemic blood flow: vigorous treatment of cardiac failure, maintenance of adequate blood and extracellular fluid volumes, correction of metabolic abnormalities, intestinal decompression, and reduction of an abnormally high hematocrit reading. Obviously, vasopressors should be avoided whenever possible and vasodilatation by serial epidural blockade may be of benefit.[18] Operation may prove necessary in a patient with nonobstructive mesenteric arterial insufficiency, but when the clinical findings indicate this diagnosis, laporatomy should be performed only if definite signs of intestinal infarction appear.

SUMMARY

A patient is described in whom nonobstructive mesenteric arterial insufficiency caused focal infarction of the bowel and liver. The precipitating cause was a strikingly diminished cardiac output, the result of rheumatic mitral stenosis and congestive heart failure. Nonobstructive mesenteric arterial insufficiency, rather than mesenteric embolus or thrombosis, was indicated by evidences of inadequate perfusion of other organ systems resulting in oliguria, hypoglycemia, and metabolic acidosis.

GENERIC AND TRADE NAME OF DRUG

Chlorothiazide—*Diuril*

REFERENCES

1. Berger, R. L., and Byrne, J. J.: Intestinal gangrene associated with heart disease, *Surg Gynec Obstct* **112**:529, 1961.
2. Ende, N.: Infarction of the bowel in cardiac failure, *New Eng J Med* **258**:879, 1958.
3. Glotzer, D. J., and Shaw, R. S.: Massive bowel infarction: An autopsy study assessing the potentialities of reconstructive vascular surgery, *New Eng J Med* **260**:59, 1960.
4. Ming, S. C., and Levitan, R.: Acute hemorrhagic necrosis of the gastrointestinal tract, *New Eng J Med* **263**:59, 1960.
5. Shaw, R. S.: Vascular lesions of the gastrointestinal tract, *Surg Clin N Amer* **39**:1253, 1959.
6. Wilson, R., and Qualheim, R. E.: A form of acute hemorrhagic enterocolitis afflicting chronically 111 individuals, *Gastroenterology* **27**:431, 1954.

7. Corday, E., et al: Mesenteric vascular insufficiency: Intestinal ischemia induced by remote circulatory disturbances, *Amer J Med* **33**:365, 1962.

8. Corday, E., and Williams, J. H.: Effect of shock and vasopressor drugs on the regional circulation of the brain, heart, kidney, and liver, *Amer J Med* **29**:228, 1960.

9. Lillehei, R.C.: The intestinal factor of irreversible hemorrhagic shock, *Surgery* **42**:1043, 1957.

10. Aklerfer, H. H., and Richardson, J. H.: Hepatic hypoglycemia and infarction of the bowel, *Arch Intern Med* **112**:96, 1963.

11. Clarke, W. T. W.: Centrilobular hepatic necrosis following cardiac infarction, *Amer J Path* **26**:249, 1950.

12. Ellenberg, M., and Osserman, K. E.: The role of shock in the production of central liver cell necrosis, *Amer J Med* **11**:170, 1951.

13. Clowes, G. H. A., Jr., et al: Effects of acidosis on cardiovascular function in surgical patients, *Ann Surg* **154**:524, 1961.

14. Huckabee, W. E.: Lactic acidosis, *Amer J Cardiol* **12**:663, 1963.

15. Litwin, M. S., et al: Acidosis and lacticacidermia in extracorporeal circulation: The significance of perfusion flow rate and the relation to preperfusion respiratory alkalosis, *Ann Surg* **149**:188, 1959.

16. Rutledge, R. H.: Superior mesenteric artery embolectomy, *Ann Surg* **159**:529, 1964.

17. Zuidema, G. D., et al: Superior mesenteric artery embolectomy, *Ann Surg* **159**:548, 1964.

18. Jackson, B. B., and Lykins, R.: Serial epidural analgesia in mesenteric arterial failure, *Arch Surg* **90**:177, 1965.

19. Bachrach, W. H., and Thorner, M. C.: Hemorrhagic enteropathy complicating myocardial infarction, *Amer J Cardiol* **11**:89, 1963.

Case 56 Roentgenogram of the Month

William C. Roberts, MD,* Gonstan VV. Berard, MD and Nina S. Braunwald, MD
Bethesda, Maryland

Benjamin Felson, M.D., Editor
Harold Spitz, M.D., Co-Editor

A 45-YEAR-OLD WHITE MAN WITH RHEUMATIC mitral stenosis and aortic regurgitation underwent replacement of both mitral and aortic valves with Starr-Edwards prostheses on April 21, 1964. In October, 1964, he developed fulminating hepatic decompensation secondary to probable serum hepatitis superimposed on cardiac cirrhosis, and was treated thereafter with high doses of a corticosteroid. In January, 1965, he developed fever, night sweats, anorexia and dyspnea. Figures 1 and 2 were obtained at that time. He died on February 27, 1965.

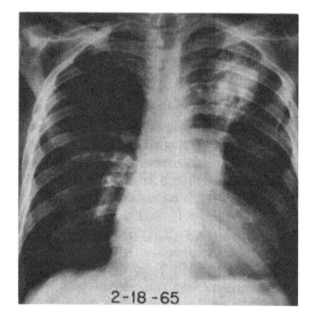

Figure 1

For reprints, please write: Dr. William C. Roberts, Laboratory of Pathology, Clinic of Surgery, National Heart Institute, National Institutes of Health, Bethesda, Maryland 20014.
* From the Clinic of Surgery, National Heart Institute and the Pathologic Anatomy Branch, National Cancer Institute, National Institutes of Health.

DOI: 10.1201/9781003409281-7

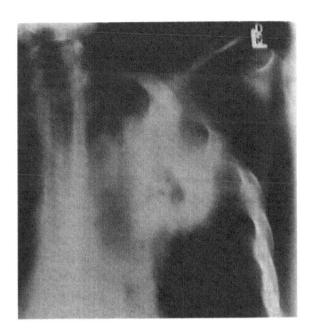

Figure 2

DIAGNOSIS: **Pulmonary Nocardiosis**

The teleoroentgenogram and tomogram demonstrate an area of consolidation with an irregular central cavity. Figure 3A is a cut surface of the left upper lobe showing the cavity. *Nocardia asteroides* organisms, which were cultured from the sputa during life and from the pulmonary cavity at necropsy, are shown in Figure 3B (Brown and Brenn stain; x1200).

Systemic nocardiosis, which is virtually always caused by *N. asteroides*, usually begins in the bronchial mucosa and spreads through the bronchial wall to the pulmonary parenchyma, resulting in extensive necrosis of tissue with the formation of confluent abscesses.[1] The infection may be chronic or acute or even fulminating.[2] *N. asteroides* are aerobic, Gram-positive and variably acid-fast, delicate, branching filamentous fungi which break up into bacillary forms of varying lengths. Pulmonary-cutaneous fistulas and granules are less common than in actinomycosis. Hematogenous spread results in metastatic lesions throughout the body, most commonly to the brain.

The diagnosis of pulmonary nocardiosis is made by staining a smear of the sputa specifically for bacterial organisms (Brown and Brenn stain). The organism grows on a variety of simple media, including blood agar, but a three to four week period is required before the typical colonies are identifiable.

Sulfonamides (4–8 gm daily in adults) constitute the treatment of systemic nocardiosis, and the therapy should be continued for two to three months after all signs and symptoms of the disease have disappeared.[2]

The nocardiosis in this patient represents an infection in one whose resistance had been lowered by a combination of chronic diseases (cardiac and hepatic) and steroid therapy, although nocardiosis may occur as a primary disease.[2,3]

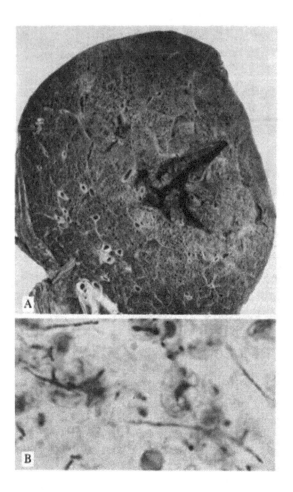

Figure 3

REFERENCES

1. WEED, L. A., ANDERSEN, H. A., GOOD, G. A. AND BAGGENSTOSS, A. H.: "Nocardiosis. Clinical, bacteriologic and pathologic aspects," *New Engl. J. Med.*, 253:1137, 1955.
2. FREESE, J. W., YOUNG, W. G., JR., SEALY, W. C. AND CONANT, N. F.: "Pulmonary infection by *Nocardia asteroides*. Findings in eleven clinical cases," *J. Thor. and Cardiovas. Surg.*, 46:537, 1963.
3. SALTZMAN, H. A., CHICK, E. W. AND CONANT, N. F.: "Nocardiosis as a complication of other diseases," *Lab. Invest.*, 11:1110, 1962.

Case 65 Quadrivalvular Rheumatoid Heart Disease Associated with Left Bundle Branch Block*

Deborah F. Carpenter, MD,† Abner Golden, MD and William C. Roberts, MD‡
Washington, D. C.

The clinical and necropsy findings are described in a sixty-five year old woman with rheumatoid arthritis and rheumatoid nodules in the heart, lungs, joints and subcutaneous tissue. Signs of aortic and mitral regurgitation, congestive cardiac failure and left bundle branch block were observed clinically and necropsy revealed numerous rheumatoid nodules in all four cardiac valves as well as in the adjacent myocardium and in the pericardium. The extensive nature of the cardiac involvement by rheumatoid granulomas is the most unusual aspect of this patient's illness.

NONSPECIFIC obliterative pericarditis is frequently observed at autopsy in patients with rheumatoid arthritis but the finding of rheumatoid nodules in the heart is unusual. Granulomas histologically indistinguishable from those of the subcutaneous tissues have been described in the pericardium, myocardium and endocardium, including the cardiac valves. They are usually few in number and involve only one valve or a limited area of myocardium or pericardium. Similar lesions have at times been described in lung, pleura, larynx, vertebrae, skeletal muscle, peripheral nerve, esophagus, kidney, spleen, eyes and dura.

Described herein are the clinical and postmortem findings in a patient with rheumatoid arthritis who had mitral and aortic valvular regurgitation, severe congestive cardiac failure and left bundle branch block. Numerous rheumatoid nodules were present in all four cardiac valves, in large areas of myocardium including the conduction system and in the pericardium.

CASE REPORT

A sixty-five year old white woman (D.Y., No. 98266) died on March 15, 1966, in congestive cardiac failure. Although she apparently had had systemic hypertension at one time, she had been well until age fifty when signs and symptoms of rheumatoid arthritis appeared, with progressive involvement of the knees, ankles, hips, wrists, shoulders and cervical vertebrae. She received adrenocorticotropic hormone, nitrogen mustard, gold, prednisone, whirlpool therapy and intra-articular hydrocortisone at various times. Approximately six months before death signs and symptoms of right- and left-sided congestive cardiac failure appeared. She lost 35 pounds, became bedridden mainly because of dyspnea, and two days before death became obtunded and was hospitalized.

On examination, the blood pressure ranged from 140/60 to 105/30 mm. Hg, the pulse was 80 per minute, respiration 12 per minute and the temperature was normal.

* From the Department of Pathology, Georgetown University School of Medicine and Medical Center, Washington, D. C. Manuscript received November 10 1966.

† Present address: Pathologic Anatomy Branch, National Cancer Institute, National Institutes of Health, Bethesda, Maryland.

‡ Present address: Laboratory of Pathology, Clinic of Surgery, National Heart Institute, National Institutes of Health, Bethesda, Maryland.

DOI: 10.1201/9781003409281-8

49

She was cachectic (weight 43 kg.), obtunded and dehydrated. There was severe limitation to passive as well as active movement of all peripheral joints and to flexion and extension of the neck. There was marked ulnar deviation of both wrists and fusiform swelling of the metacarpal-phalangeal joints. The heart was enlarged and both atrial and ventricular gallops were audible. A grade 3/6 ejection type systolic murmur which radiated into the neck was audible over the cardiac base, a grade 2/6 high-pitched blowing diastolic murmur was heard over the left sternal border and a grade 2/6 blowing pansystolic murmur which radiated into the left axilla was heard over the cardiac apex.

The blood hematocrit was 40 per cent and the white blood cell count was 8,200 per cu. mm. The serum total protein was 6.7 gm. with albumin 2.1 gm. per 100 ml. Blood electrolytes and urea nitrogen were normal. Chest roentgenogram (Figure 1) showed cardiomegaly, a small left pleural effusion and arthritic changes in the shoulders. Electrocardiogram (Figure 2) showed normal sinus rhythm, left bundle

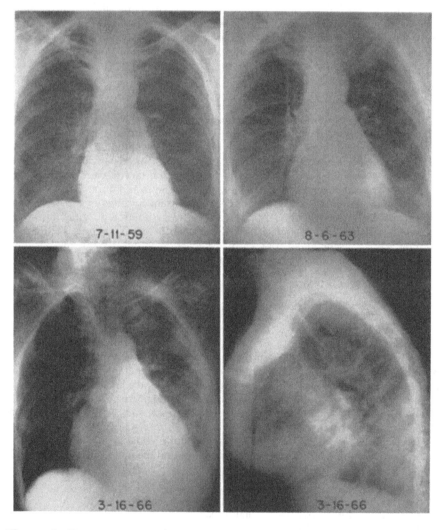

Figure 1 Roentgenograms demonstrating progressive cardiomegaly. The lower roentgenograms were made one day before death.

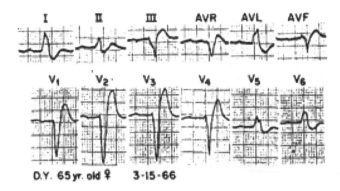

Figure 2 Electrocardiogram recorded one day before death. Left bundle branch block and first degree heart block are present.

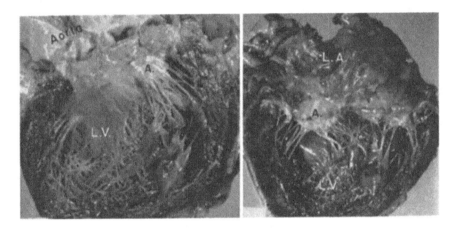

Figure 3 The opened heart. *Left*, the aortic root, aortic valve and left ventricle (L.V.) are shown. Each of the aortic valvular cusps as well as the anterior mitral leaflet (A.) is diffusely thickened. The aortic cusps also are contracted, and prolapse slightly toward the left ventricle. No lesions are present in the aorta itself. *Right*, the left atrium (L.A.), mitral valve and left ventricle (L.V.) are shown. Both anterior (A.) and posterior mitral leaflets are diffusely thickened, but the chordae tendineae are normal and neither commissure is fused. Focal areas of thickening are visible on the endocardial surface of the left atrium.

branch block and a prolonged P-R interval (0.26 second). (Electrocardiogram in August 1963 had been normal.) Breathing became labored and she died two days after admission.

At autopsy (No. 66A-129) the pericardial space was obliterated by fibrous and a few fibrinous adhesions. Within the adhesions and in the subepicardial fat numerous firm, yellow nodules measuring up to 1.5 cm. were found, and on microscopic examination these were typical rheumatoid granulomas. The heart weighed 550 gm. All chambers were dilated and the walls of both right (0.7 cm. thick) and left (1.5 cm. thick) ventricles were hypertrophied (Figure 3 through 10). The aortic and mitral valvular leaflets were markedly thickened, and the normal cuspal tissue was replaced by innumerable rheumatoid nodules. The thickening

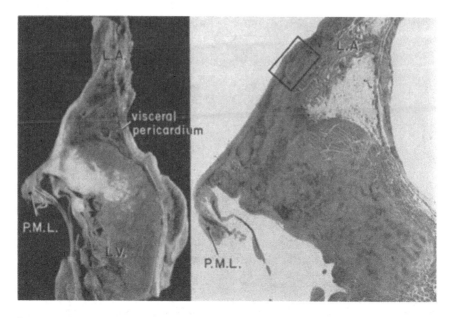

Figure 4 Gross (*left*) and histologic section (*right*) of wall of left atrium (L.A.) and left ventricle (L.V.), and posterior mitral leaflet (P.M.L.). The basal portion of the left ventricular myocardium and the caudal portion of the left atrial endocardium are replaced by rheumatoid nodules which appear white (*left*). The visceral and parietal pericardia are adherent to one another. A close-up of the area enclosed by the black-lined rectangle is shown in Figure 5. Hematoxylin and eosin stain (*right*), original magnification × 2.5.

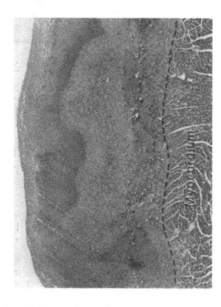

Figure 5 Left atrial wall. The endocardium is markedly thickened by the presence of rheumatoid nodules. The dashed line separates the endocardium from the myocardium. Hematoxylin and eosin stain, original magnification × 28.

of these cusps almost certainly prevented them from closing completely. Similar rheumatoid nodules were localized discretely at the basal attachments of the septal and anterior tricuspid leaflets and of two of the three pulmonic valvular cusps. Function of these right-sided valves, however, would not appear to have been altered. In addition to the rheumatoid nodules in the mitral and aortic leaflets, the process extended into the myocardium in the basal portion of the left ventricular free wall, into the adipose tissue of the left atrioventricular sulcus, and down the membranous septum to the cephalad portion of the muscular ventricular septum. Remnants of the atrioventricular bundle were found, but the proximal portion of the left bundle branch was completely interrupted by the granulomatous process.

The lungs were edematous, and firm well circumscribed yellow nodules up to 0.5 cm. in diameter were found in both lower lobes and in the middle lobe of the right lung. The nodules demonstrated the characteristic histologic features of rheumatoid granulomas.

The articular cartilages of the knee joints were destroyed and the bone on the articular surfaces of the tibial and femoral condyles was focally eroded. The

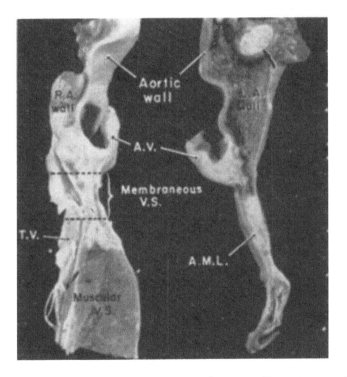

Figure 6 Cut sections depicting aortic root and surrounding structures. *Left*, this block includes an aortic valvular cusp (A.V.), membranous and muscular ventricular septa (V.S.), septal tricuspid valvular leaflet (T.V.) and portion of right atrial wall (R.A.). The entire membranous and the cephalad portion of the muscular septum are virtually replaced by rheumatoid granulomas which appear white. The granulomatous process extends into the tricuspid valve ring through the membranous septum. *Right*, this section includes an aortic valvular cusp, anterior mitral leaflet (A.M.L.), aorta and left atrial wall (L.A.). The "core" of both mitral and aortic valvular cusps are replaced by the innumerable granulomas which appear white. A circumscribed rheumatoid nodule (arrow) is located between the aortic and left atrial walls.

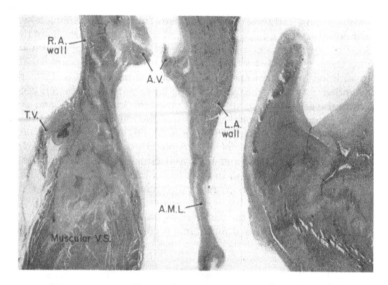

Figure 7 Histologic sections depicting extensive infiltration of the cardiac valves and adjacent structures by rheumatoid nodules. *Left*, this section was prepared from the tissue block shown in Figure 6, left. The membranous and cephalad tip of the muscular ventricular septum (V.S.) are replaced by rheumatoid granulomas. In addition, a rheumatoid nodule is present at the base of the tricuspid valve (T.V.), and others extend up the right atrial wall (R.A.). *Middle*, the aortic valvular cusps (A.V.), anterior mitral leaflet (A.M.L.) and portions of aortic and left atrial (L.A.) walls are extensively infiltrated by rheumatoid granulomas. *Right*, close-up of aortic valvular cusp shown on middle photograph. The "core" of the cusp is uniformly necrotic. The margins of the cusps are relatively well preserved. Hematoxylin and eosin stains, original magnification × 7 (*left*), × 3.5 (*middle*) and × 19 (*right*).

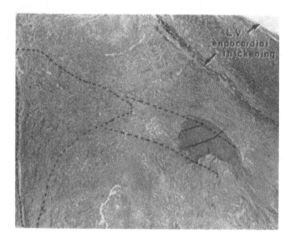

Figure 8 Close-up of most cephalad portion of ventricular septum. The area is extensively infiltrated by rheumatoid granulomas, but portions of the atrioventricular bundle (enclosed by dashed line) remain. The proximal portions of the left bundle branch (the area enclosed by dashed parallel lines), however, are completely disrupted by the granulomatous process. Elastic tissue stain, original magnification × 18.

synovia of these joints was thickened, and histologic sections disclosed organizing connective tissue containing bone chips and pigment-laden macrophages, with proliferation of villi. In addition, inactive and involuting rheumatoid nodules were identified in the synovia of the knee joints and immobile subcutaneous nodules were found over both elbows.

Special stains including Brown and Brenn, Fite, methenamine silver and stains for acid-fast organisms were applied to selected sections of heart and lung; no organisms were found.

COMMENTS

Since the first description by Baggenstoss and Rosenberg in 1941 of cardiac nodules morphologically similar to those seen in the subcutaneous tissues of patients with rheumatoid arthritis, a number of reports describing the heart in this disease have appeared.[1-27] Although specific for this condition, rheumatoid nodules are found in the heart in only 1 to 3 per cent of patients with rheumatoid arthritis who come to autopsy.[2] Other nonspecific types of cardiac lesions, however, have been observed at necropsy in these patients, including pericarditis, myocarditis, coronary arteritis and patchy valvular fibrosis (Table 1). In addition to these specific and nonspecific cardiac lesions which have been considered to be manifestations of rheumatoid disease, other types of heart disease have been identified as being more common in patients with rheumatoid arthritis than in control groups, although these lesions in themselves are not considered to be part of the rheumatoid process. Lebowitz[4] found a higher over-all incidence of cardiac disease, especially calcific aortic stenosis and valvular sclerosis, at autopsy among patients with rheumatoid arthritis than in control subjects matched for age and sex. He noted a similar incidence of arteriosclerotic heart disease, including myocardial infarction, in the two groups and a lower incidence of systemic hypertension and hypertensive heart disease among the patients with rheumatoid arthritis. There was a comparable incidence of previous rheumatic heart disease in the two groups. These observations differ from those of Sokoloff who found a higher incidence of what he called rheumatic heart disease or heart disease indistinguishable from rheumatic heart disease in patients with rheumatoid arthritis.[2] The differences in the incidences of the cardiac diseases associated with rheumatoid arthritis reported by these two investigators can probably be explained by differences in criteria used for the cardiac diagnoses. Goehrs et al.[5] found cardiac hypertrophy in twenty-five of thirty-six autopsy patients with rheumatoid arthritis, and only seven of them had systemic hypertension. Asai found that the incidence of S-T segment depression and/or inverted or flat T waves was significantly greater among 158 patients with rheumatoid arthritis than among 182 apparently healthy control subjects.[6] In those with rheumatoid arthritis changes were most marked in the patients with high levels of serum beta or gamma globulins, and he speculated that dysproteinemia could be a factor in causing the electrocardiographic abnormalities.

At least twenty-one patients with rheumatoid granulomas involving cardiac valves or valve rings have been described in the literature.[4,5,7-16] The aortic valve alone was involved in four patients, the mitral valve alone in ten and both aortic and mitral valves in three. The tricuspid valve alone was involved once, and in another patient both mitral and tricuspid valves were affected. Three valves (aortic, mitral and pulmonic) were involved in one patient and all four in another. In nine of the twelve patients in whom cardiac size was recorded the heart weighed over 300 gm.; in the other three it weighed less than 300 gm. Of the nine patients in whom blood pressure determinations were reported, three had systemic hypertension ($\geq$ 140/90 mm. Hg). The presence or absence of a precordial murmur was recorded in fifteen of these twenty-one subjects. Six

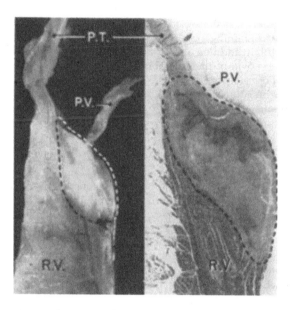

Figure 9 Gross (*left*) and histologic section (*right*) of rheumatoid nodule in right ventricular (R.V.) myocardium at the base of a pulmonic valvular cusp (P.V.). P.T., pulmonic trunk. Hematoxylin and eosin stain (*right*), original magnification × 9.

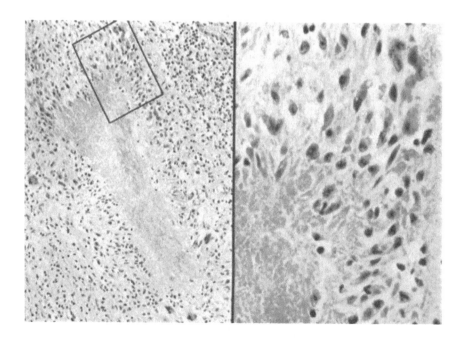

Figure 10 Close-up of cardiac rheumatoid granuloma. This nodule is representative of the many in the heart; this particular one was located at the base of a pulmonic cusp. Hematoxylin and eosin stains, original magnification × 160 (*left*), × 628 (*right*).

Table 1: Rheumatoid heart disease

Rheumatoid granulomas (3%)
   Valve rings and valve leaflets
   Myocardium

                           Complete heart block
      Ventricular septum
                           Left bundle branch block

   Pericardium
Nonspecific inflammatory lesions
   Pericarditis (40%)—Fibrous
   Myocarditis (20%)
   Coronary arteritis (20%)
   Acute and chronic valvulitis (5%)

NOTE: The percentages quoted in this table are from the paper by Sokoloff in 1953.[2]

patients had precordial murmurs which appeared to be related to the presence of granulomas in the cardiac valves, and another patient (not included in the total of twenty-one) had a murmur typical of aortic regurgitation with rheumatoid nodules in the wall of the dilated aortic root but none in the aortic valve itself.[7] In each of these six patients the murmurs were interpreted as representing either mitral regurgitation or aortic stenosis or regurgitation. Three of the other nine patients had precordial murmurs which did not appear to be caused by valvular granulomas, and six patients had no murmur despite the presence of valvular lesions at necropsy. The precordial murmurs when secondary to valvular granulomas tended to indicate that a cardiac valve was extensively involved, but did not correlate with the number of valves containing granulomas. The only patient described with rheumatoid granulomas in all four cardiac valves had no precordial murmur. The murmurs in the present patient were almost certainly the result of incompetent mitral and aortic valves which were not able to close completely because of diffuse thickening of the leaflets. There may also have been some element of aortic valvular stenosis in the present patient, the result of the inability of the thickened cusps to open properly.

The feature which distinguishes our patient from those previously described is the extent and severity of the cardiac involvement. Rheumatoid granulomas were observed in all four valves, in the mural endocardium, in the myocardium and in the pericardium. The mitral and aortic leaflets were diffusely and uniformly thickened by granulomas, but only focal lesions were observed on the tricuspid leaflets and at the base of the pulmonic valvular cusps. The rheumatoid lesions in the previously described patients were generally focal, usually small and widely scattered. The granulomatous process involved the central portion of the valvular leaflets with relative sparing of the margins. This involvement of the "core" of the valvular leaflets is in direct contrast to the valvular involvement in carcinoid heart disease in which the valve itself remains normal and the atypical fibrous tissue is deposited on the surface of the valvular cusp.

In the present patient the left bundle branch block was the result of disruption by rheumatoid granulomas of the left bundle branch as it emerged from the atrioventricular bundle. Complete heart block has been reported in at least two necropsy patients with rheumatoid arthritis, and in one a single rheumatoid nodule was located in the area of the atrioventricular bundle.[17,18] Neither of these patients had granulomas in cardiac valves and appropriate histologic sections were not prepared to determine the precise cause of the heart block.

REFERENCES

1. BAGGENSTOSS, A. H. and ROSENBERG, E. F. Cardiac lesions associated with chronic infectious arthritis. *Arch. Int. Med.*, 67: 241, 1941.
2. SOKOLOFF, L. The heart in rheumatoid arthritis. *Am. Heart J.*, 45: 635, 1953.
3. SOKOLOFF, L. Cardiac involvement in rheumatoid arthritis and allied disorders: current concepts. *Mod. Concepts Cardiovasc. Dis.*, 33: 847, 1964.
4. LEBOWITZ, W. B. The heart in rheumatoid arthritis (rheumatoid disease). *Ann. Int. Med.*, 58: 102, 1963.
5. GOEHRS, H. R., BAGGENSTOSS, A. H. and SLOCUMB, C. H. Cardiac lesions in rheumatoid arthritis. *Arthritis & Rheumat.*, 3: 298, 1960.
6. ASAI, K. Electrographic changes in rheumatoid arthritis. *Jap. Heart J.*, 6: 367, 1965.
7. WEINTRAUB, A. M. and ZVAIFLER, N. J. The occurrence of valvular and myocardial disease in patients with chronic joint deformity. *Am. J, Med.*, 35: 145, 1963.
8. BAGGENSTOSS, A. H. and ROSENBERG, E. F. Unusual cardiac lesions associated with chronic multiple rheumatoid arthritis. *Arch. Path.*, 37: 54, 1944.
9. ELLMAN, P., CUDKOWICZ, L. and ELWOOD, J. S. Widespread serous membrane involvement by rheumatoid nodules. *J. Clin. Path.*, 7: 239, 1954.
10. SCHOENE, R. H. and RISSE, G. B. Rheumatoid heart disease. *Ohio State M. J.*, 60: 377, 1964.
11. SKOGRAND, A. Visceral lesions in rheumatoid arthritis. *Acta Rheumat. Scandinav.*, 2: 17, 1956.
12. GRUENWALD, P. Visceral lesions in a case of rheumatoid arthritis. *Arch. Path.*, 46: 59, 1948.
13. BYWATERS, E. G. L. The relation between heart and joint disease including "rheumatoid heart disease" and chronic post-rheumatic arthritis (type Jaccoud). *Brit. Heart J.*, 12: 101, 1950.
14. LASSITER, G. S. and TASSY, F. T. Malignant rheumatoid disease with aortic stenosis. *Arch. Int. Med.*, 116: 930, 1965.
15. CRUICKSHANK, B. Heart lesions in rheumatoid disease. *J. Path. Bact.*, 76: 223, 1958.
16. SOKOLOFF, L. and BUNIM, J. J. Vascular lesions in rheumatoid arthritis. *J. Chron. Dis.*, 5: 668, 1957.
17. GOWANS, J. D. C. Complete heart block with Stokes-Adams syndrome due to rheumatoid heart disease. *New England J. Med.*, 262: 1012, 1960.
18. HANDFORTH, C. P. and WOODBURY, J. F. L. Cardiovascular manifestations of rheumatoid arthritis. *Canad. M. A. J.*, 80: 86, 1959.
19. HOFFMAN, F. G. and LEIGHT, L. Complete atrioventricular block associated with rheumatoid disease. *Am. J. Cardiol.*, 16: 585, 1965.
20. LEBOWITZ, W. B. The heart in rheumatoid disease. *Geriatrics*, 21: 194, 1966.
21. SINCLAIR, R. J. G. and CRUICKSHANK, B. A clinical and pathological study of sixteen cases of rheumatoid arthritis with extensive visceral involvement (rheumatoid disease). *Quart. J. Med.*, 25: 313, 1956.
22. MAHER, J. A. Dural nodules in rheumatoid arthritis. *Arch. Path.*, 58: 354, 1954.
23. CATHCART, E. S. and SPODICK, D. H. Rheumatoid heart disease. *New England J. Med.*, 266: 959, 1962.
24. CHRISTIE, G. S. Pulmonary lesions in rheumatoid arthritis. *Aust. Am. Med.*, 3: 49, 1954.
25. GRAEF, J., HICKEY, D. V. and ALTMANN, V. Cardiac lesions in rheumatoid arthritis. *Am. Heart J.*, 37: 635, 1949.
26. RAVEN, R. W., WEBER, F. P. and PRICE, L. W. The necrobiotic nodules of rheumatoid arthritis. *Ann. Rheumat. Dis.*, 7: 63, 1948.
27. PIRANI, C. L. and BENNETT, G. A. Rheumatoid arthritis. *Bull. Hosp. Joint Dis.*, 12: 335, 1951.

Case 78 Cardiac Valvular Lesions in Rheumatoid Arthritis

William C. Roberts, MD; James A. Kehoe, MD; Deborah F. Carpenter, MD; and Abner Golden, MD

Washington, DC, and Bethesda, MD

Nodules, similar to those which occur in the subcutaneous tissue, also may occur in the respiratory, intestinal hematopoietic, musculoskeletal, and cardiac systems of patients with rheumatoid arthritis (RA). Recently, we described rheumatoid nodules in all four cardiac valves of a 65-year-old woman with RA.[1] Since that report was submitted for publication, which was the first report to describe significant quadrivalvular involvement in RA, we have observed similar quadrivalvular cardiac disease in another patient who died with RA. This paper describes the cardiac lesions in the latter patient, and compares them with those found in the previously described subject and with those observed in the more frequent types of valvular heart disease.

PATIENT SUMMARY

A 72-year-old man (GMC, 12-47-82) who died Nov 28, 1966, was well until age 36 when he suddenly developed right-sided pleuritis with effusion, and several days later, swelling, redness, pain, and tenderness of both ankles and the metatarsophalangeal joints of both feet. He was treated with aspirin and the arthritis disappeared within a six-month period. Thereafter, with the exception of several approximately six-hour episodes of pain and swelling of the metatarsophalangeal joints, the patient was completely well and on no medications until age 66 (1960) when acute arthritis appeared involving initially mainly the right ankle. He was treated with phenylbutazone with considerable improvement of the joint manifestations, but signs and symptoms of an active peptic ulcer appeared and the drug was stopped. Thereafter, he had severe chronic pain, stiffness and swelling, and periodic tenderness and redness bilaterally of the metacarpo-, metatarso-, and proximal interphalangeal joints, wrists, elbows, shoulders, knees, and ankles. Despite weekly intramuscular gold injections, he did not receive complete relief from these joint manifestations.

At age 68 (February 1963) he was admitted to the Georgetown University Medical Center for further therapy. Examination disclosed fusiform swelling of the proximal interphalangeal joints of the hands, tender and swollen ankles, subcutaneous nodules over both olecranon processes, basilar pulmonary rales, atrial and ventricular diastolic gallops, and lower leg edema. The patient's blood pressure was 120/70 mm Hg, the heart was not enlarged, and a grade 1/6 systolic murmur was heard over the cardiac base and over the left sternal border. Chest roentgenogram disclosed the cardiac silhouette to be at the upper limits

Received for publication March 13, 1968; accepted May 6.

From the departments of pathology (Drs. Carpenter and Golden) and medicine (Dr. Kehoe), Georgetown University Medical Center, Washington, DC, and the Section of Pathology, National Heart Institute, National Institutes of Health, Bethesda, Md (Dr. Roberts).

Reprint requests to Section of Pathology, National Heart Institute, National Institutes of Health, Bethesda, Md 20014 (Dr. Roberts).

DOI: 10.1201/9781003409281-9

of normal; there was evidence of right pleural thickening. The blood hematocrit level was 39%; white blood cell count (WBC), 8,000/cu mm; and the differential blood smear, normal. The latex test for rheumatoid arthritis was positive (4+). The electrocardiogram showed left axis deviation and enlarged notched P waves in leads II and V_1 consistent with left atrial enlargement. He received nitrogen mustard, adrenal steroids, and weekly intramuscular gold injections; for several months he showed improvement.

At age 71 (March 1965) he was rehospitalized because of left-sided pleuritic chest pain, cough, slight orthopnea and exertional dyspnea, fever, and lower leg edema. A left-sided empyema was found and drained. The cardiac physical findings, ECG, and size of the heart on chest roentgenogram were unchanged. Fibrotic changes, congestion and hyperinflation were seen in the lung fields as well as a left pleural effusion. Because of findings suggesting cardiac failure, he was digitalized.

He was rehospitalized in May 1965 because of a fall which fractured the medial meniscus of the right knee and because of rapid worsening of the arthritis. During his 83 days in the hospital, the previously described cardiac findings persisted and, in addition, occasional premature atrial and ventricular contractions were recorded. The patient's hematocrit level was now 31% and he weighed 46.7 kg (103 lb); three months earlier he had weighed 62.1 kg (137 lb). He was discharged in August, and thereafter received weekly gold and corticosteroids intramuscularly. He was totally bedridden during his last year which was characterized by repeated episodes of pneumonia, periods of confusion and disorientation, fracture of one femur, Cushing's syndrome secondary to the corticosteroid therapy, episcleritis which progressed to scleromalacia perforans, and multiple decubiti. His severe weakness gradually progressed, and 12 hours before death he became comatose. At no time during his last year were there signs of cardiac decompensation.

At autopsy (GMC, 66A-599), severe deforming rheumatoid arthritis involved numerous joints. There was severe ulnar deviation of both hands and subluxation of the metacarpophalangeal joints and enlargement of the proximal and distal interphalangeal joints. Subcutaneous nodules were present in the areas of many joints. The pericardial and pleural spaces were obliterated by adhesions. An abscess (5 × 5 × 2 cm) was present in the lower left pleural space, and it communicated with the left lower lobe of the lung via a bronchopleural fistula. The bronchi were dilated and many were filled with purulent material. Typical rheumatoid granulomas were observed grossly and histologically in the skin and subcutaneous tissue, lungs, larynx, pleural and pericardial surfaces, splenic capsule, dura, and adventitia of the bowel at the esophagogastric junction. In addition, numerous focal yellow (rheumatoid) nodules, identical histologically to those observed in the tissues mentioned, were present in the endocardium of the right and left atria, all four cardiac valves, membraneous ventricular septum, and in the myocardium of both atria and ventricles. The cardiac lesions are described in detail in Figure 1 through 6. The heart weighed 350 gm. Both mitral and aortic valvular leaflets were considerably thickened, moderately rigid, and their orifices probably incompetent. In contrast, the focal nodules in the tricuspid and pulmonic valves almost certainly did not interfere with proper functioning of these structures. Both atria were mildly dilated. The yellow nodules located in the membraneous and upper muscular septum caused these structures to be thick and firm. Several yellow plaques were noted in the walls of the major coronary arteries, but there was no luminal narrowing.

Special stains for pyogenic and acid-fast bacteria and fungi on selected sections of heart and lung disclosed no organisms.

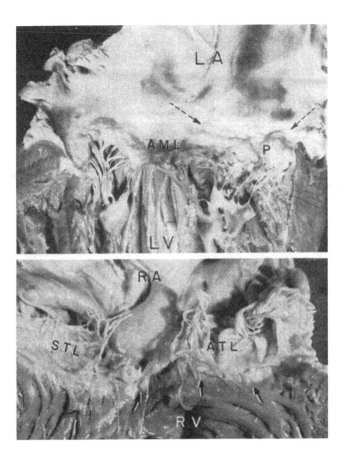

Figure 1 Atrioventricular valves. *Top*, Opened left atrium (LA), mitral valve, and left ventricle (LV). Between arrows is row of nodules at line of attachment of posterior (P) leaflet. Both anterior (AML) and posterior leaflets are diffusely thickened, but chordae tendineae are normal. *Bottom*, Opened right atrium (RA), tricuspid valve and right ventricle (RV). Leaflets have been reflected back into right atrium exposing small focal rheumatoid nodules (arrows) at line of attachment of anterior (ATL) and septal (STL) tricuspid leaflets as well as on leaflets themselves.

COMMENT

Although nonspecific forms of pericarditis, myocarditis, and coronary arteritis have been observed at necropsy in patients with rheumatoid arthritis (RA),[2,3] rheumatoid nodules (granulomas) similar to subcutaneous nodules are pathognomonic and occur in the heart in 1% of 3% of autopsied patients with this condition.[2,4] At least 22 patients with rheumatoid granulomas involving cardiac valves or valvular rings have been reported.[1] In ten subjects the mitral valve alone was involved; in four, the aortic alone; in three, both mitral and aortic; in one, the tricuspid alone; in one, both mitral and tricuspid; in three, the mitral, aortic, and pulmonic; and in two, all four valves. The order of incidence of involvement of the cardiac valves—mitral, aortic, triscuspid, and pulmonary—is as in rheumatic fever, and as in the Hurler syndrome. Seven of the 22 patients had auscultatory evidence of mitral or aortic regurgitation or both, and ten of them had hearts weighing more than 300 gm. Most

61

frequently, the valvular lesions were focal and did not appear to have interfered with valvular function. In the present patient the diffuse nature of the involvement of the mitral and aortic valvular leaflets probably rendered them incompetent. The cardiomegaly observed at necropsy and the clinical signs of cardiac dysfunction can most readily be explained on the basis of valvular cardiac disease, since there was no significant coronary arterial narrowing, no systemic hypertension, and the myocardial rheumatoid nodules do not appear to have been extensive enough to have caused these findings.

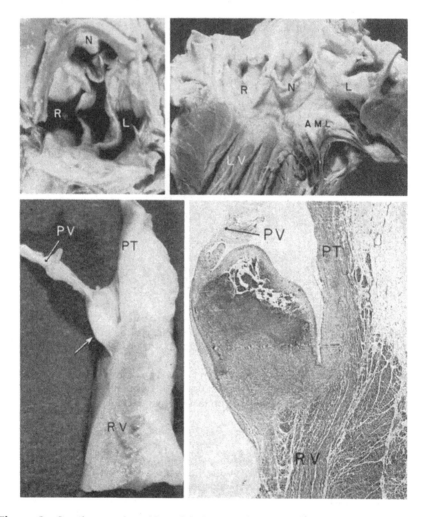

Figure 2 Semilunar valves. *Upper left*, Aortic valve as seen from above. Right (R), left (L) and noncoronary (N) cusps are diffusely thickened, and cusps are partially fused at two commissures. *Upper right*, Opened aortic valve. Diffuse thickening of anterior mitral leaflet (AML) also is apparent. LV indicates left ventricle. *Lower left*, Longitudinal section through one pulmonic valvular cusp. Nodule farrow) is present at basal attachment of this cusp, but remainder of it is normal. *Lower right*, Histologic section of pulmonic valve (PV), pulmonary trunk (PT), and right ventricle (RV). Large nodule at base of cusp is a typical rheumatoid granuloma (hematoxylin and eosin, × 20).

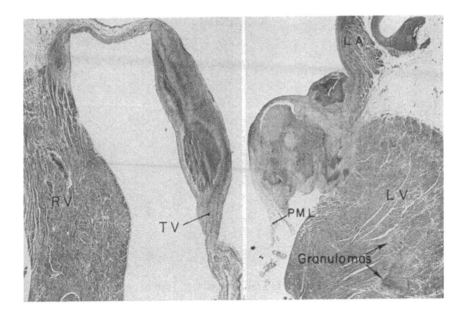

Figure 3 Atrioventricular valves. *Left,* Tricuspid valve (TV) leaflet. Typical rheumatoid granuloma is located within substance of leaflet. RV indicates right ventricle (hematoxylin and eosin, × 12). *Right,* Mitral valve. Section includes posterior mitral leaflet (PML), and adjacent portions of left atrial (LA) and left ventricular (LV) walls. Large rheumatoid granuloma is located within proximal three-fourths of posterior leaflet. Smaller nodule involves endocardium of left atrium as well. Two rheumatoid granulomas are located within left ventricular wall (hematoxylin and eosin, × 6.5).

Although rheumatoid nodules in the hearts of patients with RA have been well described, little attention has been given to the exact location of these lesions in the valve leaflets and rings. In the present patient, and in the one previously studied by us[1] with rheumatoid heart disease, the location and size of the lesions were identical in each of the respective cardiac valves. The lesions grossly were yellow, firm, smooth, and focal or diffuse. On the tricuspid valve the lesions were focal and located at the basal attachment of the septal and anterior leaflets. The posterior tricuspid leaflets were uninvolved. A single nodule was present at the basal attachment of a pulmonic valvular cusp. These right-sided cardiac lesions did not interfere with valvular function since most of the valve tissue was uninvolved. In contrast to these right-sided lesions, those on the left-sided cardiac valves were diffuse; nearly all areas of both mitral and aortic leaflets were thickened.

Histologically, the lesions were located *within* the valve leaflets leaving a thin border of fibrous tissue to enclose the necrotic material (Figure 6). This thin fibrous capsule probably represents the original and uninvolved valve tissue, and prevents the necrotic debris within the valve leaflets from being extruded into the circulation. It appears from the study of the cardiac valves in these two patients that the process begins as a reaction within the core or central portion of the valve leaflet preserving the peripheral portions. The valvular involvement in rheumatoid heart disease thus is in direct contrast to that in carcinoid heart disease, in which the valve itself remains normal and atypical fibrous tissue is deposited on the surface of the valvular cusp (Figure 7). Also, it differs from rheumatic valvular disease in which

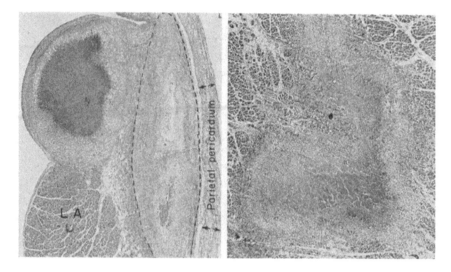

Figure 4 Myocardial rheumatoid granulomas. *Left,* Typical nodule replaces portion of left atrial (LA) wall. Parietal pericardium was adherent to epicardium diffusely in this patient, obliterating pericardial sac. Enclosed by dashed lines is cholesterol granuloma which lies beneath rheumatoid granuloma (hematoxylin and eosin, × 22). *Right,* Close-up of a left ventricular rheumatoid granuloma. Central portion consists of necrotic debris which is surrounded by pleomorphic collection of cells, mainly histiocytes, which are arranged perpendicular to border of necrotic material (hematoxylin and eosin, × 37).

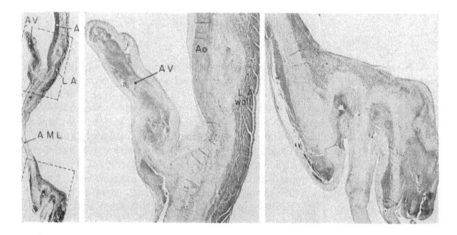

Figure 5 Aortic and mitral valves. *Left,* Section includes aortic valve (AV) cusp, anterior mitral leaflet (AML) adjacent aorta (A), and left atrial (LA) wall (hematoxylin and eosin, × 2.5). Middle and right photographs are close-up views of areas shown in brackets. *Center,* Necrotic debris is within core of valvular cusp, and is surrounded by border of thin fibrous tissue, which probably represents remaining original valvular tissue. Rheumatoid granulomas also are present between media of ascending aorta (Ao) and the left atrial (La) wall (hematoxylin and eosin, × 11). *Right,* Distal margin of anterior mitral leaflet contains several rheumatoid granulomas (hematoxylin and eosin, × 11).

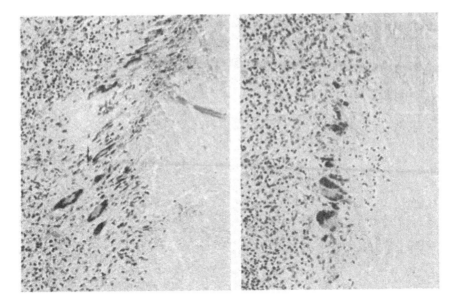

Figure 6 Portions of rheumatoid nodules in an aortic valve cusp (left) and in membraneous ventricular septum (right). Langhans and foreign-body type giant cells as demonstrated here were observed in many of the cardiac rheumatoid nodules. Necrotic central portion is on right of each photomicrograph (hematoxylin and eosin, × 160).

the *entire leaflet*, both its central and peripheral portions, is involved, often leaving no residual normal or near-normal valvular tissue.

The reason the cardiac valves are involved at all in HA is unclear. If vasculitis is considered to be an intrinsic part of the development of the subcutaneous nodules, as proposed by Sokoloff et al,[5] then involvement of valvular blood vessels must occur. The cardiac valves, however, contain few blood vessels. Certainly, if vasculitis predisposes to the development of rheumatoid granuloma, these lesions might be expected to be much more frequent in the myocardium than in the endocardium (valves), although this does not appear to be the situation.

SUMMARY

The clinical and necropsy findings are described in a 72-year-old man with severe deforming rheumatoid arthritis and rheumatoid cardiac nodules. The nodules were located in all four cardiac valves, as well as in the pericardium and myocardium. Rheumatoid nodules occur infrequently (3%) in the hearts of subjects with rheumatoid arthritis, but the type of involvement is pathognomonic. The nodules, when present in a cardiac valve, are located in the "core" or central portions of the leaflets, and may cause them to be incompetent. Involvement of the left-sided cardiac valves in this condition is more frequent and more extensive than involvement of the right-sided valves.

ACKNOWLEDGMENTS

Mr. Larry D. Ent prepared the histologic sections and Mr. Gebhard Gsell took the photomicrographs.

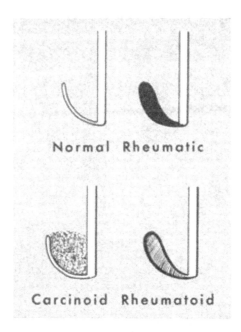

Normal   Rheumatic

Carcinoid   Rheumatoid

Figure 7 Similunar valvular cusp in various cardiac diseases. A normal cusp is on top left for comparison. Normal components of rheumatically diseased cusp are replaced by uniform dense fibrous tissue. In carcinoid heart disease, valve cusp remains normal, and atypical fibrous tissue is simply superimposed on it. In rheumatoid heart disease, peripheral portions of original cusp remain, but central portions are replaced by rheumatoid granulomas.

GENERIC AND TRADE NAME OF DRUG

Phenylbutazone—*Butazolidin.*

REFERENCES

1. Carpenter, D.F.; Golden, A.; Roberts, W.C.: Quadrivalvular Rheumatoid Heart Disease Associated with Left Bundle Branch Block, *Amer J Med* 43:922–929 (Dec) 1967.
2. Sokoloff, L.: Cardiac Involvement in Rheumatoid Arthritis and Allied Disorders: Current Concepts, *Mod Conc Cardiov Dis* 33:847–850 (April) 1964.
3. Lebowitz, W.B.: The Heart in Rheumatoid Arthritis (Rheumatoid Disease), *Ann Intern Med* 58:102–123 (Jan) 1963.
4. Baggenstoss, A.H.; Rosenberg, E.F.: Cardiac Lesions Associated with Chronic Infectious Arthritis, *Arch Intern Med* 67:241–258 (Feb) 1941.
5. Sokoloff, L.; McCluskey, R.T.; Bunim, J.J.: Vascularity of the Early Subcutaneous Nodule of Rheumatoid Arthritis, *Arch Path* 55:475–495 (June) 1953.

Case 89 Fatal Acute Rheumatic Fever in Childhood Despite Corticosteroid Therapy

A Note on the Spectrum of Childhood Rheumatic Fever

D. Luke Glancy, M.D*, Rashid A. Massumi, M.D.**, William C. Roberts, M.D.***
Bethesda, MD., and Washington, D.C.

The incidence of death in childhood from rheumatic heart disease has been declining in the United States for 3 decades.[1] The role of adrenocorticotrophic hormone and adrenal corticosteroids in the continuing decline in the mortality rate during the past 2 decades has been debated widely and remains uncertain. Nevertheless, death from rheumatic carditis is now uncommon in children treated with these agents and is rare during an initial attack of rheumatic fever.[2] Such occurred, however, in 2 children recently studied by us. Each died of different causes, which represent widely separate bands in the spectrum of rheumatic heart disease in children.

REPORT OF PATIENTS

Patient 1. A 3-year-old girl was hospitalized following an upper respiratory infection because of a skin rash, which had features of both erythema marginatum and urticaria, and arthritis of both ankles. Fever (101° F), pharyngitis, and a systolic, ejection-type murmur at the left sternal edge were present. A leukocyte count was 22,000 per cubic millimeter; anti-streptolysin 0 titer, 625 Todd units; corrected sedimentation rate, 32 mm. per hour; and C-reactive protein, reactive. In the hospital, the temperature rose to 103° F., arthritis of both knees developed while that of the ankles subsided, and the systolic murmur became loudest at the cardiac apex and radiated to the left axilla and back. The fever and arthritis responded favorably to aspirin and prednisolone (50 mg. per day), but on her eighteenth day of hospitalization, the twentieth day of illness, she developed dyspnea, tachypnea, tachycardia (170 per minute), a ventricular gallop, hepatomegaly, and died.

Necropsy (A67–286) disclosed generalized cardiomegaly (weight, 105 grams; expected weight, 60 grams), slight thickening of all 4 cardiac valves, and histologically pancarditis with numerous Aschoff bodies (Figures 1 and 2).

Patient 2. A 9-year-old girl was well until 1/2 years before death when she developed typical signs and symptoms of acute rheumatic fever. She remained in the hospital during the entire 1½-year period. A loud murmur typical of mitral regurgitation was heard when she was first examined and remained thereafter. Congestive cardiac failure was present throughout the illness, but it appeared to be

---

Received for publication Feb. 12, 1968.

* Staff Associate, Section of Pathology, National Heart Institute, National Institutes of Health, Bethesda, Md. 20014.

** Cardiologist, District of Columbia General Hospital, and Chief, Cardiopulmonary Laboratory, George Washington University Division of Medicine, District of Columbia General Hospital, Washington, D. C.

***Chief, Section of Pathology, National Heart Institute, National Institutes of Health, Bethesda, Md.

DOI: 10.1201/9781003409281-10

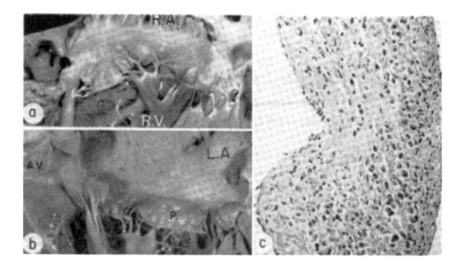

Figure 1 The heart of Case 1. *a*, Opened right atrium *(R.A)*, right ventricle *(R.V.)*, and slightly but diffusely thickened tricuspid valve. *b*, Opened left atrium *(L.A.)*, left ventricle *(L.V.)*, and slightly but diffusely thickened aortic *(A.V.)* and mitral valves. Above the posterior mitral leaflet *(P.)* the left atrial endocardium is thickened and irregular (MacCallum's plaque). *c*, Photomicrograph showing pleomorphic infiltrate with large mononuclear cells, similar to those in Aschoff bodies, in a pulmonic valve cusp. (Hematoxylin and eosin stain, × 208.)

less severe when the child was receiving prednisone (up to 40 mg., daily) and more severe when this medication was discontinued. First degree heart block was present until the last weeks of life when atrial fibrillation developed. She died unexpectedly.

Necropsy (A67–185) disclosed generalized cardiomegaly (weight, 320 grams; expected weight, 115 grams); severe fibrosis of the mitral valve with a fixed, severely incompetent orifice; a left atrial jet lesion; normal aortic, tricuspid and pulmonic valves; and normal pericardium. Histologically, most myocardial fibers of each cardiac chamber were hypertrophied, but no inflammatory cells or Aschoff bodies were found (Figure 3).

COMMENT

Although acute rheumatic fever occurs in patients under 4 years of age,[3] it does so infrequently, and we are aware of only 14 children[4–13] who, like Patient 1, died of acute rheumatic fever before 4 years of age and who were found at necropsy to have Aschoff bodies. Photomicrographic demonstration of the Aschoff bodies was presented in 5 of them.[4-7] Aschoff bodies are said to be absent during the first few weeks of acute rheumatic fever,[14] and adrenal corticosteroids have been reported to decrease markedly the cellular reaction in rheumatic myocarditis.[15] The heart of Patient 1, however, contained numerous, typical Aschoff bodies and an exuberant cellular reaction despite a total symptomatic illness of only 20 days and treatment with large doses of prednisolone.

In contrast to Patient 1, whose death was primarily due to acute rheumatic myocarditis, Patient 2 died of severe mitral regurgitation. Although it is reasonable to believe that acute rheumatic carditis was present at the beginning of her illness, no inflammatory lesions were present at necropsy 1½ years later, and except for hypertrophy, the myocardium was normal. Cardiac failure in children with

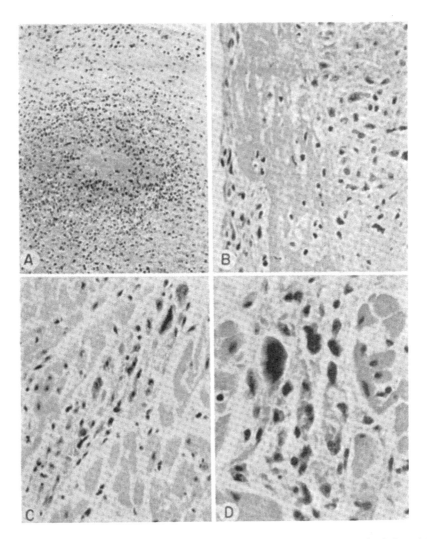

Figure 2 Photomicrographs in Case 1. *A*, Inflammatory nodule in the left atrial endocardium, consisting of a necrotic center surrounded by large mononuclear cells and a peripheral zone of polymorphonuclear neutrophils. *B*, Posterior mitral leaflet containing fibrinoid material, polymorphonuclear neutrophils, and large mononuclear cells. *C* and *D*, Aschoff bodies consisting of altered collagen surrounded by large, mononuclear (Anitschkow) cells, and giant cells. (Hematoxylin and eosin stains; *A*, ×160, *B* and *C*, ×400, and *D*, ×628; each reduced by 25 per cent.)

rheumatic heart disease suggests that the rheumatic carditis is still active,[16] and in Patient 2 this suggestion was supported by the transient, but apparently beneficial effects of prednisone. Her cardiac failure, however, was due to an operatively correctable mechanical defect, mitral incompetence, and mitral valve replacement might have been lifesaving. Rheumatic mitral regurgitation has been considered a benign lesion in certain selected groups of patients,[17] but in Patient 2 it caused death 1½ years after the initial episode of acute rheumatic fever.

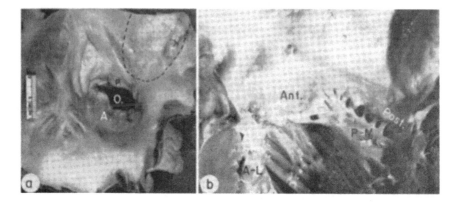

Figure 3 Interior of heart of Case 2. *a*, Opened left atrium showing the incompetent mitral valve orifice (*O.*) and the contracted anterior (*A.*) and posterior (*P.*) leaflets. The dashed line encloses an area of thickened endocardium on the posterior wall. This lesion almost certainly resulted from the impact of a jet of blood regurgitated through the incompetent mitral orifice from the left ventricle during ventricular systole. The myocardium beneath this lesion showed histologic features of severe degeneration, but this was the only portion of myocardium that showed changes other than hypertrophy. *b*, Close-up of the opened mitral valve. Both leaflets and the chordae tendineae are thick and shortened. No calcium deposits are present. *Ant.* and *Post.*, anterior and posterior leaflets, respectively; *A-L* and *P-M*, anterolateral and posteromedial papillary muscles, respectively.

REFERENCES

1. Massell, B. F., Amezcua, F., and Pelargonio, S.: Evolving picture of rheumatic fever: Data from 40 years at the House of the Good Samaritan, J.A.M.A. **188**:287, 1964.
2. A joint report by the Rheumatic Fever Working Party of the Medical Research Council of Great Britain and the Subcommittee of Principal Investigators of the American Council of Rheumatic Fever and Congenital Heart Disease, American Heart Association. The evolution of rheumatic heart disease in children. Five-year report of a cooperative clinical trial of ACTH, cortisone, and aspirin, Circulation **22**:503, 1960.
3. Logue, R. B., and Hurst, J. W.: Rheumatic fever during the first few years of life, and its differentiation from endocardial fibrosis, Am. J. M. Sc. **223**:648, 1952.
4. McIntosh, R., and Wood, C. L.: Rheumatic infections occurring in the first three years of life, Am. J. Dis. Child. **49**:835, 1935.
5. Fischer, V. E.: Rheumatic heart disease at one year, Am. J. Dis. Child. **48**:590, 1934.
6. Schwarz, H.: An unusual case of acute rheumatic fever in an infant, *in* Contributions to the medical sciences in honor of Dr. Emanuel Libman, New York, 1932, The International Press, vol. 3, p. 1061.
7. Murphy, G. E.: The characteristic rheumatic lesions of striated and of non-striated or smooth muscle cells of the heart, Medicine **42**:73, 1963.
8. Eigen, L. A.: Juvenile rheumatic fever: Report of a case in an infant two years of age, Am. Heart J. **16**:363, 1938.
9. White, P. D.: The incidence of endocarditis in earliest childhood, Am. J. Dis. Child. **32**:536, 1926.

10. Denzer, B. S.: Rheumatic heart disease in children under two years of age: Report of three cases, J.A.M.A. **82**:1243, 1924.
11. Schroeder, L. C.: Observations on the etiology and pathology of chorea minor, J.A.M.A. **79**:181, 1922.
12. Friedberg, C. K.: Diseases of the heart, 3rd ed., Philadelphia, 1966, W. B. Saunders Company, p. 1321.
13. Smith, A. deG.: Rheumatism and its manifestations in children under five years, Arch. Pediat. **39**:799, 1922.
14. Baggenstoss, A. H., and Saphir, O.: Rheumatic disease of the heart, *in* Gould, S. E., editor: Pathology of the heart, 2nd ed., Springfield, IL, 1960, Charles C Thomas, Publisher, p. 655.
15. Gulden, A., and Hurst, J. W.: Alterations of the lesions of acute rheumatic myocarditis during cortisone therapy, Circulation **7**:218, 1953.
16. Massell, B. F., Fyler, D. C., and Roy, S. B.: The clinical picture of rheumatic fever: Diagnosis, immediate prognosis, course, and therapeutic implications, Am. J. Cardiol. **1**:436, 1958.
17. Jhaveri, S., Czoniczer, G., Reider, R. B., and Massell, B. F.: Relatively benign "pure" mitral regurgitation of rheumatic origin: A study of seventy-four adult patients, Circulation **22**:39, 1960.

Case 97 Clinical Pathologic Conference

Gordon A. Ewy, MD*, Myron Lotz, MD, Michael Gèraghty, MD,
Frank I. Marcus, MD, William C. Roberts, MD
Washington, DC and Bethesda, MD

CLINICAL ABSTRACT

O.C., a 41-year-old Negro cook, was admitted to the District of Columbia General Hospital for the first time on Jan. 7, 1968, complaining of weakness. She had been in good health until six weeks earlier when she developed a sore throat. She was again asymptomatic for the next three weeks. Thereafter she noted the insidious onset of fatigue, weakness, and general malaise which was accompanied by swelling and tenderness of her left knee. Subsequently, dyspnea on exertion, orthopnea, and paroxysmal nocturnal dyspnea developed. The patient visited a private physician who found bilateral basilar râles and ankle edema. During the next week she was treated by mercurial injection, parenteral corticosteroids, digitalis, thiazides, expectorants, and tetracycline. Despite some subjective improvement she continued to have paroxysmal nocturnal dyspnea, weakness, and edema of the hands and ankles.

On admission she was found to be well developed, moderately obese, apprehensive, pale, and sweating. The pulse was 80 beats per minute; blood pressure measured 120/80 mm. Hg; respirations were 24 per minute; rectal temperature was 99° F. The breath sounds were decreased in the bases of both lungs. The heart sounds were somewhat distant. There were no audible precordial murmurs, gallops, or rubs. There was no evidence of hepatomegaly or splenomegaly. Minimal pitting edema was present in the lower extremities. The joints appeared normal. The hematocrit was 32 per cent, white blood cell count was 12,300 per cubic millimeter, 70 per cent of which were polymorphonuclear cells. The urine had a specific gravity of 1.010, was free of glucose, acetone, erythrocytes, and casts, contained 2+ protein (later only trace) and 2 to 4 leukocytes per high-power field of sediment. The blood urea nitrogen was 38, creatinine 2.3, total bilirubin 4.3 with direct reacting 2.5, and glucose 225 mg. per cent. The serum sodium was 130, potassium 4.2, chloride 88, and carbon dioxide 25 mEq. per liter. The total protein was 7.4 with albumin 4.5 Gm. per cent. Serum protein electrophoresis revealed a discrete increase in the alpha-2 globulin fraction. Alkaline phosphatase was 30.9 King-Armstrong units. The serum glutamic oxalacetic transaminase was 170 units. The lactic dehydrogenase was 720 units. Prothrombin time was 17 seconds (control 14 seconds). The antistreptolysin-0 titer was 833 Todd units. Normal flora was cultured from the throat. Bentonite flocculation, lupus erythematosus (LE), and antinuclear antibody preparations were negative. The peripheral venous pressure was 11 cm. of water and the sodium dehydrocholate arm-to-tongue circulation time was 11 seconds. The electrocardiogram revealed a sinus rate of 75 beats per minute. The mean QRS axis, the QRS duration, the P-R interval, and the Q-T interval were normal. There was T-wave inversion in Leads aVF and V_1 through V_4. Chest roentgenogram on admission showed

From the Georgetown University School of Medicine, Georgetown University Medical Division, District of Columbia General Hospital, Washington, D. C., and the Section of Pathology, National Heart Institute, National Institutes of Health, Bethesda, Md.

* Reprint requests to: Dr. Ewy, Georgetown University Medical Division, District of Columbia General Hospital. Washington. D. C. 20003.

DOI: 10.1201/9781003409281-11

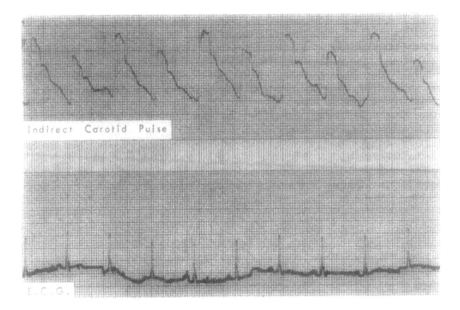

Figure 1 Indirect carotid pulse tracing showing pulsus alternans with reference Lead H electrocardiogram.

"blunting" of the costophrenic angles bilaterally, but no parenchymal infiltrates. There was no cardiomegaly.

On the second hospital day the patient developed migratory polyarthritis involving the ankles, knees, wrists, metatarsal phalangeal, and the inter-phalangeal joints. Even though aspirin therapy brought prompt relief to the joint symptoms, she developed spiking fever to 103° and progressive deterioration with delirium. On the third hospital day a ventricular diastolic gallop was heard along with alternation of the intensity of the cardiac sounds. Pulsus alternans was demonstrated (Figure 1). At no time was a precordial murmur heard. Prednisolone, 100 mg. per 24 hours, was started on the sixth hospital day. On the seventh hospital day she was semicomatose. Determinations on blood drawn at this time showed blood urea nitrogen of 143 and glucose 1,320 mg. per cent. The serum sodium was 160, chloride 114, potassium 5.3, and carbon dioxide 13 mEq. per liter. The serum osmolality was 445 milliosmoles per liter. Serum and urine acetone determinations were negative. Despite intensive therapy with fluids, electrolytes, and insulin, she died on the eighth hospital day.

DISCUSSION

Dr. Marcus: This 41-year-old woman dated the onset of her illness to six weeks before admission when she had pharyngitis. There was an interval of three weeks when she felt well, only to be followed by a severe, unremitting illness ending in death three weeks later. The terminal illness was characterized by involvement of multiple organs including the liver, joints, heart, kidneys, and central nervous system. The antistreptolysin-O (ASO) titer of 833 Todd units was definitely elevated. At this age, this value should not be greater than 100 to 150 units.[1] Since the ASO titer began to rise within a week after a streptococcal infection and reached a peak within 3 to 5 weeks,[2] the titer found in this patient was consistent with a streptococcal pharyngitis six weeks previously. It is not clear, however, whether

73

the pharyngitis was at all related to subsequent events. There is laboratory evidence documenting impairment of hepatic and renal function. Her arthritis was consistent with that found in acute rheumatic fever because of its migratory nature and prompt response to salicylates. The symptoms of orthopnea, paroxysmal nocturnal dyspnea, and edema suggest left ventricular failure. However, on admission, gallop rhythm was not heard, nor was the venous pressure or circulation time elevated. Nevertheless, when she was seen by a cardiologist (Dr. Gordon A. Ewy) on the third hospital day, heart failure was documented by the presence of ventricular diastolic gallop as well as pulsus alternans (Figure 1). The heart failure seemed to be secondary to myocardial rather than valvular dysfunction since no murmur was heard.

The differential diagnosis here is extensive. The most likely cause of this patient's illness is systemic lupus erythematosus because of the multiple-system involvement including arthritis in a 41-year-old woman. Several LE preparations, however, were negative. The marked increase in the alpha-2 globulin on serum electrophoresis was suggestive of a monoclonal spike, as may be found in multiple myeloma. Increases of the alpha-2 globulin, however, are nonspecific[3] and bone marrow aspiration did not show any abnormality. Thrombotic thrombocytopenic purpura is possible but unlikely in the absence of thrombocytopenia. Several unusual infectious diseases should be considered. I cannot exclude toxoplasmosis which can present in many forms including one characterized by multiple system involvement.[4] Leptospirosis is usually associated with severe headache and myalgias—symptoms not present in this patient.[5] I would be reluctant to make the diagnosis of either bacterial endocarditis or acute rheumatic carditis in the absence of an organic murmur. It is conceivable that she could have had a combination of both acute poststreptococcal glomerulonephritis and rheumatic carditis. My final diagnosis, however, would be *lupus erythematosus.*

During the last two days of life she developed coma and hyperglycemia without acetonemia. This combination has been characterized as hyperosmolar coma and will be discussed by Dr. Myron Lotz.

Dr. Lotz: On the final day of life the patient became progressively obtunded and was found to have marked hyperglycemia and hyperosmolarity in the absence of ketosis. By definition she had the *syndrome of hyperglycemia, hyperosmolar, nonketotic coma* of which some 130 cases have been described since the original report by Sament and Schwartz in 1957.[6] Other features usually present are dehydration, hypernatremia, and azotemia. Acidosis, when present, is usually mild.[7] The mortality rate in these patients approaches 60 to 70 per cent, a fate unfortunately shared by our patient despite vigorous therapy with hypotonic fluids, insulin, and potassium.[7]

This syndrome may occur in the following settings: (1) during convalescence from burns when on a high carbohydrate diet;[8] (2) during peritoneal dialysis[9] and hemodialysis;[10] (3) during therapy with thiazide diuretics; (4) during both long- and short-term corticosteroid therapy;[7] (5) during nonspecific stress, i.e., infections, trauma; and (6) without known precipitating cause.

Patients with this syndrome generally have the following characteristics: (1) They are usually elderly, but the syndrome has been reported in patients of 18 months[11] and 16 years of age;[12] (2) they may or may not be known diabetics and following recovery some patients remain diabetic while others regain normal glucose tolerance;[7] (3) upon recovery, the diabetes, when present, is usually easily controlled with small doses of insulin;[7] and (4) with one exception, a 24-year-old woman with ketosis-prone juvenile diabetes whom we saw recently, the syndrome has not occurred in a ketosis-prone individual.

The syndrome has been reported[13, 14] in seven patients receiving corticosteroid therapy. The mechanism by which corticosteroids precipitate this syndrome is unknown. Corticosteroids facilitate gluconeogenesis, impair sensitivity of peripheral tissue to insulin, and are antiketotic. Although diabetes develops in 5 to 7 per cent of patients on corticosteroids, it is usually mild. To my knowledge, no patient with this syndrome has had evidence of adrenal hyperfunction. The pathogenesis of hyperglycemia and the reason for the absence of ketosis is unclear.

Therapy for this syndrome includes fluids, preferably hypotonic, either intravenously or by gastric tube, potassium, and insulin. The insulin requirement is usually about 200 to 300 units but can vary enormously; some patients have required more than 13,000 units,[9] while one patient recovered without any insulin.[15] The high mortality (60 to 70 per cent) has been attributed to rupture of cerebral veins resulting from the hyperosmolarity. At necropsy, pathological findings are usually minimal and nonspecific.

There remains a great deal to learn about the pathogenesis and therapy of this entity which seems to have been the major cause of death in this patient.

Dr. William C. Roberts will discuss the pathologic findings.

Dr. Roberts: From the numerous abnormal clinical and laboratory findings, multiple organ systems appear to have been involved, including kidneys, heart, liver, and blood. Terminally, the blood urea nitrogen was 143 mg. per cent, and the specific gravity of the urine was never over 1.012. The kidneys were of normal size, their surfaces smooth, but each was severely congested (Figure 2). Histologic examination of the kidneys disclosed no abnormalities other than congestion. Thus, the azotemia was "prerenal."

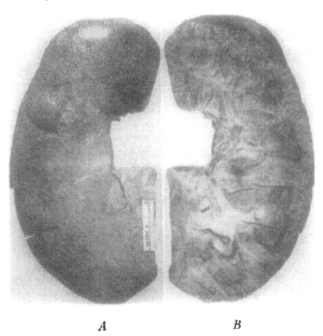

A　　　　*B*

Figure 2　Kidney. It is of normal size, and the external surface is smooth *(A)*. The discoloration of both external and cut *(B)* surfaces resulted from severe congestion of the renal vessels. The parenchyma was normal histologically.

The cardiac necropsy findings are especially interesting in view of the absence of precordial murmur and friction rub. The parietal pericardium was firmly adherent to the visceral pericardium by fibrofibrinous adhesions (Figure 3). Thus, diffuse pericarditis, which had obliterated the pericardial space, was present. Histologic examination of the pericardium disclosed inflammatory cells, consisting mainly of mononuclear cells, but occasionally a few polymorphonuclear leukocytes, in addition to fibrin and fibrous tissue. The heart weighed 400 grams. The mitral valve leaflets were diffusely thickened, but the chordae tendineae were probably normal (Figure 4). Thus, the mitral valve was anatomically abnormal, yet functionally normal. Grossly, the left atrial endocardium and atrial and ventricular myocardium appeared normal. The aortic valve cusps were slightly, but diffusely, thickened. In addition, a small verruca was present on the ventricular aspect of each of the three aortic valve cusps (Figure 4). Verrucae were located at the points of contact of the cusps during ventricular diastole. Histologic study of the verrucae disclosed that they consisted primarily of fibrin, but numerous inflammatory cells were present in the aortic cusps adjacent to, as well as at a distance from the verrucae (Figure 5). No organisms were present in the verrucae (Brown and Brenn and periodic acid-Schiff stains). A large number of inflammatory cells, mainly mononuclear but a few polymorphonuclear cells, were present throughout the entire aortic valve cusps. In addition, the cusps were edematous and contained numerous vascular channels. Similar inflammatory cells were present in the mitral and tricuspid valve leaflets (Figure 5).

The specific diagnosis in this patient was obtainable by examination of histologic sections of myocardium. All sections of myocardium disclosed Aschoff bodies (Figure 6). Thus, this patient had *acute rheumatic fever*. The myocardial fibers appeared

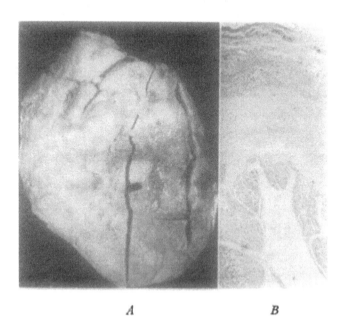

A   *B*

Figure 3 Pericardium. *(A)* Anterior surface of the heart showing diffuse pericardial disease. The visceral and parietal pericardia were adherent to one another. *(B)* Section of right atrium showing obliteration of the pericardial space. (Hematoxylin and eosin stain; ×25.)

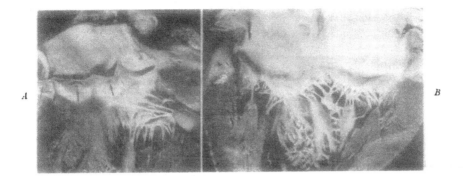

Figure 4 Interior of the left side of the heart. *(A)* Opened aorta, aortic valve and left ventricle. A small verruca (arrows) is present on each of the three aortic valve cusps which are mildly but diffusely thickened. *(B)* Opened left atrium, mitral valve, and left ventricle. Both mitral leaflets are diffusely thickened, and the ventricular wall is mildly thickened.

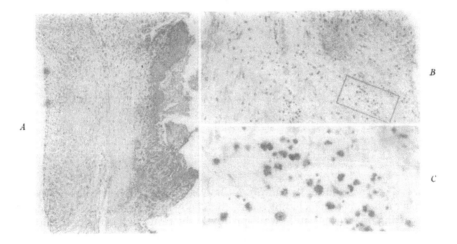

Figure 5 Portions of aortic and tricuspid valvular leaflets. *(A)* Verruca on aortic valvular cusp. *(B)* Section through tricuspid valve leaflet. Grossly this valve appeared normal, but histologically it was edematous and contained many acute and chronic inflammatory cells. *(C)* A close-up of the polymorphonuclear leukocytes in the brackets is shown in the photomicrograph. (Hematoxylin and eosin stains on each; *(A)* ×81, *(B)* ×160, *(C)* ×628.)

hypertrophied and focally degenerated. In addition to foci of mononuclear cells in the myocardium, there were also foci consisting mainly of polymorphonuclear leukocytes. Thus, the myocarditis was acute as well as chronic. The inflammation was seen in the walls of all four cardiac chambers, but primarily in the ventricular myocardium. A few foci of replacement fibrosis, often adjacent to Aschoff bodies, were present in sections of the myocardial wall (Figure 6). The coronary arteries were normal.

Elevation of the blood sugar and total bilirubin levels in this patient requires explanation. Sections of the liver showed centrolobular hemorrhage and degeneration of mild to moderate severity. The cause of these changes is uncertain,

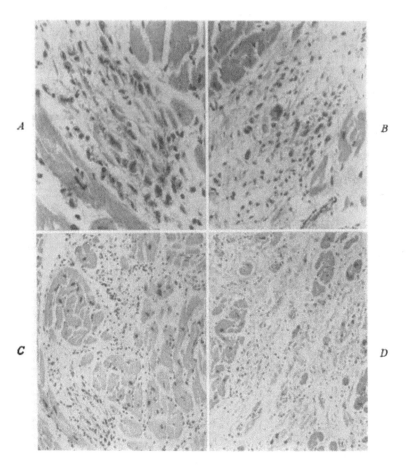

Figure 6 Myocardium. *(A)* and *(B)*: Aschoff bodies in left ventricular walls. *(C)*: Extensive inflammation including one Aschoff body in another area of left ventricle. *(D)*: Scarring of left ventricular wall apparently the result of healing of the inflammatory process. A single healing Aschoff body is present.

but acute hepatic arterial hypoxia is a possible explanation. It is well appreciated that central venous congestion may be the cause of centrolobular hepatic hemorrhage and necrosis, but these changes may also result from arterial hypoxia of the liver. Ligation of the hepatic artery probably produces the same anatomic lesion as occurs after ligation of the hepatic vein just as it enters the vena cava. However, the presence of hyperglycemia raises doubts regarding the possibility of hepatic arterial hypoxia causing the changes in the liver. There is suggestive evidence that hypoglycemia, not hyperglycemia, is a consequence of hepatic hypoxia.[16] Prolonged hepatic ischemia may have caused the hyperbilirubinemia.

The bone marrow was extremely hyper-cellular, but the increase in cells appeared to have been the result of an increase in all three blood elements. The brain was grossly edematous and histologic sections did not show any abnormality.

In summary, this patient had *acute rheumatic fever* with *pancarditis* (pericarditis, myocarditis, and endocarditis). The disease in this patient was unusual in the following respects: (1) the patient was 41 years of age when the initial clinical attack of acute rheumatic fever occurred; (2) the course of the illness was fulminant since she had been well seven weeks before death; (3) despite gross anatomic involvement of two cardiac valves and histologic involvement of three, no precordial murmur was heard; (4) although there was extensive pericarditis, a precordial friction rub was not heard; and (5) the severe functional impairment of the kidneys and liver was apparently secondary to severely decreased cardiac output, which in turn was the result of the rheumatic myocarditis.

REFERENCES

1. Rantz, L. A., Randall, E., and Rantz, H. H.: Antistreptolysin "O." A study of this antibody in health and in hemolytic streptococcus respiratory disease in man, Am. J. Med. **5**:3, 1948.
2. McCarty, M.: The antibody response to streptococcal infections, *in* McCarty, M., editor: Streptococcal infections, New York, 1954, Columbia University Press, p. 130.
3. Spiro, R. G.: Glycoproteins: structure, metabolism and biology, New England J. Med. **269**:566, 616, 1963.
4. Remington, J. S., Jacobs, L., and Kaufman, H. E.: Toxoplasmosis in the adult, New England J. Med. **262**:180, 237, 1960.
5. Edwards, G. A., and Domm, B. M.: Human leptospirosis, Medicine **39**:117, 1960.
6. Sament, S., and Schwartz, M.: Severe diabetic stupor without ketosis, South African M. J. **31**:893, 1957.
7. Schwartz, T. B., and Apfelbaum, R. I.: Nonketotic, Chicago, 1966, Year Book Medical Publishers, Inc., p. 165.
8. Rosenberg, S. A., Frief, D. K., Kinney, J. M., Herrera, M. G., Wilson, R. E., and Moore, F. D.: The syndrome of dehydration, coma, and severe hyperglycemia without ketosis in patients convalescing from burns, New England J. Med. **272**:931, 1965.
9. Boyer, J., Gill, G. N., and Epstein, F. H.: Hyperglycemia and hyperosmolality complicating peritoneal dialysis, Ann. Int. Med. **67**:568, 1967.
10. Potter, D. J.: Death as a result of hyperglycemia without ketosis—a complication of hemodialysis, Ann. Int. Med. **64**:399, 1966.
11. Ehrlich, R. M., and Bain, H. W.: Hyperglycemia and hyperosmolarity in an eighteen-month-old child, New England J. Med. **276**:683, 1967.
12. Seftel, H. C., Goldin, A. R., and Rubenstein, A. H.: Hyperosmolar non-ketotic coma, Lancet **2**:1042, 1967.
13. Boyer, M. H.: Hyperosmolar anacidotic coma in association with glucocorticoid therapy, J. A. M. A. **202**:1007, 1967.
14. Kumar, R. S.: Hyperosmolar non-ketotic coma, Lancet **1**:48, 1968.
15. Hayes, T. M., and Woods, C. J.: Hyperosmolar non-ketotic coma, Lancet **1**:209, 1968.
16. Brawley, R. K., Roberts, W. C., and Morrow, A. G.: Intestinal infarction resulting from nonobstructive mesenteric arterial insufficiency with a note on hepatic hypoglycemia as a possible aid in diagnosis, Arch. Surg. **92**:374, 1966.

Case 114 Lethal Ball Variance in the Starr-Edwards Prosthetic *Mitral* Valve

William C. Roberts, MD; Gilbert E. Levinson, MD; and Andrew G. Morrow, MD
Bethesda, MD

Lethal degeneration of a silicone rubber ball of a Starr-Edwards *mitral* prosthesis implanted for 78 months occurred. Variance of mitral silicone rubber poppets requires longer periods of implantation than required for degeneration of aortic poppets. Syncope or near syncope and congestive cardiac-failure appearing more than four years after mitral replacement with a silicone rubber poppet suggests ball variance. Alterations in intensity of the opening sound of the mitral prosthesis in the absence of arrhythmias further suggests this diagnosis.

Degeneration or variance of the silicone rubber poppet is now a well-recognized late complication of aortic valve replacement with a caged-ball prosthesis.[1,2] Constant trauma of the ball against the metallic struts and valve base by the high pressures of both systole and diastole is considered of importance in causing degeneration. In contrast to its common occurrence in the aortic position, degeneration of a silicone rubber poppet of a *mitral* caged-ball prosthesis thus far has been rare. Recently, however, severe degeneration of the silicone rubber ball was observed in a woman who had had isolated mitral valve replacement at the National Heart and Lung Institute with a Starr-Edwards prosthesis 78 months before death. Observations in this patient are described in this report.

PATIENT SUMMARY

A 41-year-old woman who died on Nov 17, 1969, underwent mitral valve replacement with a 3M Starr-Edwards prosthesis on May 21, 1963. The immediate postoperative course was uneventful and the patient was considerably improved. A grade 1–2/6 apical systolic murmur was heard initially 18 months after operation and persisted thereafter. The murmur was described as pansystolic by some and as ejection type by others. In addition, a grade 1–2/6 diastolic blowing murmur along the left sternal border was audible during the three years before death. Sudden transient unilateral hemiplegia occurred three years after operation, despite warfarin sodium therapy. Five years postoperatively dermal petechiae and menometrorrhagia appeared leading to iron deficiency anemia. Six years postoperatively hysterectomy was performed. Overt congestive cardiac-failure and hemolytic anemia (direct Coombs' test positive) occurred in the early postoperative period. The opening and closing sounds of the mitral prosthesis appeared normal. Six months later, or two months before death, the patient had returned to near normal status. The blood hematocrit reading and reticulocyte count were normal and easy fatiguability was the patient's

Received for publication April 3, 1970; accepted May 20.

From the Section of Pathology and the Clinic of Surgery, National Heart and Lung Institute, Bethesda, Md, and the Division of Cardiovascular Diseases, Department of Medicine, New Jersey College of Medicine and Dentistry, Newark.

Reprint requests to Section of Pathology, National Heart and Lung Institute, Bethesda, Md 20014 (Dr. Roberts).

80

DOI: 10.1201/9781003409281-12

only symptom. A month later epigastric discomfort appeared and 26 days later, or four days before death, hematemesis (600 ml) occurred and anemia (hematocrit value, 32%) reappeared. The prothrombin time was 130 seconds (control, 12) and the hypoprothrombinemia was attributed to documented excessive salicylate ingestion. No recurrence of bleeding occurred (vitamin K therapy) but her condition steadily worsened. Alteration in the intensity of the opening sound of the prosthesis was detected by auscultation during this hospitalization. Tachycardia, fever, pallor, and a right upper lobe pulmonary infiltrate appeared, and the patient was found dead in bed.

At autopsy, the pulmonary infiltrate was typical of lobar pneumonia. The viscera was congested. The silicone rubber ball of the mitral prosthesis showed evidence of severe degeneration (Figure 1). It was uniformly yellow, fractured at two

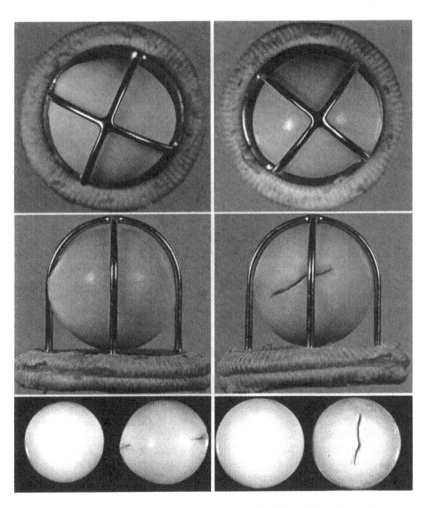

Figure 1 Prosthetic mitral valve in patient described. Top, Two views of prosthesis from above. When ball is in position shown on the left it is immobile. Middle, Two views from side. On the left ball is immobile. Bottom, White poppet is a normal 3M Starr-Edwards ball for comparison with yellow, fractured, swollen, and deformed poppet of present patient, also size 3M originally. Two fractures are visible on view on left, and the length of one fracture is visible in view on right.

sites, and swollen in an oblong manner. Neither a peribasilar left ventricular atrial communication nor antemortem prosthetic thrombus was present.

COMMENT

It is disappointing indeed to observe degeneration of the silicone rubber ball of the Starr-Edwards mitral prosthesis in the patient described. The degeneration of the poppet in this patient may well prove not to be an isolated occurrence but an indication of other such events to come. When degeneration of the silicone poppet of the Starr-Edwards prosthetic aortic valve was first observed, investigators attributed ball variance to associated peribasilar aortic left ventricular leaks, to antemortem thrombus on the prosthesis, to elevated blood lipid levels, or to chronic alcoholism. Rapidly, however, it became apparent that the silicone rubber in the aortic prosthetic cage could not withstand the trauma of contact against the metallic struts and ring under systemic pressure, whether or not associated lesions, particularly peribasilar leaks, were present.

At the National Heart and Lung Institute we have examined the silicone rubber poppets in 68 patients who died after one month (range 1.3 to 78 months [average, 20]) of replacement of one or more cardiac valves with Starr-Edwards prostheses. Degeneration of the prosthetic poppet was not observed in any of the 43 patients who died less than 24 months after valve replacement. Of the 25 patients who died 24 months or longer after valve replacement, 17 patients had had only the aortic valve replaced, four had had only the mitral valve replaced, and four had had both mitral and aortic valves replaced. Of the 21 aortic valve poppets examined, 17 showed degeneration. In ten patients the balls were discolored, swollen, grooved, and impacted in the cage, and caused prosthetic stenosis (implantation period 24 to 67 months [average, 45 months]). In six patients the balls were fractured or atrophied, and had dislodged from the cage causing fatal aortic regurgitation (implantation period 28 to 37 months [average, 33 months]); interestingly, all six of the patients in whom the ball dislodged underwent valve replacement in 1965, and all six died in 1967. In the 17th patient the aortic ball was discolored but not grooved, swollen, or fractured and it functioned normally for 65 months. Of the remaining four aortic poppets examined no gross ball degeneration was present (implantation period, 27 to 45 months [average, 36 months]). Of the eight mitral poppets examined, seven were normal (implantation period, 28 to 68 months [average, 43 months]) and only in the patient described herein did the ball show severe degeneration.

Degeneration of silicone rubber poppets of caged ball mitral prostheses has occurred in at least nine other patients: four in SCDK-Cutter[3–5] and five in Starr-Edwards[6] type prostheses. Sanderson et al[4] described swelling, softening, and "light canary-yellow" discoloration of the silicone rubber poppet of a Cutter mitral prosthesis inserted 37 months earlier. Chemical analysis of the ball revealed cholesterol and triglyceride deposits. Changes in the intensity and timing of the opening and closing clicks of the prosthesis were noted before reoperation in this patient who was in "moderate" congestive cardiac-failure. Leatherman et al[3] described two patients who had mitral valve replacements with Cutter prostheses eight and ten months, respectively, before reoperation, which was performed because of the sudden appearance of syncope or presyncope in both patients. The prosthetic sounds in each patient were of variable intensity and irregular, despite sinus rhythm. At reoperation, the mitral poppet in each patient was white and swollen, and movement of the poppet in the cage was impaired. Connolly and associates[6] described swelling (16% increase from original weight and 5% increase from original dimensions), yellow discoloration, and grooving of the silicone rubber ball of a mitral Starr-Edwards prosthesis (model 6000) implanted 50 months earlier. Muffling and finally disappearance of the opening sound of the prosthesis, along with acute pulmonary edema, suggested the diagnosis of mitral ball variance in their patient. At reoperation the swollen poppet moved only with difficulty and then only for a short distance within the cage, "obviously causing severe obstruction." In addition to the mitral poppet in the patient described by Connolly et al, P. E. Chappell, Jr. (written communication, January 1970) described four other Starr-Edwards mitral valve poppets (all of the model 6000 series) returned to the laboratory because of ball variance. The period of implantation in the four patients varied from 50 to 67 months. All four poppets were discolored and each showed slight loss of weight. One showed minor surface damage, and one was split. No prosthetic dysfunction occurred in any of the four patients. With the probable exception of the fractured poppet and of the swollen ball in the patient described by Connolly et al, none of the other seven mitral poppets mentioned were degenerated to the degree present in the present patient. The poppet in her was oblong, and when its longest diameter was at a right angle to the metallic struts of the cage, movement of the ball could occur only with manual pressure. When the long diameter of the ball was parallel with the struts, however, the ball moved well when the cage was tilted back and forth; soon the poppet's axis would change, and then it could neither extend fully to the apex of the cage nor seat completely. It seems likely, therefore, that valve function was normal with some beats and abnormal with others. It is probable that death occurred when the ball was made immobile for a brief period in the cage. In addition to the variance of the caged mitral silicone rubber ball, we have observed severe degeneration of the silicone rubber in a Hufnagel discoid mitral as well as Hufnagel discoid aortic prosthesis in a heart from a 23-year-old man operated on elsewhere. The prostheses had been implanted 33 months earlier. In contrast to the severe degeneration of the silicone rubber portion of each of these disks, the polypropylene portions of the disks were intact.

It is clear that the incidence of degeneration of the silicone rubber of mitral prostheses is low at this time, compared to the incidence of degeneration of the silicone rubber in the aortic valve position. This difference is further emphasized by the fact that the total number of Starr-Edwards mitral prostheses and aortic prostheses supplied to surgeons is approximately equal (30,000 of each type). Differences in aortic and mitral valvular blood velocities are probably the explanation. Typically, the orifice diameters of aortic prostheses are smaller than those of mitral prostheses, and the time of ventricular systole is approximately half that of ventricular diastole for a patient at rest. The velocity of flow through the orifice of the average aortic prosthesis is at least three times greater than the velocity through the orifice of the average mitral prosthesis. Also, the aortic ball contacts both the valve ring and the apex of the cage under high pressure, whereas the mitral ball contacts only the ring under high pressure (except in the Cutter prosthesis) since the ball passes to the apex of the cage during ventricular diastole.

The period of implantation necessary to produce significant mitral poppet degeneration is unknown at present. In our patient the period was 78 months, but much shorter periods have been observed. Peribasilar leaks or prosthetic thrombus may shorten this period. The presence or absence of peribasilar leaks was not mentioned in the nine other patients described with variant mitral balls. The shortest implantation period in which severe aortic poppet degeneration was observed was 24 months. This patient also had a peribasilar communication.[1]

Clinical features of *aortic* ball variance are variable, but this diagnosis must be suspected in any patient in whom a prosthesis containing silicone rubber has been in place 24 months or longer. When the aortic ball swells, congestive cardiac-failure usually ensues and alterations of prosthetic sounds are often apparent. Dislodgement of the aortic ball from the cage has not been preceded by symptoms of cardiac dysfunction in the six patients studied by us. The clinical features resulting from severe degeneration of the silicone rubber *mitral* poppet also are variable, and consist of syncope or near syncope, congestive heart-failure, and alterations in prosthetic sounds. Sanderson et al[4] in their patient with a variant mitral Cutter ball showed that the interval between aortic closure and mitral opening sound varied from 0.10 to 0.62 seconds (normal, 0.07 to 0.15 seconds), and the opening sound disappeared in the patient described by Connolly et al[6] and varied in our patient. Mitral ball degeneration should thus be considered in any patient doing poorly four or more years after mitral replacement, and reoperation may be necessary in many of these patients. It is hoped that the hollow metal ball in Starr-Edwards prostheses of current design will not degenerate. This newer prosthesis, introduced in 1967, had yet to be tested adequately, however, and no conclusions concerning its superiority are yet justified.

REFERENCES

1. Roberts WC, Morrow AG: Fatal degeneration of the silicone rubber ball of the Starr-Edwards prosthetic aortic valve. *Amer J Cardiol* **22**:614–620, 1968.
2. Hylen JC, et al: Aortic ball variance: Diagnosis and treatment. *Ann Intern Med* **72**:1–8, 1970.
3. Leatherman LL, et al: Malfunction of mitral ball-valve prosthesis due to swollen poppet. *J Thorac Cardivvasc Surg* **53**:398–400, 1967.
4. Sanderson RG, Hall AD, Thomas AN: The clinical diagnosis of ball variance in a mitral valve prosthesis. *Ann Thorac Surg* **6**:473–475, 1968.
5. Beall AC Jr, et al: Prosthetic replacement of cardiac valves: Five and one-half years' experience. *Amer J Cardiol* **23**:250–257, 1969.
6. Connolly DC, Harrison CE Jr, Ellis FH: Ball variance in a Starr-Edwards prosthetic mitral valve causing acute pulmonary edema (diagnosis by auscultation before onset of symptoms). *Mayo Clin Proc* **45**:20–24, 1970.

Case 156 Hemodynamic Confirmation of Obstruction to Left Ventricular Inflow by a Caged-Ball Prosthetic Mitral Valve

Richard L. Shepherd, D. Luke Glancy, Edward B. Stinson, and William C. Roberts
Bethesda, MD

It is now generally recognized that insertion of a large caged-ball mitral prosthesis into a relatively small-sized left ventricular cavity may lead to obstruction of the left ventricular inflow or outflow or both.[1-4] Recently, routine postoperative cardiac catheterization was performed on a patient who had undergone double valve replacement for combined mitral and aortic stenosis 6½ months earlier. A significant pressure gradient between the left atrium and left ventricle was documented at catheterization, and its mechanism was later established by necropsy. Pertinent clinical and anatomic features of the mitral obstruction by the mitral prosthesis in this patient are presented in this report.

CASE REPORT

L. K., a 58-year-old man, was evaluated at the National Heart and Lung Institute in July, 1971, because of a 1 year history of progressive fatigue, orthopnea, frequent paroxysms of nocturnal dyspnea, and one episode of pulmonary edema. Physical examination revealed a markedly prolonged carotid upstroke, an aortic ejection murmur, a diastolic blowing murmur along the left sternal margin, and a diastolic rumble at the apex. The electrocardiogram indicated left ventricular hypertrophy with "strain." Chest roentgenograms showed left ventricular and left atrial enlargement and dilatation of the ascending aorta. Fluoroscopy revealed extensive calcific deposits on the aortic valve. Cardiac catheterization data are summarized in Table 1.

On July 29, 1971, the aortic valve was replaced with a 9A, Model 2320 Starr-Edwards prosthesis, and the mitral valve was exchanged for a 4M, Model 6320 Starr-Edwards prosthesis. The immediate postoperative period was complicated by mild low-output syndrome treated with isoproterenol. The patient was discharged on Aug. 15, 1971, on a regimen of digoxin, furosemide, and warfarin. In November he voluntarily discontinued warfarin, and 2 weeks later he suddenly developed transient right-sided hemiparesis and dizziness; warfarin therapy was reinstituted. At the time of readmission to the National Heart and Lung Institute in February, 1972, the patient was nearly asymptomatic. Neurologic examination revealed normal findings. The prosthetic valve sounds were crisp, and no murmurs were heard. Postoperative cardiac catheterization data are shown in Table 1. Five days after catheterization he died suddenly while still in the hospital.

At necropsy, the heart was enlarged (total weight 450 grams), but neither ventricle was dilated. Each of the four struts of the mitral prosthetic cage were in contact with endocardium of left ventricle, and the mitral poppet was prevented from descending fully by ventricular septum which protruded into the cage (Figure 1).

From the Cardiology Branch, Clinic of Surgery, and Section of Pathology, National Heart and Lung Institute, Bethesda, Md. 20014.

Received for publication July 19, 1972.

Address for reprints: Richard L. Shepherd, M.D., Cardiology Branch, National Heart and Lung Institute, Bldg. 10, 7B-15, Bethesda, Md. 20014.

DOI: 10.1201/9781003409281-13

Table 1: Catheterization data*

Parameter	July 5, 1971 (24 days before operation)	Feb. 7, 1972 (6½ months after operation)
Pulmonary artery (mm. Hg)	38/18 (26)	34/16 (22)
Pulmonary artery wedge (mm. Hg)	(16)	(14)
Left ventricle (mm. Hg)	205/30	125/6
Left brachial artery (mm. Hg)	102/55 (70)	125/70 (90)
Left ventricle-pulmonary artery wedge (mm. Hg)†	7	11
Cardiac output (L./ min.)	3.48	4.87
Aortic valve area (sq. cm.)	0.32	
Mitral valve area (sq. cm.)	1.96	1.59

*Figures in parentheses are mean values.
†Mean diastolic gradient.

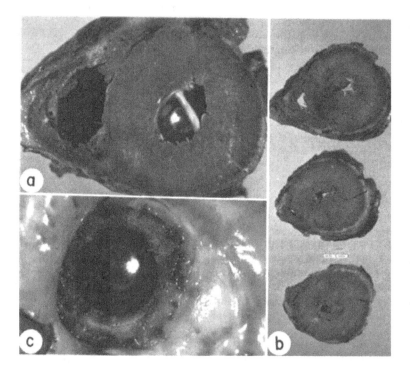

Figure 1 *a*, Transverse section of the ventricles shows that the Starr-Edwards mitral prosthesis fills the entire left ventricular cavity at this level. The poppet was prevented from descending completely by the ventricular septum which bulged into the cage. The cloth-covered struts, which are visible in this view, are completely covered by collagen. The left ventricular wall is hypertrophied. Other transverse sections caudal to this one are shown in *b*. The left ventricular cavity is extremely small. *c*, View of mitral prosthesis from left atrium. The entire "floor" of this chamber is occupied by the prosthesis.

Collagen deposits covering the struts of the mitral prosthesis were thin and did not inhibit free movement of the poppet. No thrombus was present in the primary orifice or on the struts of the mitral prosthesis. There was no thrombus on the aortic prosthesis, and the aortic poppet moved freely. The left ventricle showed no foci of fibrosis or necrosis. There was no evidence of a recent systemic or pulmonary embolus.

COMMENTS

The patient described above died 6½ months after aortic and mitral valve replacement for severe aortic stenosis and mild-to-moderate mitral stenosis. In retrospect, it would appear that the 4M Starr-Edwards mitral prosthesis was too large for this patient's normal-sized left ventricular cavity; the obstruction associated with the prosthesis was more severe than that caused by the excised mitral valve.

The cause of sudden death 5 days after cardiac catheterization is uncertain, but it is highly probable that stenosis of the prosthetic mitral valve was a contributing cause. Necropsy showed that the prosthetic obstruction was due to protrusion of the interventricular septum into the cage of the mitral prosthesis, which prevented free descent of the poppet. It has been postulated[5] that a caged-ball mitral valve prosthesis may be too large for the left ventricle into which it is inserted, but hemodynamic and anatomic confirmation of this concept has previously been lacking. More severe forms of prosthetic dysfunction probably result in low-output syndrome and early postoperative death, and the increased mortality rate which has been reported in patients with small left ventricles[6] may be due in part to dysfunction of the prosthesis.

REFERENCES

1. Morrow, A. G., Clark, W. D., Harrison, D. C., and Braunwald, E.: Prosthetic Replacement of the Mitral Valve: Operative Methods and the Results of Preoperative and Postoperative Hemodynamic Assessments, Circulation **29**: 2, 1964 (Suppl.).
2. Morrow, A. G., Oldham, H. N., Elkins, R. C., and Braunwald, E.: Prosthetic Replacement of the Mitral Valve. Preoperative and Postoperative Clinical and Hemodynamic Assessment in 100 Patients, Circulation **35**: 962, 1967.
3. Glancy, D. L., O'Brien, K. P., Reiss, R. L., Epstein, S. E., and Morrow, A. G.: Hemodynamic Studies in Patients With 2M and 3M Starr-Edwards Prostheses: Evidence of Obstruction to Left Atrial Emptying, Circulation **29, 30**: 113, 1969 (Suppl. I).
4. Reis, R. L., Glancy, D. L., O'Brien, K. P., Epstein, S. E., and Morrow, A. G.: Clinical and Hemodynamic Assessments of Fabric-Covered Starr-Edwards Prosthetic Valves, J. Thorac. Cardiovasc. Surg. **59**: 84, 1970.
5. Roberts, W. C., and Morrow, A. G.: Mechanisms of Acute Left Atrial Thrombosis After Mitral Valve Replacement: Pathologic Findings Indicating Obstruction to Left Atrial Emptying, Am. J. Cardiol. **18**: 497, 1966.
6. Terzaki, A. K., Cokkinos, D. V., Leachman, R. D., Meade, J. B., Hallman, G. L., and Cooley, D. A.: Combined Mitral and Aortic Valve Disease, Am. J. Cardiol. **25**: 588, 1970.

Case 182 Combined Mitral and Aortic Regurgitation in Ankylosing Spondylitis

Angiographic and Anatomic Features

William C. Roberts, MD, Jefferson F. Hollingsworth, MD*,
Bernadine H. Bulkley, MD, Richard B. Jaffe, MD‡, Stephen E. Epstein, MD
and Edward B. Stinson, MD*
Bethesda, Maryland

Clinical and cardiac morphologic features are described in a man with combined aortic and mitral regurgitation associated with ankylosing spondylitis. Although aortic regurgitation is a recognized accompaniment of ankylosing spondylitis, the occurrence of hemodynamically-significant mitral regurgitation in this arthritic condition has not been documented previously. Histologic study disclosed changes in the anterior mitral leaflet identical to those observed in the wall of the aorta and base of the aortic valve cusps in patients with ankylosing spondylitis. Thus, ankylosing spondylitis may be associated with characteristic lesions in anterior mitral leaflet in addition to those in the ascending aorta and aortic valve. The subaortic bump at the base of the anterior mitral leaflet, the most characteristic cardiovascular lesion of ankylosing spondylitis, may be visualized during life by left ventricular angiography, and its identification allows proper etiologic diagnosis of the valvular regurgitation.

Aortic regurgitation has been reported in 3 to 10 per cent of patients with ankylosing spondylitis.[1-3] Mitral regurgitation, in contrast, has rarely been described in association with this arthritic condition. Both valvular lesions, however, occurred in the patient described herein. In addition, the unique cardiovascular lesion of ankylosing spondylitis, namely, a subaortic bump or ridge,[4] was demonstrated during life for the first time by left ventricular angiography and confirmed by cardiac operation and histologic study.

CASE REPORT

This 57 year old man (W.S., 9-11-06) was admitted to the National Heart and Lung Institute in January 1972 because of mitral and aortic regurgitation. He had had arthritis of the ankles, knees, hands and wrists since age 38 (1943), and cervical and thoracic spondylitis since age 52 (1967). He never was known to have had rheumatic

From the Section of Pathology, Clinic of Surgery, and Cardiology Branch, National Heart and Lung Institute, and the Diagnostic Radiology Department, Clinical Center, National Institutes of Health, Bethesda, Maryland 20014. Requests for reprints should be addressed to Dr. William C. Roberts, Bldg. 10A, Rm. 3E30, NHLI-NIH, Bethesda, Maryland 20014. Manuscript accepted September 17, 1973.

* Present address: Department of Surgery, Stanford University, Palo Alto, California.

† Present address: University of Utah Medical Center, 3621 Golden Hills Avenue, Salt Lake City, Utah 84121.

DOI: 10.1201/9781003409281-14

fever. In January 1971 (age 56) he noted the onset of exertional dyspnea, which became nocturnal within a month. In August 1971 he noted angina pectoris, which in December 1971 also became nocturnal.

On examination, he had joint manifestations, including posture and gait, typical of ankylosing spondylitis. The peripheral pulses were bounding. The anteroposterior diameter of the chest was increased. The precordial cardiac impulse was diffuse and sustained. A grade 4/6 systolic ejection type murmur was audible over the cardiac base and neck. A grade 3/6 diastolic decrescendo murmur was heard over the cardiac base and over both sternal borders, loudest over the right one. A grade 2/6 pansystolic blowing murmur was present over the cardiac apex, and it radiated well into the left axilla. A third heart sound was present.

The blood hematocrit value was 35 per cent, leukocyte count 8,100/mm³ and erythrocyte sedimentation rate 102 mm in 1 hour. Urinalysis disclosed proteinuria (2+). The blood urea nitrogen was 53 and 37 mg/100 ml, and the uric acid 9.9 mg/100 ml. Serum calcium, phosphorus, alkaline phosphatase and protein levels were normal, and tests for the rheumatoid factor and syphilis (VDRL) were either negative or nonreactive. Electrocardiogram disclosed a prolonged (0.24 sec) P-R interval and left ventricular hypertrophy with strain. Skeletal roentgenograms revealed characteristic lesions of ankylosing spondylitis with bilateral fusion of the sacroiliac joints, extensive syndesmyophytes of the entire thoracolumbar spine, and healed periostitis of the posterior calcanei and ischial tuberosities (Figure 1). The articular surfaces of the knees and hands were eroded, and the joint spaces were narrowed. Chest roentgenograms demonstrated distention of the pulmonary veins in the upper lobes and marked cardiomegaly (Figure 2). No calcific deposits were observed in the chest on fluoroscopy. Pressures obtained at cardiac catheterization are shown in Table 1. Left ventricular angiocardiography showed a dilated chamber with hypokinetic but symmetric contractions. Mitral regurgitation (2+ to 4+) was present (Figure 3). The aortic valve cusps were thickened, and their mobility was decreased. A discrete nodule contiguous with the anterior mitral leaflet was

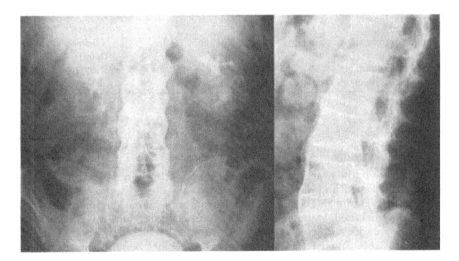

Figure 1 Roentgenogram of pelvis and lower vertebral column showing typical changes of ankylosing spondylitis.

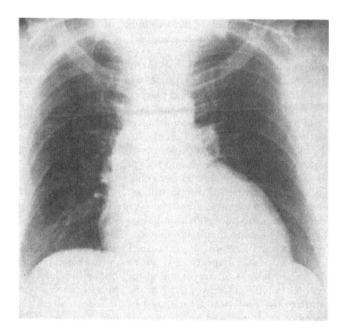

Figure 2 Chest roentgenogram showing considerable cardiomegaly.

Table 1: Hemodynamic data

	Operation		
	1/27/72	2/16/72	9/5/72
Pulmonary artery (mm Hg)	60/30		26/15
Right ventricle (mm Hg)	60/12		26/7
Right atrium	Mean 8		Mean 8
Pulmonary artery wedge (mm Hg)	Mean 28 V wave 50		Mean 14 V wave 15
Left ventricle (mm Hg)	176/16		160/16
Brachial artery (mm Hg)	195/45		130/80
Cardiac index (liters/min/m²)	3.6		2.3

observed immediately below the aortic valve (Figures 3 and 4). Injection of contrast material into the ascending aorta demonstrated aortic regurgitation (3+ to 4+) and a normal sized aortic root.

At operation, the heart was huge, the coronary ostia were normal, the wall of aorta was thickened, and each of the three aortic valve cusps was fibrotic, thickened and retracted (Figure 5). The mitral valve leaflets and chordae tendineae also were fibrotic and thickened (Figures 6 through 8). A firm nodular ridge was present at the base of the anterior mitral leaflet. The aortic valve was replaced by a Starr-Edwards prosthesis (size 9A, model 2320), and the mitral valve by a porcine heterograft (size 31 mm) (Hancock Laboratories). The postoperative course was smooth.

Histologic study of the excised aortic valve cusps disclosed that they were thickened by fibrous tissue devoid of inflammatory cells except just at their bases. The anterior mitral leaflet was thickened by similar fibrous tissue, which contained

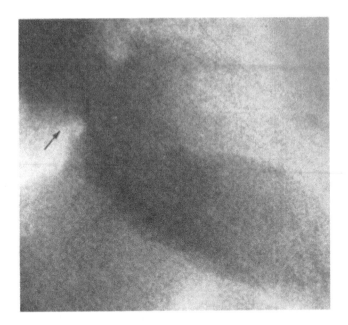

Figure 3 One frame of the left ventricular cineangiogram showing a discrete bump (arrow) just below the aortic valve. This bump corresponds to the subaortic ridge observed in necropsy patients with ankylosing spondylitis.[4]

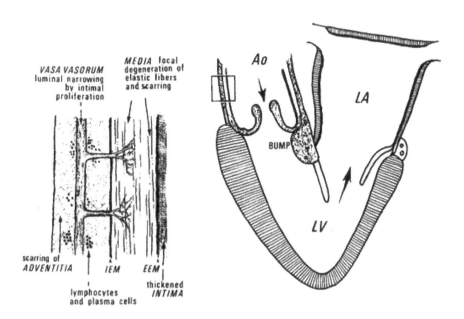

Figure 4 Diagram depicting the characteristic changes observed in ascending aorta, aortic valve and anterior mitral leaflet in ankylosing spondylitis.

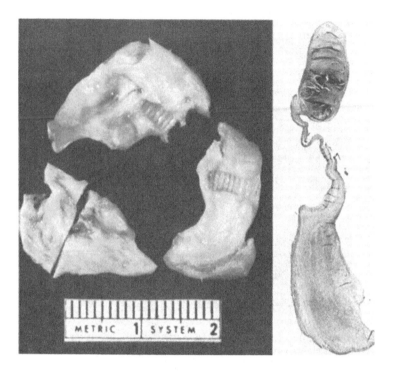

Figure 5 Excised aortic valve **(left)** (S72–4034) and photomicrograph **(right)** of section through one aortic valve cusp in the patient described. Hematoxylin and eosin stain; original magnification × 8 (right).

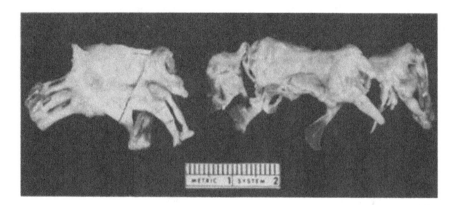

Figure 6 Atrial aspect of the excised mitral valve (S72–4034) in the patient described. Both anterior and posterior leaflets are thickened as are most of the chordae tendineae. Collections of plasma cells were present in the anterior leaflet but not in the similarly thickened posterior leaflet or in the thickened chordae tendineae. The reason for the thickening of the posterior leaflet and of the chordae tendineae is uncertain.

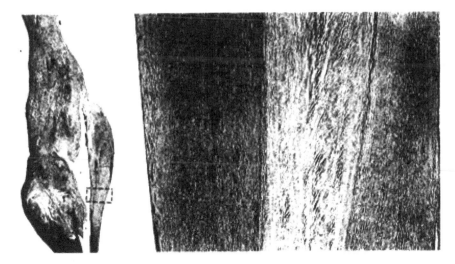

Figure 7 Photomicrographs of a portion of the thickened anterior mitral leaflet **(left)** and a chorda tendineae **(right).** The normal portion of the chorda is clearly separated from the overlying fibrous tissue by an elastic membrane. Elastic van Gieson stains; original magnification × 5 (left), × 40 (right), reduced by 25 per cent.

many collections of plasma cells (Figure 8). The inflammatory cells were present throughout the anterior mitral leaflet but were present in largest numbers near its base. Neither the thickened chordae tendineae nor the thickened posterior mitral leaflet contained inflammatory cells. Both mitral and aortic valve leaflets contained increased numbers of vascular channels.

When studied 7 months after operation, the patient was free of exertional dyspnea and chest pain despite nearly normal physical activities. There were no physical signs of congestive cardiac failure. A grade 1 to 2/6 systolic ejection murmur was audible over the lower cardiac base and a grade 2/6 diastolic murmur was audible over the lower left sternal border. The blood hematocrit value was 39 per cent. The blood urea nitrogen was 17 mg/100 ml and the uric acid 4.0 mg/100 ml. The urine was free of abnormal quantities of protein. The electrocardiogram and chest roentgenogram were unchanged compared to the preoperative studies. The results of cardiac catheterization are shown in Table 1.

COMMENTS

Although a number of reports have described structural alterations in the ascending aorta and aortic valve in patients with combined aortic regurgitation and ankylosing spondylitis, the specifics of the cardiovascular lesions in this arthritic condition have only recently been described.[4] Cardiovascular ankylosing spondylitis is limited largely to the area immediately above and below the aortic valve. The wall of aorta behind and immediately above the sinuses of Valsalva is thickened by dense adventitial scarring which is relatively acellular except for collections of lymphocytes and plasma cells around some vasa vasora, many of which are narrowed. The aortic intima is thickened, but less densely than adventitia, by rather cellular fibrous tissue. The aortic media is focally scarred and many of its elastic fibers are degenerated. Thus, the lesion in the aortic wall up to this point is identical to syphilis, indeed it is often mistaken for syphilis, but it is distinctly different from that resulting from the Marfan or Marfan-like syndromes or from atherosclerosis. In contrast to syphilis,

93

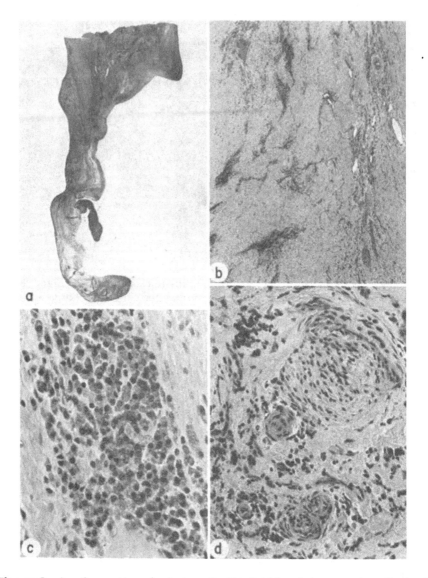

Figure 8 Another section of anterior mitral leaflet (a) and close-up views (b, c and d) of its detailed structure. **a,** the anterior leaflet is diffusely thickened. **b,** portion of leaflet showing large collections of cells and many vascular channels. **c,** the collections are mainly plasma cells. **d,** many of the vascular channels within the leaflet are thick-walled and have narrowed lumens. Hematoxylin and eosin stains; original magnification × 6.5 (a), × 40 (b), × 400 (c), × 250 (d), reduced by 26 per cent.

however, the lesion in the aortic wall in ankylosing spondylitis rarely extends more than a centimeter or so above the sinotubular junction (a level corresponding to the most cephalad extension of the aortic valve cusps), whereas in syphilis the process often spares the wall of aorta behind the sinuses of Valsalva and always involves the wall above the sinuses. Furthermore, in syphilis only the distal margins of the aortic valve cusps are thickened, whereas in ankylosing spondylitis the more basal portions of the cusps also are always thickened. In ankylosing spondylitis the endocardium in the immediate subaortic area is thickened by dense fibrous tissue, identical to and continuous with that in the adventitia of aorta. This subaortic extension, which never occurs in syphilis, is a distinctive cardiovascular lesion of ankylosing spondylitis, and results in a ridge or bump at the base of the anterior mitral leaflet. The anterior mitral leaflet is normal except for this bump or ridge near its basal attachment. The entire posterior mitral leaflet and all mitral chordae tendineae are usually normal.

The unusual features of the patient described herein were as follows: (1) diagnosis of the subaortic bump or ridge by left ventricular cineangiography, and subsequent confirmation by histologic examination that the cardiovascular changes were those characteristic of ankylosing spondylitis. (2) Extension of the subarotic fibrosing process to involve the entire anterior mitral leaflet, not just its basal portion. Histologic study demonstrated changes in the entire anterior mitral leaflet similar to those characteristically observed only in its basal portion and in the adventitia of aorta. Collections of plasma cells throughout the entire anterior mitral leaflet, not just at its base, identical to those present in the adventitia of ascending aorta are unique and not previously described. (3) Although it has been briefly mentioned in a few previously reported patients with aortic regurgitation and ankylosing spondylitis, mitral regurgitation was always mild and often associated with a history of rheumatic fever.[1-3] Among 25 necropsy patients with ankylosing spondylitis and aortic regurgitation,[4-11] however, mitral regurgitation was described in only 1.[11] In this patient both mitral leaflets were thickened, but inflammatory infiltrates were not present in the leaflets. Thus, our patient appears to be the first reported with cardiovascular ankylosing spondylitis in whom mitral regurgitation was documented in life, and the mitral leaflets were diffusely thickened and contained collections of plasma cells. The mitral regurgitation in our patient, however, was of less severity than the aortic regurgitation.

REFERENCES

1. Graham DC, Smythe HA: The carditis and aortitis of ankylosing spondylitis. Bull Rheum Dis 9: 171, 1958.
2. Gamp A, Ogorrek I: Beteiligung des Herzens bei der Spondylarthritis ankylopoetica. Z Rheumaforsch 17: 53, 1958.
3. Julkunen H: Rheumatoid spondylitis—clinical and laboratory study of 149 cases compared with 182 cases of rheumatoid arthritis. Acta Rheum Scand 172 (suppl 4): 24, 1962.
4. Bulkley BH, Roberts WC: Ankylosing spondylitis and aortic regurgitation. Description of the characteristic cardiovascular lesion from study of eight necropsy patients. Circulation 48: 1014, 1973.
5. Clark WS, Kulka PJ, Bauer W: Rheumatoid aortitis with aortic regurgitation. An unusual manifestation of rheumatoid arthritis (including spondylitis). Am J Med 22: 580, 1957.
6. Schilder DP, Harvey WP, Hufnagel CA: Rheumatoid spondylitis and aortic insufficiency. N Engl J Med 255: 11, 1956.
7. Ansell BM, Bywaters EGL, Doniach I: The aortic lesion of ankylosing spondylitis. Brit Heart J 20: 507, 1958.
8. Toone EC, Pierce EL, Hennigar GR: Aortitis and aortic regurgitation associated with rheumatoid spondylitis. Am J Med 26: 255, 1959.
9. Weed CL, Kulander BG, Mazarella JA, Decker JL: Heart block in ankylosing spondylitis. Arch Intern Med 117: 800, 1966.
10. Liu SM, Alexander CS: Complete heart block and aortic insufficiency in rheumatoid spondylitis. Am J Cardiol 23: 888, 1969.
11. MacMahon HE, Magendantz H, Brugsch HG, Patterson JF: Clinicopathologic conference. Bull Tufts-N Engl Med Center 1: 50, 1955.

Case 231 Cocking of a Poppet-Disc Prosthesis in the Aortic Position

A Cause of Intermittent Aortic Regurgitation

William J. Hammer, MD,* Michael J. Heame, MD, and William C. Roberts, MD,**
Washington, D. C.

Intermittent aortic regurgitation due to cocking is described for the first time after replacement of the aortic valve with a poppet-disc prosthesis. A combination of disc grooving and strut thrombus produced the cocking with resultant aortic regurgitation.

Among patients with prosthetic cardiac valves, a common cause of both early and late death is prosthetic dysfunction.[1] Auscultation and phonocardiographic abnormalities in these patients often are clues to such dysfunction.[2-4] Peribasilar communications or improper seating of the poppet as a result of thrombus or variance are the usual causes of regurgitant type murmurs. This report was prompted by observing intermittent aortic regurgitation after aortic valve replacement with a poppet disc prosthesis. The mechanism of the regurgitation has not been recorded previously after aortic valve replacement.

CASE REPORT

A 51-year-old man had been well during the first 6½ years after aortic valve replacement with a 16.5 mm. Hufnagel disc prosthesis.[5] Evidence of left ventricular failure then appeared and gradually progressed. Precordial auscultation 7 years after valve replacement disclosed distinct opening and closing prosthetic sounds: a Grade 4/6, harsh, basal systolic murmur and, along the left sternal border, a high-frequency decrescendo murmur, which varied from Grade 1/6 to 3/6 in intensity in successive cardiac cycles (Figure 1). Before cardiac catheterization could be performed, the patient suddenly died.

Necropsy (74A-347) disclosed multiple notches on the margins of the aortic prosthetic disc (Figures 2 and 3) and thrombus bordering the primary orifice and surrounding two of the four prosthetic struts. No peribasilar communications were present.

COMMENTS

Variance of the silicone rubber poppet of a caged-ball prosthetic cardiac valve is well known and usually is characterized by discoloration, grooving, swelling, or shrinkage.[1] Decreased mobility may be the consequence of the poppet's swelling or shrinkage. Either may lead to regurgitation. Grooving of the disc margins is a

From the Department of Medicine (Cardiology) and Pathology, Georgetown University Medical Center, Washington, D. C.

Received for publication May 28, 1975.

* Present address: Division of Cardiology, Department of Medicine, Temple University Health Science Center, Philadelphia, Pa.

** Present address: Section of Pathology, National Heart and Lung Institute, National Institutes of Health, Bethesda, Md.

DOI: 10.1201/9781003409281-15

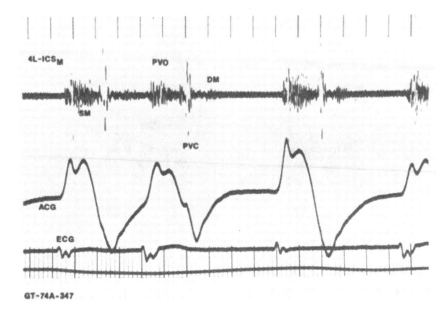

GT-74A-347

Figure 1 Phonocardiogram in the patient described showing a prominent systolic murmur *(SM)* and a diastolic murmur *(DM)* of varying intensity. The prosthetic valve opening *(PVO)* and closing *(PVC)* sounds are distinct. This recording was made over the fourth left intercostal space *(ICS)*, at medium *(M)* frequency, and simultaneously an apex cardiogram *(ACG)* and electrocardiogram *(ECG)* (Lead II) were recorded. The latter shows atrial fibrillation and left bundle branch block.

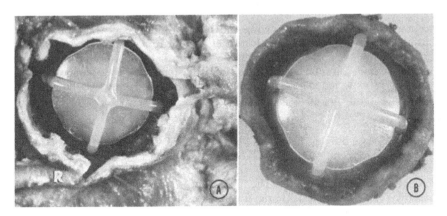

Figure 2 Views of the aortic disc prosthesis from above. *A,* While situated within the ascending aorta. *R,* Right coronary artery. *L,* Left coronary artery. *B,* After removal of the prosthesis from the aorta. The indentations of the margins of the disc are easily seen.

common late finding after replacement of either mitral or aortic valves with a caged-disc prosthesis. It may cause both fixed and intermittent regurgitation with the prosthesis in the mitral position.[6] Cocking of a disc in the aortic position, however, has not been described. Disc variance, as occurred in our patient, is probably the major cause of such cocking because it allows the disc to stick to one or two of the

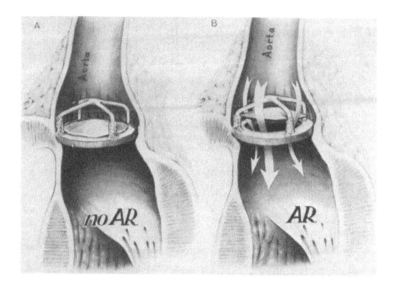

Figure 3 Drawing showing thrombus on two of the four struts and indentations on the margins of the disc. *A*, The appearance of the prosthesis when the disc is seated properly and there is no aortic regurgitation *(AR)*. *B*, The appearance of the prosthesis when disc-cocking has occurred, allowing aortic regurgitation.

struts and thereby prevents proper seating.[6] Our patient, who had no peribasilar communication at necropsy, had an obvious aortic regurgitant murmur *of varying intensity* that developed late after valve replacement. Not only were the margins of the disc grooved on our patient, but thrombus surrounded two of the four struts. The combination of poppet grooving and strut thrombus appears responsible for causing the disc to seat differently during each cardiac cycle. Thus there were varying amounts of aortic regurgitant flow (Figure 3). Because both thrombus and disc variance are common late findings after valve replacement, cocking of a poppet disc might be expected to be more common. A poppet-disc prosthesis, however, has been used infrequently in the aortic position.[6]

REFERENCES

1. Roberts, W. C., Bulkley, B. H., and Morrow, A. G.: Pathologic Anatomy of Cardiac Valve Replacement: A Study of 224 Necropsy Patients, Progr. Cardiovasc. Dis. **15:** 539, 1973.
2. Allen, P., and Robertson, R.: The Significance of Intermittent Regurgitation in Aortic Valve Prosthesis, J. Thorac. Cardiovasc. Surg. **54:** 549, 1967.
3. Hylen, J. C., Kloster, F. E., Starr, A., and Griswald, H. E.: Aortic Ball Variance: Diagnosis and Treatment, Ann. Intern. Med. **72:** 1, 1970.
4. Hildner, F. J.: Detection of Prosthetic Valve Dysfunction by Bedside and Laboratory Evaluation, Cardiovasc. Clin. **5:** 289, 1973.
5. Hufnagel, C. A., and Conrad, P. W.: A Comparative Study of Some Prosthetic Valves for Aortic and Mitral Replacement, Surgery **57:** 205, 1965.
6. Roberts, W. C., Fishbein, M. C., and Golden, A.: Cardiac Pathology After Valve Replacement Using Disc Prosthesis: A Study of 61 Necropsy Patients, Am. J. Cardiol. **35:** 740, 1975.

Case 243 Combined Acute Rheumatic Fever and Congenitally Bicuspid Aortic Valve

A Hitherto Unconfirmed Combination

*Richard. A. McReynolds, MD,*** Nayab Ali, MD,[†] Michael Cuadra, MD;[‡] and William C. Roberts, MD, F.C.C.P.[§]*

An 18-year-old man is described in whom rheumatic heart disease, as evidenced by the presence of classic Aschoff bodies, occurred in combination with a congenitally bicuspid (purely incompetent) aortic valve. To our knowledge, this is the first report documenting the presence of rheumatic heart disease and congenitally bicuspid aortic valve in the same patient.

Although fusion of two of three aortic valve cusps (one of three commissures) causing "acquired" bicuspid valve is common in rheumatic heart disease, the occurrence of a congenitally bicuspid aortic valve in a patient with unequivocal rheumatic disease, *ie*, with Aschoff bodies present, has not been reported. The report which follows describes this association in the same patient.

CASE REPORT

An 18-year-old black man was well until two years before death when he developed flank pain for which he was hospitalized. Examination at that time disclosed blood pressure of 140/80 mm Hg, collapsing peripheral pulses, and grade 3/6 basal systolic and diastolic precordial murmurs consistent with aortic "stenosis" and regurgitation. Electrocardiogram (Figure 1) and chest roentgenogram (Figure 2) showed cardiomegaly. After several days, the flank pain subsided; its etiology was never determined. Infective endocarditis was ruled out by repeatedly negative blood cultures. After discharge, he remained well and active until he suddenly collapsed and died while at work.

At necropsy the heart weighed 800 gm. Both ventricular cavities were dilated and their walls hypertrophied (Figure 3). Neither atrial cavity was dilated. No foci of myocardial fibrosis or necrosis were noted grossly. The aortic valve was congenitally bicuspid. Each cusp was diffusely fibrotic and retracted but mobile, and devoid of calcium (Figure 3). The valve orifice was not stenotic, but it was incompetent. Both coronary arteries arose in front of the anterior cusp, which contained a raphe. The mitral leaflets were mildly but diffusely thickened by fibrous tissue, but the

From the Section of Pathology, National Heart and Lung Institute, National Institutes of Health, Bethesda, Maryland and the Cardiac Laboratory, Howard University Medical Service, and the Department of Pathology, D.C. General Hospital, Washington, D.C.

** Presently Assistant Professor of Pathology, University of Alabama School of Medicine, Birmingham.

† Assistant Professor of Medicine, Howard University School of Medicine; Cardiologist, D.C. General Hospital.

‡ Chief, Autopsy Service, D.C. General Hospital, Washington, D.C.

§ Chief, Section of Pathology, National Heart and Lung Institute, National Institutes of Health, Bethesda.

Reprint requests: Dr. Roberts, NIH Bldg 10A, Room 3E20, Bethesda, 20014

DOI: 10.1201/9781003409281-16

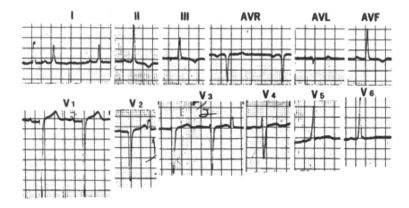

Figure 1 Electrocardiogram showing left ventricular hypertrophy and sinus rhythm.

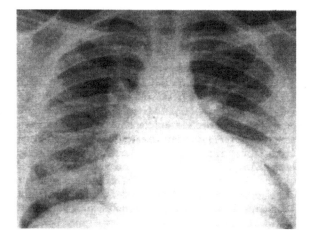

Figure 2 Chest roentgenogram showing considerable cardiomegaly of the left ventricular type.

chordae tendineae were normal. The tricuspid and pulmonic valves were normal. The left ventricular endocardium was diffusely opaque, and the right ventricular endocardium was focally opaque. Histologic examination disclosed multiple typical Aschoff bodies in the endocardium of both atria and in the endocardium and interstitium of both ventricles (Figure 4).

COMMENTS

Although each is a fairly common condition, a congenitally bicuspid aortic valve and rheumatic heart disease have not previously been clearly demonstrated to be present simultaneously in the same patient. Previous studies[1-3] from this laboratory have shown that congenitally bicuspid aortic valves may occur in as high as 2 percent of the population, and the incidence of rheumatic heart disease clinically has been reported to be as high as 6 percent of the population.[4] Thus, it is surprising that the two conditions have not been described previously in the same

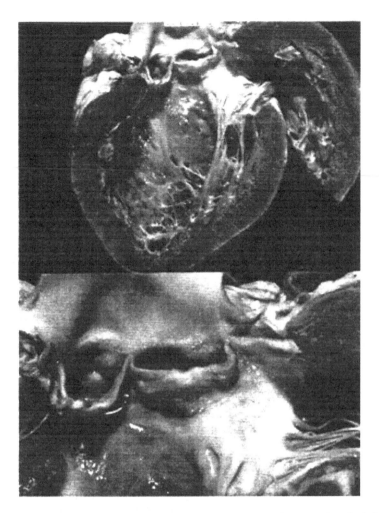

Figure 3 Heart. *Upper:* Opened aorta, aortic valve, and left ventricle. The left ventricular cavity is quite dilated, its endocardium mildly thickened, and its wall, very thick. *Lower.* Close-up view of the opened aortic valve. The anterior cusp, the one containing the raphe, has been severed during the opening of the valve. The posterior cusp, from which no coronary arteries arose, is intact. The anterior leaflet of the mitral valve (shown here) also is thickened by fibrous tissue. No inflammatory cells were found in histologic sections of any of the four cardiac valves.

patient. One of the reasons for this discrepancy may be different criteria utilized for defining the congenitally bicuspid condition of the aortic valve and for designating valvular disease as rheumatic in type. Our criteria for designating an aortic valve as congenitally bicuspid have been delineatéd elsewhere.[1] In essence, there are only two aortic valve cusps, only two true commissures, and, in about half of the cases, a false commissure or raphe also is present. The cusps are oriented either anteriorly and posteriorly (and if a raphe is present it is always in the anterior cusp) or right and left (and if a raphe is present it is always in the right cusp). The distance circumferentially between any two true commissures is always greater than

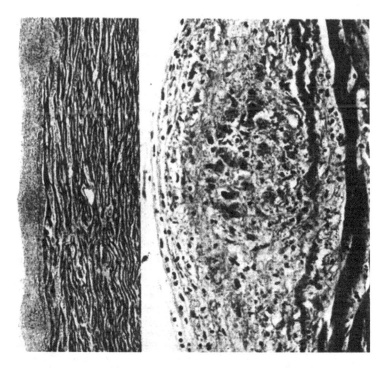

Figure 4 Left ventricular endocardium with multiple typical Aschoff bodies. *Left:* Low-power (x55) view showing three discrete Aschoff bodies in the thickened endocardium. *Right:* Close-up (x350) view of one of the Aschoff bodies (hematoxylin and eosin stains).

between a true and a false commissure. The raphe rarely extends as far cephalad in the aorta as do the true commissures.

The only unequivocal criterion of rheumatic heart disease is the presence of Aschoff bodies. Although a number of different stages of Aschoff bodies have been described,[5] only in the granulomatous stage can an Aschoff body be unequivocally identified.[6] In our laboratory, we have found Aschoff bodies at necropsy or in biopsies of atrial appendages[7] or papillary muscles obtained at operation only in patients with diffuse disease, nearly always stenosis, of the mitral valve. About 5 percent of our patients with fatal mitral valve disease studied at necropsy had Aschoff bodies.[8] We have never observed an Aschoff body in the heart of a patient with anatomically isolated aortic valve disease, *ie*, an anatomically normal mitral valve, and indeed we have been unable to find any report demonstrating an Aschoff body in the heart of a patient with isolated aortic valve disease, irrespective of the number of aortic valve cusps present. Among approximately 200 adult patients with congenitally biscuspid aortic valves studied by us at necropsy, only the patient described herein had an Aschoff body in his heart.

At least two previous authors, however, have mentioned the occurrence of Aschoff bodies in patients with bicuspid aortic valves. Gross[9] described Aschoff bodies in 5 of 16 hearts with "so-called congenital bicuspid aortic valve." It is clear from study of his paper, however, that his criteria for Aschoff bodies were extremely loose, indeed unacceptable, and furthermore that several of his patients almost surely had acquired bicuspid aortic valves rather than congenital malformations. Hall and

Ichioka[10] found Aschoff bodies in five of eight patients with "bicuspid aortic valves." Three of these five patients were over 65 years of age and a fourth was 53. Thus, three of their patients may have had aortic valve disease of the elderly, probably degenerative in origin,[3] rather than congenital malformations. These authors also used the loose, nonspecific criteria of Gross and Ehrlich[5] for identification of Aschoff bodies. In addition, none of their five patients had anatomic disease of the mitral valve. To reemphasize, we have never observed an Aschoff body, using the criteria defined by Saphir,[6] in a patient without anatomic disease of the mitral valve. Almost surely in years past there has been an "over-diagnosis" of Aschoff bodies at necropsy, using loose criteria which may include nonspecific inflammatory lesions of the heart.

Our patient had a classic congenitally bicuspid aortic valve and numerous classic Aschoff bodies in the heart at necropsy. To our knowledge, this combination has neither been clearly documented nor illustrated previously.

REFERENCES

1. Roberts WC: The congenitally bicuspid aortic valve. A study of 85 autopsy cases. Am J Cardiol 26:72–83, 1970
2. Roberts WC: The structure of the aortic valve in clinically-isolated aortic stenosis. An autopsy study of 162 patients over 15 years of age. Circulation 42:91–97, 1970
3. Roberts WC, Perloff JK, Constantino T: Severe valvular aortic stenosis in patients over 65 years of age. A clinicopathologic study. Am J Cardiol 27:497–506, 1971
4. Marienfield CJ, Robins M, Sandidge RP, et al: Rheumatic fever and rheumatic heart disease among U.S. college freshmen, 1956–60. Pub Health Rep 79:789–811, 1964
5. Gross L, Ehrlich JC: Studies on the myocardial Aschoff body: Descriptive classification of lesions. Am J Pathol 10:467–488, 1934
6. Saphir O: The Aschoff nodule (editorial). Am J Clin Pathol 31:534–539, 1959
7. Vermani R, Roberts WC: Incidence and significance of Aschoff bodies in atrial appendages removed at operation: An analysis of 800 patients. (In preparation)
8. Roberts WC: Anatomically isolated aortic valvular disease. The case against its being of rheumatic etiology. Am J Med 49:151–159, 1970
9. Gross L: So-called congenital bicuspid aortic valve. Arch Pathol 23:350–362, 1937
10. Hall EM, Ichioka T: Etiology of calcified nodular aortic stenosis. Am J Pathol 16:761–785, 1940

Case 267 Clinical Pathologic Conference

A Conversation on Prosthetic Valve Endocarditis

Ernest N. Arnett, MD*, David G. Kastl, MD, A. Julian Garvin, MD, PhD, and William C. Roberts, MD
Bethesda, MD

Dr. Roberts: The starting point for this discussion on prosthetic valve endocarditis will be a description of a patient with this fatal complication of cardiac valve replacement.

Dr. Kastl: This 47-year-old man (J.G. #1123701) was in good health until 11 months before death when symptoms of fatigue and exertional dyspnea appeared four weeks after a dental procedure. Hospitalization four months after onset of symptoms (seven months before death) revealed anemia, a colonic filling defect, periodic fever, and *Streptococcus bovis* in several blood cultures. Penicillin, 20 million units intravenously per day, was administered for six weeks; the fever rapidly disappeared, but murmurs of mitral and aortic regurgitation and signs of congestive heart failure appeared. Digoxin and diuretic therapy resulted in transient improvement of the congestive heart failure, and the colonic mass, which proved to be a benign polyp, was resected. He returned home, but heart failure quickly returned and he was hospitalized, now in functional Class IV (New York Heart Association classification), 55 days before death. Digoxin, furosemide, and aldactone produced a 20 pound weight loss. Subsequently, at cardiac catheterization, the pressures in mm. Hg were: pulmonary artery wedge mean 35, a wave 35, v wave 55; pulmonary artery 60/35 (mean 50); right ventricle 60/15; and right atrial mean 15, a wave 22, and v wave 17. Multiple blood cultures during that hospitalization were negative. He was transferred to the National Heart, Lung and Blood Institute (NHLI) 37 days before death.

The blood pressure was 140/70 mm. Hg, cardiac rate, 90 beats per minute, and respiratory rate, 20 breaths per minute. The jugular venous pressure was elevated, and the carotid upstroke was rapid but weak. Basilar râles were present in both lungs. The second heart sound split paradoxically and both third and fourth heart sounds were present. A Grade 3/6 decrescendo diastolic murmur was present along the left sternal border, and a Grade 2/6 holosystolic murmur and a Grade 2/6 middiastolic rumbling murmur were present at the apex. The anteroinferior edge of the liver was palpable 4 cm. below the right costal margin. Chest roentgenograms

From the Pathology Branch and Clinic of Surgery, National Heart, Lung and Blood Institute, and the Laboratory of Pathology, National Cancer Institute, National Institutes of Heaíth, Bethesda, Md.

Received for publication June 9, 1976.

Reprint requests: W. C. Roberts, M.D., Bldg. 10A Rm 3E-30, National Institutes of Health, Bethesda, Maryland 20014.

* Present address: Department of Medicine, The Johns Hopkins Hospital, Baltimore, Maryland.

DOI: 10.1201/9781003409281-17

(Figure 1) showed marked cardiac enlargement and electrocardiogram (Figure 2*a*) showed left ventricular hypertrophy. The hematocrit was 37 per cent, and the white blood count 11,900 per cubic millimeter. Simultaneous aortic and left ventricular pressures were 120/50 and 120/30 mm. Hg, respectively. Cineangiography revealed severe aortic and mitral valve regurgitation, but good left ventricular function.

The aortic valve was replaced with a No. 10A model 2320, Starr-Edwards prosthesis and the mitral valve, with a 33 mm. Hancock xenograft 28 days before death. Both the excised aortic valve and the excised mitral valve (Figure 3) contained one or more perforations in the cusps. Histologic examination of the excised valves revealed no evidence of active infection.

During the first 24 hours postoperatively, excessive bleeding necessitated repeat thoracotomy. Although no specific bleeding sites were found, a large quantity (2,000 ml.) of blood was evacuated from the mediastinum. Oxacillin, 4 Gm. intravenously per day, and streptomycin, 1 Gm. intramuscularly per day, were started at the time of the initial operation and continued for 10 and 7 days, respectively. All chest tubes were removed on the fourth postoperative day. Two days later fever (38.5° C.) was noted but he otherwise appeared to be doing well. Nine days postoperatively ventricular fibrillation occurred, but electroshock was successful in restoring sinus rhythm. Electrocardiograms following this episode showed diffuse nonspecific ST segment and T wave abnormalities. Over the ensuing 4 days, he continued to have frequent ventricular premature beats. On the 17th postoperative day his temperature rose to 39.5° C., the white blood cell count was 14,500 per cubic millimeter, and blood cultures were positive for *Staphylococcus epidermidis*. Oxacillin, 12 Gm. intravenously per day, was reinstituted. The following day the blood pressure dropped to 95/70 mm. Hg and the electrocardiogram (Figure 2*b*) showed changes of an acute anterolateral myocardial infarction. On the nineteenth postoperative day, splinter hemorrhages were noted, the white blood cell count was 17,000 per cubic millimeter,

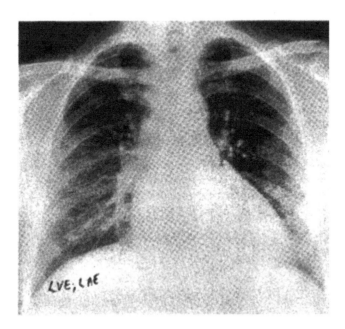

Figure 1   Posteroanterior chest roentgenogram 4 days before valve replacement.

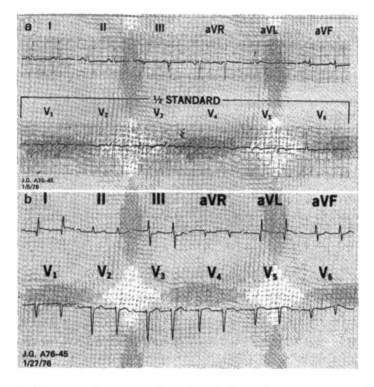

Figure 2 Electrocardiograms. *a*, Four days before valve replacements showing changes of left ventricular hypertrophy and left atrial enlargement. *b*, Eighteen days postoperatively (10 days before death). Q waves are present in Leads I, aVR, aVL and V_e, the R waves in the precordial leads are of markedly diminished amplitude, and the ST segments are elevated in Leads I, aVL and V_4 through V_6. In addition, the P-R interval is prolonged.

and blood cultures again were positive for *S. epidermidis*, resistant to penicillin but sensitive to both oxacillin and cephalosporin. On the twenty-first postoperative day he lost consciousness, his temperature rose to 39° C., and his systolic blood pressure fell to 90 mm. Hg. During insertion of a catheter into a jugular vein, a collection of pus was entered, and Gram stain and culture of the aspirated material disclosed *S. epidermidis*. Exploration of the mediastinum revealed no focal collections of pus. Oxacillin was stopped and cephalosporin, 12 Gm. intravenously per day, was started. Over the next four days consciousness returned, the blood pressure rose to 110/60 mm. Hg, but the white blood count was 27,000 per cubic millimeter, and fever and positive blood cultures continued. On the twenty-seventh postoperative day, his blood pressure suddenly dropped and he died the next day.

Dr. Garvin: Necropsy (A76–45) disclosed no residual pus in the chest. The heart weighed 660 Gm., and the anterolateral left ventricular wall from midportion to apex was necrotic. Large vegetations closed the primary orifice of the aortic valve prosthesis, and a fibrin thrombus was present at the apex of its cage (Figure 4). Although the aortic prosthesis remained attached, the site of attachment of the prosthesis was necrotic. Necrosis of the valve anulus, however, was apparent only after removal of the prosthesis (Figure 5). The ring infection extended through the

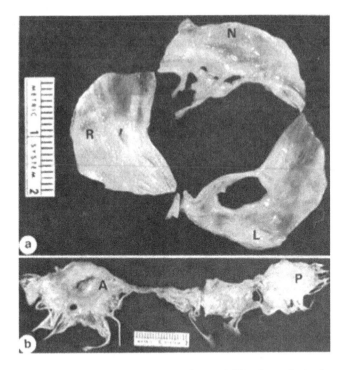

Figure 3 Operatively excised aortic *(a)* and mitral *(b)* valves. A single perforation is present in the left *(L)* and right *(R)* coronary cusp, and multiple ones are present in the noncoronary *(N)* cusp. A perforation is present in the anterior *(A)* mitral leaflet, and several chordae tendineae from the posterior *(P)* mitral leaflet are absent.

atrial septum into the right atrium and into the adjacent portion of the prosthetic mitral anulus. Histologic sections from the site of attachment of the aortic prosthesis revealed numerous colonies of Gram-positive cocci. Examination of subserial sections of the extramural coronary arteries revealed total obstruction of the lumen of the left anterior descending coronary artery by a septic embolus (Figure 6). Sections of myocardium showed numerous foci of suppurating and nonsuppurating inflammation. The lungs were edematous and contained foci of acute inflammation. The walls of the small muscular pulmonary arteries were thick. Both the liver (2,600 grams) and spleen (670 grams) were enlarged, and multiple infarcts were present in the spleen. Focal collections of mononuclear cells were present in the renal interstitium, but otherwise the kidneys were normal.

Dr. Roberts: The above-described patient provides an opportunity to apply information previously derived from a study of 22 necropsy patients with fatal prosthetic valve endocarditis to the present patient.[1] To begin this discourse, Dr. Arnett, how do you define "Prosthetic Valve Endocarditis?"

Dr. Arnett: "Prosthetic valve endocarditis" is an infection involving a prosthetic cardiac valve in a patient in whom no active infective endocarditis was present at the time of prosthetic valve insertion. In other words, the infection was acquired after valve replacement. Although the present patient's valvular disease resulted from infective endocarditis, the infection was healed at the time of valve replacement.

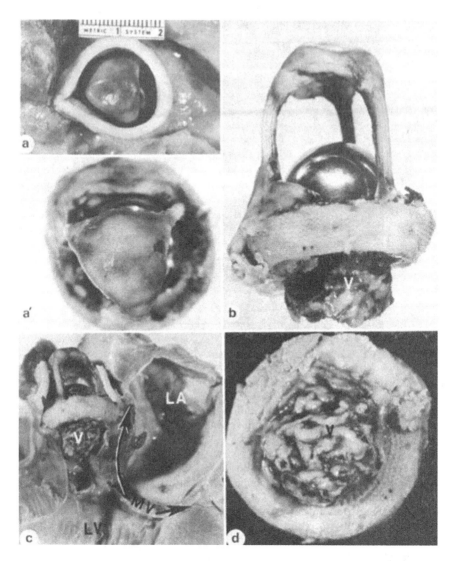

Figure 4 Infected aortic valve prosthesis. *a*, Prosthesis, viewed from above, in place, and *a′* after removal. Thrombus covers the apex of the cage. *b*, Excised prosthesis viewed laterally. *c*, Longitudinal section showing aortic prosthesis in place. The mitral valve prosthesis has been excised. The aortic "anulus" is necrotic and so is the adjacent portion of mitral anulus. A large vegetation *(V)* is present in the primary orifice of the prosthesis; its obstructive nature is better seen in *d*, a view of the prosthesis from the left ventricular *(LV)* aspect. *LA* = left atrium.

Dr. Roberts: Dr. Kastl, in your presentation of this patient, you mentioned that the cause of this patient's infective endocarditis, which had involved presumably both anatomically and functionally normal valves, was *Streptococcus bovis*. The cause of the prosthetic valve endocarditis in him, however, was *Staphylococcus epidermidis*. Dr. Arnett, could you summarize the organisms found in our previous 22 patients with prosthetic valve endocarditis?

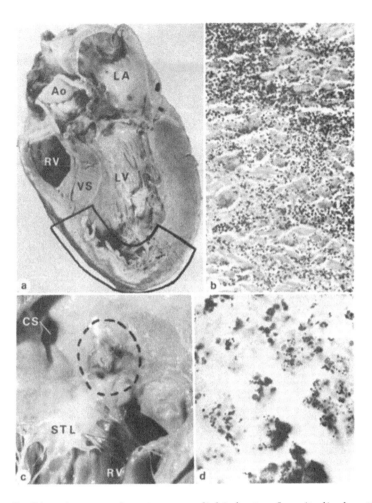

Figure 5 Ring abscess and acute myocardial infarct. *a*, Longitudinal section of heart showing the ring abscess involving the entire aortic "anulus" and the portion of mitral anulus adjacent to the aortic valve. A large transmural infarct is present in the anterior wall of left ventricle (in brackets). *Ao* = aorta; *LA* = left atrium; *LV* = left ventricle; *RV* = right ventricle; *VS* = ventricular septum. *b*, Histologic section of the anterior left ventricular wall. The myocardial cells are necrotic and numerous polymorphonuclear leukocytes are present. (Hematoxylin and eosin stain; × 330). *c*, Opened right atrium, tricuspid valve, and right ventricle *(RV)*. The aortic ring abscess has extended through the adjacent atrial septum and is visible in right atrium *(dashed circle)*. *CS* = ostium of coronary sinus; *STL* = septal tricuspid leaflet. *d*, Histologic section showing colonies of Gram-positive cocci in the necrotic aortic valve anulus (Brown and Brenn stain; × 880).

Dr. Arnett: Among our 22 previous necropsy patients with prosthetic valve endocarditis, *Staphylococcus (epidermidis* in 10 and *aureus* in three) caused the infection in 13 (59 per cent.) In the other nine patients, nine different organisms caused the infection. Of these later nine organisms, three were Gram-negative bacteria, and two were fungi.

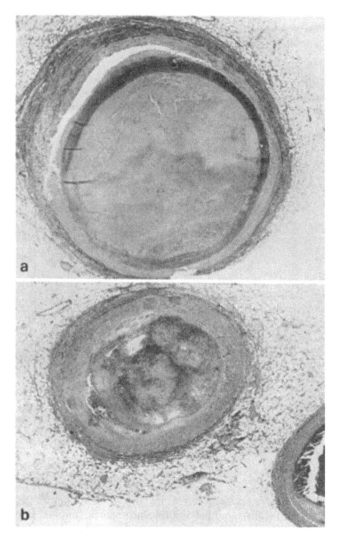

Figure 6 Left anterior descending coronary artery. *a*, Proximal 1 cm. and *b*, a distal branch. The lumen is totally obstructed by a septic embolus. (*a*, Elastic van Gieson stain; *b*, hematoxylin and eosin stain; both × 12.)

Dr. Roberts: We have found it useful to subdivide patients with prosthetic valve endocarditis into those with early infection, i.e., appearing within two months of valve replacement, and those with infection appearing later, i.e., those with signs of cardiac infection appearing longer than two months after operation. Dr. Arnett, have there been any differences in the types of infecting organisms in patients with early prosthetic valve endocarditis as contrasted to those in whom the infection appeared months or years after valve replacement?

Dr. Arnett: Among patients with early prosthetic valve endocarditis, *Staphylococcus epidermidis* has been the most frequent causative organism.[2-4] Among patients with late prosthetic valve endocarditis both staphylococci and streptococci have been frequent causes; however, the former have caused most cases of necropsy-proven late prosthetic valve endocarditis, and the latter, relatively few.

Dr. Roberts: Among patients with early prosthetic valve endocarditis it is presumed that the infection either was incurred at operation or resulted from a wound infection. The former may result from contamination of cardiopulmonary bypass equipment.[5,6] Dr. Arnett, what have been the predisposing factors in patients with late prosthetic valve endocarditis?

Dr. Arnett: Late prosthetic valve endocarditis presumably results from transient bacteremia, and the source of the bacteremia is often obscure.[3,7] Among our previous 22 necropsy patients with prosthetic valve endocarditis, 14 had the onset of symptoms of prosthetic endocarditis longer than two months after operation. Predisposing factors were apparent in only five of them: dental procedures in two, and in one patient each, skin graft infection, prolonged use of an intravenous catheter, and prolonged use of a transthoracic pacing wire.

Dr. Roberts: Dr. Arnett, you mentioned a similarity between early and late prosthetic endocarditis in regard to the types of infecting organisms. Are there distinct clinical differences between patients with prosthetic valve endocarditis appearing early after operation as contrasted to those with infection appearing late?

Dr. Arnett: Prosthetic valve endocarditis occurring in the early postoperative period is often more difficult to diagnose.[7] Signs of prosthetic infection may be masked by other more common postoperative complications, and transient bacteremia may be attributed to another cause. That was the situation in the present patient: persistent staphylococcal bacteremia was attributed to the known mediastinal infection and the diagnosis of prosthetic valve endocarditis was never established during life. When fever and bacteremia appear suddenly in an otherwise well patient months or years after cardiac valve replacement, however, a diagnosis of prosthetic valve endocarditis is usually made quite readily.

Dr. Roberts: It is worth emphasizing, however, that the combination of fever and positive blood culture in a patient with a prosthetic cardiac valve, especially in the early postoperative period, does not always indicate the presence of prosthetic valve endocarditis.[8] We recently studied at necropsy a patient who was diagnosed during life as having mitral prosthetic valve endocarditis on the basis of fever, cerebral episodes consistent with emboli, and a blood culture which grew *Staphylococcus epidermidis*. She received antibiotics during most of her four-month postoperative period and, at necropsy, no prosthetic valve endocarditis was found. A left ventricular aneurysm, however, was present immediately caudal to the mitral anulus and a thrombus, which presumably had been infected at one time, was present in the aneurysm. The latter appeared to have been the source of cerebral emboli.

Although the present patient's aortic valve prosthesis was almost totally obstructed by vegetative material, a diagnosis of endocarditis was never established, presumably because signs of prosthetic dysfunction were absent. Dr. Arnett, do patients with prosthetic valve endocarditis usually have signs of prosthetic dysfunction?

Dr. Arnett: This patient was somewhat unusual. Infection of an aortic valve prosthesis usually results in detachment of the prosthesis, not obstruction, and signs of aortic regurgitation are usually present. Eleven of our previous 15 necropsy patients with aortic prosthetic infection had signs of aortic regurgitation, and in each of them the prosthesis was at least partially detached. Only one previous patient had aortic prosthetic obstruction from infection, and he had clinical signs of aortic valve obstruction. In contrast to aortic prosthetic infection, mitral infection usually

111

causes obstruction of the prosthesis, but signs of mitral obstruction usually are not detected. None of our seven patients with mitral prosthetic endocarditis had clinical signs of prosthetic dysfunction, but at necropsy five of them had large vegetations obstructing the orifice of the prosthesis.

Dr. Roberts: This patient had infection behind the site of attachment of the prosthesis, i.e., in the valve ring. Dr. Arnett, would you comment on the frequency of ring abscess among necropsy patients with prosthetic valve endocarditis?

Dr. Arnett: Infection behind the sewing ring, or ring abscess, is a consistent morphologic feature of prosthetic valve endocarditis. Ring abscess was present in each of our 22 previous patients, all of whom had rigid-framed prosthesis. In two thirds of them the entire circumference of the valve anulus was necrotic. Extension of the ring infection into adjacent cardiac structures also is common, especially in the patients with an infected aortic prosthesis. In nine of our previous 15 patients with aortic prosthetic valve endocarditis, the ring abscess burrowed through the cardiac septum into ring atrium, just as it did in the present patient.

Dr. Roberts: Thus ring abscess is to be expected in patients with infection involving rigid-frame prostheses. Indeed, the infection in these patients nearly always involves the site of attachment of the prosthesis, and this is why patients with prosthetic valve endocarditis are so difficult to treat. If the infection was limited to the prosthesis, an infected prosthesis could be excised and replaced with another prosthesis. In the present patient, as in most of the others, the entire valve anulus was necrotic, and although he had received appropriate antibiotic therapy, intravenously for four weeks, numerous colonies of viable-appearing Gram positive cocci were present in the valve ring at necropsy. This patient developed prolongation of the PR interval, presumably from extension of the aortic ring abscess into the cephalad portion of the ventricular septum. Dr. Arnett, how common are atrioventricular conduction defects in patients with aortic prosthetic endocarditis?

Dr. Arnett: Among our previous 15 patients with aortic valve prosthetic endocarditis, five developed complete heart block and two others developed left bundle branch block. In each of these patients the ring abscess had extended into the basal portion of the ventricular septum.

Dr. Roberts: The present patient had multiple infarcts in the spleen as well as a transmural acute myocardial infarct. Are systemic emboli common in patients with prosthetic valve endocarditis?

Dr. Arnett: Fourteen of our 22 previous necropsy patients (64 per cent) had gross infarcts in other organs. The organs most frequently involved were: spleen (12 patients), kidney (7 patients), and brain (7 patients). Only one of the previous 22 patients, however, had a transmural acute myocardial infarct from a coronary arterial embolus.

Dr. Roberts: We have not touched on the frequency of prosthetic valve endocarditis. We have examined at necropsy approximately 450 patients in whom one or more cardiac valves had been replaced by prostheses. Twenty-three of them (5 per cent), including the patient described herein, had infection involving a prosthetic valve. Thus, although prosthetic valve endocarditis is a devastating complication of cardiac valve replacement, fortunately, it is infrequent. Although its exact frequency is uncertain, it may be less than 1 per cent per year among patients with prosthetic cardiac valves. In the early days of cardiac valve replacement, prosthetic infection in the early postoperative period was more common than in the late postoperative period. Now, however, it is likely that infection occurring late is more common than that occurring early, simply because there are large numbers of patients with prosthetic valves.

Dr. Arnett and I have studied 74 patients with active infective endocarditis involving natural left-sided cardiac valves. Dr. Arnett, would you summarize the major differences between our patients with prosthetic endocarditis and those with natural valve infective endocarditis.

Dr. Arnett: Comparison of observations in the 22 patients with prosthetic valve endocarditis to those in the 74 patients with active left-sided valvular endocarditis revealed two major differences. *Ring abscess* was present in each of the patients with prosthetic valve endocarditis, regardless of the site of the prosthesis. Among the patients with natural valve endocarditis, ring abscess was common only in patients with aortic valve infection.[9] Because heart block in patients with infective endocarditis is usually due to extension of ring abscess into the ventricular septum, it is more frequent in patients with prosthetic endocarditis than in patients with natural valve endocarditis.

The second major difference between patients with prosthetic endocarditis, and those with natural valve endocarditis is the frequency of *valvular obstruction* from infective endocarditis. The hemodynamic consequence of natural valve endocarditis is almost always regurgitation; valvular obstruction is rare.[10,11] The hemodynamic consequence of prosthetic valve infection often is obstruction, especially when a mitral prosthesis is infected.

REFERENCES

1. Arnett, E. N., and Roberts, W. C.: Prosthetic valve endocarditis. A clinico pathologic analysis of 22 necropsy patients with comparison of observations to 74 necropsy patients with active infective endocarditis involving natural left-sided cardiac valves, Am. J. Cardiol. **38**:281, 1976.

2. Slaughter, L., Morris, J. E., and Starr, A.: Prosthetic valvular endocarditis. A 12-year review, Circulation **47**:1319, 1973.

3. Dismukes, W. E., Karchmer, A. W., Buckley, M. J., Austen, W. G., and Swartz, M. N.: Prosthetic valve endocarditis. Analysis of 38 cases, Circulation **48**:365, 1973.

4. Wilson, W. R., Jaumin, P. M., Danielson, G. K., Giuliani, E. R., Washington, J. A., and Geraci, J. E.: Prosthetic valve endocarditis, Ann. Intern. Med. **82**:751, 1975.

5. Ankeney, J. L., and Parker, R. F.: Staphylococcal endocarditis following open heart surgery related to positive intraoperative blood cultures, *in* Prosthetic heart valves, edited by Brewer, L. A., III, Springfield, IL, 1969, Charles C Thomas, Publisher, pp. 719–730.

6. Blakemore, W. S., McGarrity, G. J., Thurer, R. J., Wallace, H. W., MacVaugh, H., III, and Coriell, L. L.: Infection by air-borne bacteria with cardiopulmonary bypass, Surgery **70**:830, 1971.

7. Kloster, F. E.: Diagnosis and management of complications of prosthetic heart valves, Am. J. Cardiol. **35**:872, 1975.

8. Sande, M. A., Johnson, W. D., Jr., Hook, E. W., and Kaxe, D.: Sustained bacteremia in patients with prosthetic cardiac valves, N. Engl. J. Med. **286**:1067, 1972.

9. Arnett, E. N., and Roberts, W. C.: Valve ring abscess in active infective endocarditis. Frequency, location, and clues to clinical diagnosis from study of 95 necropsy patients, Circulation **54**:140, 1976.

10. Roberts, W. C., Ewy, G. A., Glancy, D. L., and Marcus, F. I.: Valvular stenosis produced by active infective endocarditis, Circulation **36**:449, 1967.

11. Arnett, E. N., and Roberts, W. C.: Active infective endocarditis. A clinico pathologic analysis of 137 necropsy patients. Current Concepts in Cardiology **1**:2–76, 1976.

Case 274 A Hitherto Undescribed Cause of Prosthetic Mitral Valve Obstruction

Ancil A. Jones, MD, John B. Otis, MD, Gerald F. Fletcher, MD, and William C. Roberts, MD
Bethesda, MD

A case is described in which severe prosthetic mitral valve obstruction was produced by entanglement of sutures across the central axis of the prosthesis on its ventricular side. The entangled sutures prevented the tilting disc occluder from falling into the left ventricular cavity during ventricular diastole.

Obstruction to a prosthetic cardiac valve is a well-recognized complication of cardiac valve replacement, particularly with rigid-framed prostheses. The usual causes of prosthetic valve stenosis are *prosthetic disproportion*, i.e., too large a prosthesis for the cardiac ventricle or aorta into which the prosthesis is inserted, and *prosthetic thrombosis*.[1-3] Although other causes of prosthetic obstruction have been described, suture entanglement beneath a prosthetic mitral valve occluder has not been described previously. Such was the case in the patient to be described briefly.

CASE REPORT

C. S., a 36-year-old woman, was in good health until 4 weeks before death, when fever and chills appeared. She was admitted to a hospital in her city 2 weeks later, at the time of an embolus to one leg. Blood cultures grew beta-hemolytic Streptococcus, Group B, a diagnosis of active infective endocarditis was made, and she was treated with antibiotics. Precordial systolic and diastolic murmurs were heard and congestive cardiac failure developed. The latter rapidly progressed and, on the day of her death, necessitated mitral and aortic valve replacements. At operation, both the mitral and aortic valves were purely incompetent from vegetations which had destroyed portions of the leaflets and chordae tendineae. Both valves were replaced with Björk-Shiley prostheses: No. 29 mm. in the mitral position and No. 25 mm. in the aortic position. She was weaned from cardiopulmonary bypass with difficulty, and a counter-pulsation balloon was inserted in the descending thoracic aorta. Although she manifested features of severely depressed cardiac output, she lived nearly 12 hours after completion of operation.

At necropsy, the heart weighed 320 grams. (She weighed about 95 pounds.) The occluder of the mitral prosthesis was unable to fall more than 2 mm. toward the left ventricular cavity. Examination of the left ventricular aspect of the mitral prosthesis disclosed that three sutures had become entangled across its central axis, preventing the occluder from falling into the left ventricular cavity and thereby producing severe prosthetic obstruction (Figure 1).

From the Pathology Branch, National Heart, Lung and Blood Institute, National Institutes of Health, Bethesda, Md. 20014.

Received for publication Feb. 3, 1977.

Accepted for publication March 21, 1977.

Address for reprints: William C. Roberts, M.D., Bldg. 10A, Rm. 3E-30, NIH, Bethesda, Md. 20014.

DOI: 10.1201/9781003409281-18

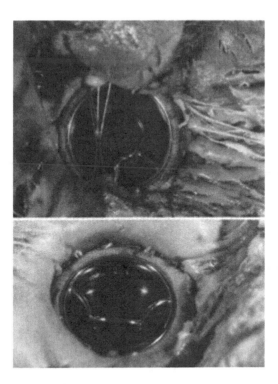

Figure 1 Mitral prosthesis in the patient described. *Top*, As viewed from the left ventricular aspect. The entangled sutures are obvious. A portion of the aortic valve prosthesis is visible in the upper left portion of the photograph. *Bottom*, As viewed from the left atrium. The disc is prevented from falling more than about 2 mm. by the entangled sutures which are visible through the residual prosthetic orifice.

COMMENTS

Two errors in technique were made in this case. One was the tangling of sutures beneath the mitral occluder during insertion of the mitral prosthesis. The second was the closing of the left atriotomy incision before checking whether or not the mitral occluder would fall normally into the left ventricular cavity. Necropsy disclosed that the mitral occluder would fall only about 2 mm. toward the left ventricle with pressure applied to it from its left atrial aspect. This report, therefore, emphasizes the importance of carefully checking the mitral occluder to ensure its free mobility before closing the atriotomy incision.

REFERENCES

1. Roberts, W. C., and Morrow, A. G.: Causes of death and other anatomic observations after cardiac valve replacement, *in* Advances in Cardiology: Long-Term Prognosis Following Valve Replacement, Second Conference on Cardiovascular Disease, vol. 7, Basel, 1972, S. Karger, pp. 226–247.
2. Roberts, W. C., Fishbein, M. C., and Golden, A.: Cardiac pathology after valve replacement by disc prosthesis: A study of 61 necropsy patients, Am. J. Cardiol. **35**: 740, 1975.
3. Roberts, W. C., and Hammer, W. J.: Cardiac pathology after valve replacement with a tilting disc prosthesis (Björk-Shiley type): A study of 46 necropsy patients and 49 Björk-Shiley prostheses, Am. J. Cardiol. **37**: 1024, 1976.

Case 301 *Prosthetic-Valve Endocarditis Due to Listeria Monocytogenes*

Robert H. Breyer, MD, Ernest N. Arnett, MD, Thomas L. Spray, MD, and William C. Roberts, MD

Clinical and necropsy observations in the case of a patient with prosthetic-valve endocarditis due to *Listeria monocytogenes* are presented. Although rare cases of *L. monocytogenes* infection of natural cardiac valves have been reported, this represents the first known case of infection of a prosthetic cardiac valve by this organism. (Key words: Prosthetic heart valves; Endocarditis; *Listeria monocytogenes*.)

PROSTHETIC-VALVE ENDOCARDITIS has been caused by a variety of unusual organisms, but, to our knowledge, there has been no report of its being caused by *Listeria monocytogenes*. Such was the case, however, in the patient to be described herein.

REPORT OF A CASE

A 64-year-old man who died November 13, 1974, had had his heavily calcified, stenotic, tricuspid aortic valve replaced with a Starr-Edwards prosthesis on January 11, 1973 (22 months before death). His early postoperative course had been complicated by temporary paresis of the right arm. Although the patient had had transient cerebral signs and symptoms 3 months after operation, he had been in functional class II status (New York Heart Association classification) until March 1974 (8 months before death) when he had noticed increasing exertional fatigue.

On September 24, 1974, the patient had had fever and sweats, and two days later he had been hospitalized. Oral temperature at that time was 39.2 C. Examination disclosed the expected prosthetic valve opening and closing sounds and a basal systolic ejection murmur. The leukocyte count was 17,000 cu mm. *Listeria monocytogenes* was grown from each of ten blood cultures of samples drawn serially over a two-day period. The organism was identified and speciated according to growth characteristics standardized by the Center for Disease Control. Minimal inhibitory concentrations (MIC) of antibiotics against this organism were (all in μg/ml): penicillin 0.2, ampicillin 0.2, cephalothin 1.6, erythromycin <0.4, tetracycline <0.4, kanamycin 3.0, gentamicin 1.6. Intravenous administration of penicillin, 20 million units daily, was begun, and within 24 hours the fever had subsided. Serum bactericidal titers confirmed the adequacy of the antibiotic therapy (>99.9% bactericidal at 1:8 dilution 30 minutes before the scheduled dose of penicillin; 100% bactericidal at 1:32 dilution 10 minutes after the intravenous penicillin injection).

On October 13, 1974, however, the patient suddenly vomited, and had a severe headache. Two hours later, acute pulmonary edema appeared, followed by shock

Received November 29, 1976; received revised manuscript January 25, 1977; accepted for publication January 25, 1977.

From the Clinic of Surgery and the Pathology Branch, National Heart, Lung and Blood Institute, National Institutes of Health, Bethesda, Maryland.

Address reprint requests to Dr. Roberts: Chief, Pathology Branch, National Heart, Lung and Blood Institute, National Institutes of Health, Bethesda, Maryland 20014.

DOI: 10.1201/9781003409281-19

and finally, cardiac arrest. Although resuscitated, the patient never fully regained consciousness, and he died 30 days later. He had received penicillin intravenously during the entire period, and all further blood cultures were negative.

At necropsy (A74–296), thrombus rimmed the primary orifice of the Starr-Edwards aortic prosthesis (Figure 1). The site of attachment of the prosthesis was focally necrotic and the prosthesis partially detached (Figure 1). The necrotic process had burrowed through the wall of the aorta into the space between the

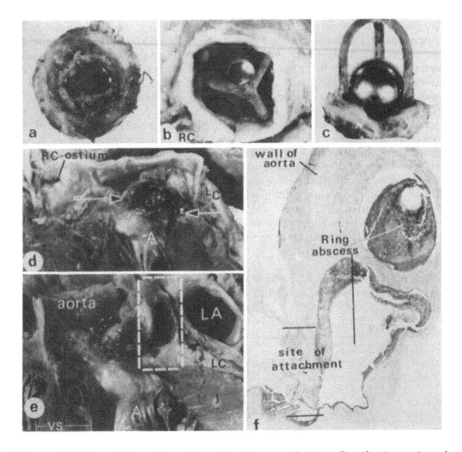

Figure 1 Infected Starr-Edwards aortic valve prosthesis. *a*, Prosthesis as viewed from left ventricle. Thrombus devoid of organisms and inflammatory cells is present on the margins of the primary orifice. *b*, Prosthesis as viewed from above. RC = right coronary artery. *c*. Prosthesis as viewed laterally. The struts are devoid of thrombus. *d*, Opened aortic valve after removal of the prosthesis. A ring abscess (between the arrows) involves nearly half of the former site of attachment of the prosthesis. A = anterior mitral leaflet; LC = left coronary artery. *e*. Longitudinal cut through the ring abscess, showing extension through the full thickness of the wall of the aorta. Extravasation of blood did not occur because of marked fibrous thickening of the aortic adventitia. LA = left atrium; VS = ventricular septum. *f*, Histologic section through the area enclosed by dashed lines in *e*. Histologic section through the ring abscess, which represents an extension from the site of attachment of the prosthesis. No colonies of organisms were seen in the ring abscess or in the prosthetic anulus. Brown and Brenn stain: ×6.2.

117

aorta and left atrium. Histologic examination of the site of prosthetic attachment disclosed polymorphonuclear leukocytes and fibrin, but no colonies of organisms, and cultures of cardiac blood were negative. Examination of the brain at necropsy revealed subarachnoid hemorrhage over the right cerebellar hemisphere and cavitary lesions in the left frontal and right parietal lobes.

COMMENTS

Although *Listeria monocytogenes* is an infrequent cause of human infection, it is known to cause infection of the meninges and the female pelvic organs. It also may produce infection in newborns and in patients who have lymphoreticular malignancies.[3] This organism is a rare cause of infective endocarditis; only 12 patients with *L. monocytogenes* endocarditis involving native cardiac valves have been reported.[2] Before the infection, five of the 12 patients had had normal cardiac valves, five others were known to have underlying valvular disease, and in two cases the status of the valve before the infection was not mentioned. None had a debilitating disease.

In our patient, the infection was present behind the site of attachment of the prosthesis but colonies of organisms were absent, and postmortem heart blood cultures were negative, presumably because of the intravenous administration of antibiotic therapy for more than 40 days. Organisms may be absent, however, in patients with fatal prosthetic valve endocarditis treated with antibiotics.[1] Although clinical signs of aortic regurgitation were never apparent, partial detachment of the prosthesis occurred. Our patient died, however, not from the effect of prosthetic endocarditis on the heart, but as a result of a central nervous system catastrophe, presumably due to an embolus from the infected prosthetic valve.

REFERENCES

1. Arnett EN, Roberts WC: Prosthetic valve endocarditis: A clinicopathologic analysis of 22 necropsy patients with comparison of observations to 74 necropsy patients with active infective endocarditis involving natural left-sided cardiac valves. Am J Cardiol 38:281–292, 1976
2. Bassan R: Bacterial endocarditis produced by *Listeria monocytogenes*. Am J Clin Pathol 63:522–527, 1975
3. Buckner LH, Schneierson SS: Clinical and laboratory aspects of *Listeria monocytogenes* infection. Am J Med 45:904–921, 1968

Case 369 Marfan Cardiovascular Disease Without the Marfan Syndrome

Fusiform Ascending Aortic Aneurysm with Aortic and Mitral Valve Regurgitation

Bruce F. Waller, MD.; Robert L. Reis, MD, F.C.C.P.; Charles L. McIntosh, MD; Stephen E. Epstein, MD; and William C. Roberts, MD, F.C.C.P.

Dr. William C. Roberts: Herein we will discuss findings in a man with a fusiform aneurysm of the proximal ascending aorta, aortic-valve regurgitation, mitral-valve regurgitation, an anomalously arising left main coronary artery, and survival for 12 years after replacement of the aortic valve and partial replacement of the ascending aorta. Dr. Waller will describe the patient.

Dr. Bruce F. Waller: A 69-year-old Jamaican man had been asymptomatic until age 44 years. At age 17 (1927), however, a precordial murmur was heard. At age 44 (1954), he developed infective endocarditis after extraction of a tooth, and he was treated with penicillin for four weeks. Thereafter, he had exertional dyspnea which gradually progressed. At age 50 (1960), he had the sudden onset of sub-sternal chest pain, but its etiology was never determined. Because of worsening dyspnea, he was started on a regimen of digitalis. At age 52 (1962), frequent premature ventricular beats were noted, and quinidine sulfate therapy was started. He underwent his first of four cardiac catheterizations at this time (Table 1).

Three years later, the exertional chest pain increased in frequency, the exertional dyspnea worsened, and he was admitted to the National Heart Institute (February 1956). A grade 4/6 murmur of aortic regurgitation, louder over the right than over the left sternal border, and a grade 2/6 holosystolic murmur at the apex were heard. The heart was big (Figure 1). Aortogram (Figure 1) showed a huge aortic root aneurysm and severe aortic regurgitation. An ECG (Figure 2) disclosed sinus tachycardia, left ventricular hypertrophy with strain, and left atrial abnormality. On July 20, 1966, a cardiac operation was performed.

Dr. Roberts: Dr. Reis, would you describe your findings at operation?

Dr. Robert L. Reis: Each of the three aortic-valve sinuses of Valsalva and the proximal tubular portion of ascending aorta were massively dilated. The distal portion of ascending aorta was of normal or near normal size. Each of the three aortic valve cusps was delicate and each appeared to prolapse toward the left ventricle. Only one coronary arterial ostium was present, and that was located in the aortic wall behind the right sinus. The aortic valve (Figure 3) was replaced with a size 9 Starr-Edwards prosthesis, and the aneurysmal wall which involved the tubular portion of ascending aorta was excised and replaced with a Teflon graft. His early postoperative period went smoothly.

From the Pathology, Surgery and Cardiology Branches, National Heart, Lung and Blood Institute, National Institutes of Health, Bethesda.

Reprint requests: Dr. Roberts, NIH-NHLBI, Building 10A, Room 3E30, Bethesda, 20205

Reprinted from CHEST

Vol. 77, p. 533–540, April 1980 Issue

Table 1: Hemodynamic and angiographic data (pressures in mm hg) at rest*

	Age 52 (1962)	Age 56 (1966)	Age 57 (1967)	Age 69 (1978)
Right atrium (mean)	1	1	–	3
Right ventricle (s/d)	28/2	26/3	–	45/8
Pulmonary artery (s/d [mean])	28/5 [10]	26/10 [16]	–	45/20 [30]
Pulmonary wedge				
a wave	3			
v wave	10	–	–	27
mean	10	8	–	14
Left ventricle (s/d)	–	135/20	160/9	160/12
Systemic artery (s/d)	100/40	155/45	147/78	155/80
Aorta (s/d)	115/85	135/40	–	160/80
CO (CI) (L/min/sq m)	–	3.9 (2.2)	7.8 (4.4)	4.9 (2.7)
AA angiogram	–	+	+	+
AR	–	4+/4 +	0	0
AA aneurysm	–	+	+	+
LV angiogram	–	–	+	+
MR	–	–	4+/4 +	4 + /4 +

*AA indicates ascending aorta; AR, aortic regurgitation; CI, cardiac index; CO, cardiac output; LV, left ventricular; MR, mitral regurgitation; and s/d, peak systole/end-diastole.

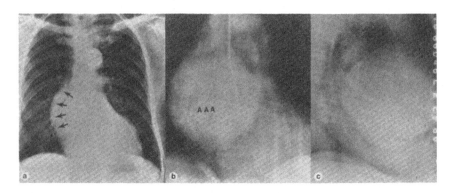

Figure 1 Preoperative posteroanterior chest roentgenogram showing huge ascending aortic aneurysm (AAA) and cardiomegaly. Anteroposterior (b) and lateral (c) aortic root angiograms demonstrate the large aneurysm.

Dr. Roberts: The excised portion of ascending aorta *(Figure 3)* had several intimal and medial tears and a thinner wall than normal. Histologically, there was massive loss of elastic fibers in the aortic media. Less than 10 percent of the expected number of elastic lamellae remained in the media, and those remaining were fragmented. The amount of acid mucopolysaccharide material in the media was focally increased. The margins of each of the three aortic valve cusps were thickened but the remaining portions were normal. The amount of acid mucopolysaccharide material was increased.

Dr. Waller, what happened to the patient after the operation?

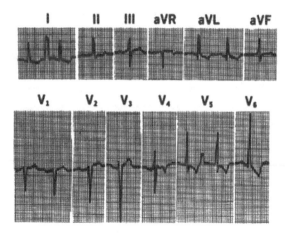

Figure 2 Electrocardiogram recorded immediately before first cardiovascular operation.

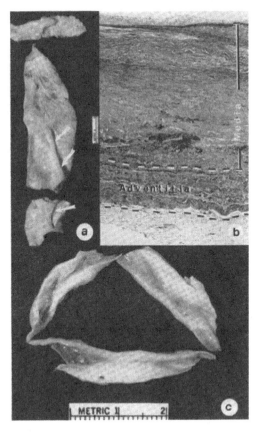

Figure 3 Excised portions of ascending aorta (a and b) and aortic-valve cusps (c). Intimal and medial tears (*arrows*) are present in aorta. Histologically, medial layer shows severe loss of elastic fibers (stained black). (Movat stain [b], original magnification × 40).

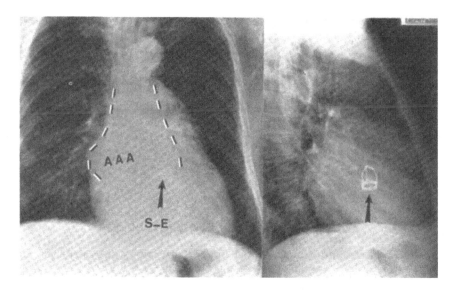

Figure 4 Postoperative posteroanterior and lateral chest roentgenograms showing generalized cardiomegaly, ascending aortic aneurysm (*AAA*) (outlined in dashed lines), and Starr-Edwards (*S-E*) aortic valve prosthesis.

Dr. Waller: The patient was re-evaluated nine months after the operation and was asymptomatic. The apical systolic murmur was now grade 4/6 in intensity, and it radiated into the left axilla. Aortography disclosed no aortic regurgitation but a small (13 mm Hg) peak systolic pressure gradient between left ventricle and aorta (presumably at the level of the caged-ball prosthesis) and severe (4+/4+) mitral regurgitation (Table 1). He remained asymptomatic for another seven years, until age 64 (1974), when mild exertional dyspnea and chest pain reappeared. Because of gradual worsening of the dyspnea and the appearance of considerable fatigue, he was reevaluated in October 1978 when he was 69 years old (12 years after the aortic operation). He was unable to walk more than one flat block because of dyspnea. Precordial examination was unchanged. Repeat chest roentgenograms disclosed the cardiac silhouette to be about the same size as it was on the preoperative roentgenogram, but the left atrial cavity was larger (Figure 4). The ECG was unchanged. Echocardiogram (Figure 5) disclosed the aortic "root" to be much larger than the left atrial cavity, and the aortic-valve prosthesis to be eccentrically located. Repeat catheterization (Table 1) and angiography showed massive mitral regurgitation and elevation of pulmonary arterial pressures. A second cardiac operation was done.

Dr. Roberts: Dr. McIntosh, would you describe your operative findings?

Dr. Charles L. McIntosh: The second operation was to replace the severely regurgitant mitral valve via a transatrial septal approach. The anterior leaflet had protruded toward left atrium, and both leaflets were mildly thickened. The anulus was severely dilated. The mitral valve was replaced with a porcine prosthesis (size 31 mm). No calcific deposits or ruptured chordae tendineae were found. The wall of left atrium was firmly adherent to the thin aneurysmal wall of the ascending aorta, and during valve replacement, a retractor tore the atrial wall and the aortic aneurysmal wall. Repeated attempts to close the atrial and aortic wall tears were unsuccessful.

Dr. Roberts: The excised mitral valve disclosed an entirely normal posterior leaflet and chordae tendineae. The anterior leaflet, in contrast, was thickened by

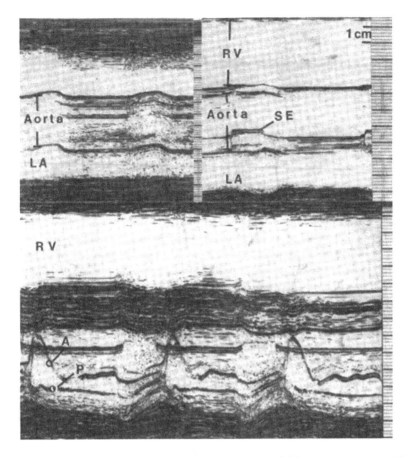

Figure 5 Postoperative echocardiogram. Top, view of dilated aortic root with its eccentrically healed Starr-Edwards (*S-E*) prosthesis and left atrium (*LA*). Right ventricular *(RV)* cavity is dilated and anterior (*A*) and posterior (*P*) mitral leaflets are normal.

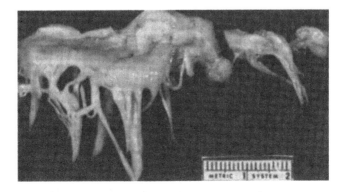

Figure 6 Excised mitral valve. Anterior leaflet and its chordae tendineae are thickened by fibrous tissue.

123

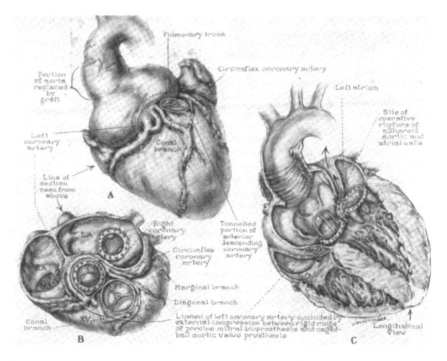

Figure 7 Drawing showing external anterior view of the heart (A), the anomalously arising left main coronary artery from the right coronary artery, and a longitudinal view (C) showing site of operative rupture of aorta and left atrium.

fibrous tissue, and its basal to distal margin was shorter than normal (Figure 6). Several of its attached chordae also were thicker than normal. Histologically, the amcunt of acid mucopolysaccharide material in it was not increased.

Dr. Waller, could you summarize the cardiovascular findings at necropsy?

Dr. Waller: The tear in the wall of left atrium and aorta was readily apparent (Figures 7 and 8). The heart weighed 750 g. The aortic root aneurysm measured 9 × 7 × 5 cm (Figure 9). The poppet of the aortic valve prosthesis was yellow, but its surface was smooth and intact. The prosthesis was free of thrombus. The left main coronary artery arose as the first branch of the right coronary artery, and after coursing behind the aorta, it branched into the left anterior descending and left circumflex arteries (Figure 7). A large conus artery also connected the right and left anterior descending coronary arteries.

Dr. Roberts: The above described patient with cardiovascular features of the Marfan syndrome but without the Marfan syndrome is unusual for several reasons, as follows: (1) He lived a long life, namely 69 years and 57 of those were before a cardiovascular operation. The average age of death in patients with the Marfan syndrome is 35 years, and nearly all die from cardiovascular complications.[1,2] (2) Our patient lived 12 years after replacement of the aortic valve and a portion of ascending aorta, a very long survivor with this type operation. (3) He developed severe mitral regurgitation, severe enough to warrant mitral valve replacement. It is well known that patients with the cardiovascular disease of the Marfan syndrome often have mitral regurgitation, but usually the mitral regurgitation is not severe enough to warrant valve replacement.[2] (4) His aortic

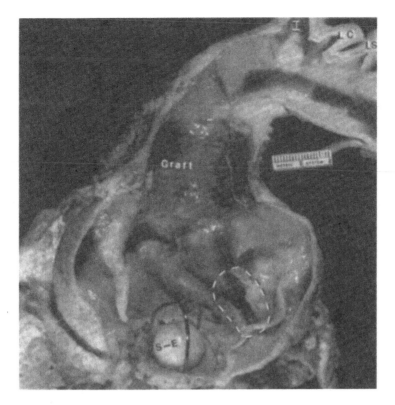

Figure 8 View of ascending aortic aneurysm and the Starr-Edwards (*S-E*) prosthetic valve. CAD (*dashed area*) designates site of operative rupture. *I* indicates innominate artery; *LC*, left common carotid artery; and *LS*, left subclavian artery.

root aneurysm was extremely large, much larger than in most patients with the Marfan type cardiovascular disease. (5) He also had a congenital anomaly of the coronary arteries, namely only one aortic ostium with origin of the left main from the right coronary artery.

Dr. Epstein, you have studied clinically many patients with aortic root aneurysms of the Marfan type. What factors determine whether or not you recommend aortic valve replacement or aortic resection or both in these patients?

Dr. Stephen E. Epstein: In patients with aortic root aneurysms of the Marfan type, but without aortic regurgitation, operation is recommended under the following circumstances: (1) the patient develops, even in the absence of medical treatment, paroxysmal nocturnal dyspnea, an episode of pulmonary edema, angina pectoris, or near syncope or syncope; (2) the patient has dyspnea or fatigue that seriously interferes with his (her) normal daily living; or (3) there is evidence of left ventricular systolic dysfunction at rest, demonstrated by echocardiographic, radionuclide or catheterization studies. It is not necessary, in my view, however, that any of these three criteria of left ventricular dysfunction be present to recommend operation in a patient with an aortic root aneurysm of the Marfan type associated with aortic regurgitation. When aortic root aneurysm is suspected clinically because of an atypical location of the aortic regurgitant murmur (to the right rather than to the left of the sternal border), or an inappropriately dilated ascending aorta is observed on chest roentgenogram or echocardiogram, aortic root angiography is recommended. If a dilated aortic root with effaced sinuses is demonstrated, the patient is an operative candidate regardless of symptomatic status or degree of left ventricular dysfunction. The reason for this view is that the presenting manifestation of the Marfan-type aortic disease can be aortic dissection or rupture, both of which can cause sudden death or make subsequent operation impossible or extremely difficult.

Dr. Roberts: Possibly in the asymptomatic individual with a relatively small aortic root aneurysm of the Marfan type without or with only minimal aortic regurgitation, operatively *wrapping the ascending aorta* with a synthetic cloth (Teflon) might be considered. This procedure might prevent the development of aortic regurgitation or possibly prevent or delay its progression. Furthermore, the wrapping might prevent additional aneurysmal dilatation of the aorta. Moreover, the wrapping procedure might stimulate the formation of considerable fibrous tissue around the aorta and this in turn might prevent aortic rupture.

Dr. Waller, the present patient had an echocardiogram which showed the ascending aorta to be much larger than the left atrium. In addition, the aortic valve prosthesis occupied a very small portion of the aortic root area, and it was very eccentrically located in the aorta. Can you summarize echocardiographic findings in patients with the Marfan type aortic root aneurysm?

Dr. Waller: Echocardiographic findings in patients with the cardiovascular disease associated with the Marfan syndrome or its form fruste varieties include the following: (1) dilatation of the aortic root; (2) mitral leaflet prolapse; (3) diastolic fluttering of the anterior mitral leaflet (if aortic regurgitation is present); and (4) dilatation of both ventricles and of the left atrium. Of 35 patients with the Marfan syndrome reported by Brown and associates,[3] 21 (60 percent) had dilated aortic roots (using at least two or three of the following criteria: absolute aortic dimensions >3.7 cm; body surface area correction for aortic diameter > 2.2 cm/sq m, and left atrial/aortic ratio < 0.7) and 32 (91 percent) had prolapsed mitral leaflets. Payvandi and colleagues[4] found aortic root dilatation in five of nine patients with the Marfan syndrome and in seven (18 percent) of 40 relatives; mitral leaflet prolapse was present in all nine patients and in 13 (33 percent) of the 40 relatives. Neither of these studies, however, had angiographic documentation of aortic root enlargement or mitral leaflet prolapse.

The severe eccentric location of our patient's aortic valve prosthesis within the aorta on the echocardiogram deserves comment. To my knowledge, this echocardiographic eccentricity of an aortic prosthesis has not been described previously in a patient with the Marfan syndrome or its forme fruste variety. The posterior location of the prosthesis within the aorta suggests that the ascending aortic aneurysm protruded more anteriorly than posteriorly. This feature, however, could not be confirmed at necropsy. The recorded echoes of the aortic prosthesis itself appear to represent both anterior and posterior surfaces of the silicone rubber poppet, which was present in our patient, in addition to the prosthetic struts.[5-7] Most current models of the caged-ball prostheses contain hollow metal poppets, and in them only, the anterior surface of the poppet can be visualized echocardiographically.

Dr. Roberts: Dr. McIntosh, what type of operation is preferred today for the aortic disease of the Marfan or Marfan type syndromes?

Dr. McIntosh: The initial operative treatment for aortic root aneurysm of the Marfan type was replacement of most or all of the ascending aorta above the sinuses of Valsalva by a graft with or without the addition of nylon or Teflon aortic wrapping.[7-8] Later, aortic-valve replacement in addition was added.[9] These procedures, however, were associated with a high frequency of postoperative

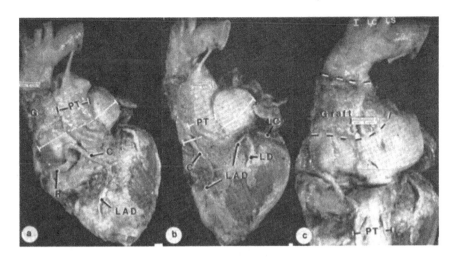

Figure 9 Exterior views of the heart at necropsy. a, Anterior view, b, left lateral view, and c, anterior view with pulmonary trunk (*PT*) retracted. The *white solid and dashed line* shows dimensions of aortic aneurysm. *C* indicates conal branch of right coronary artery; *R*, right coronary artery; *LAD*, left anterior descending coronary artery; *LD*, left diagonal coronary artery; *LC*, left circumflex coronary artery; *I*, innominate artery; *LC*, left common carotid artery; and *LS*, left subclavian artery.

bleeding, and the diseased wall of aorta behind the sinuses of Valsalva was not excised. The next major operative advancement in treatment of aortic root aneurysm of the Marfan type with aortic regurgitation and the one preferred today is insertion of an aortic graft-aortic valve composite unit after excision of the aortic valve with or without excision of the ascending aorta.[10-13] The problem of restoring coronary flow has been handled by implanting the native coronary ostia into side holes of the composite graft or attaching saphenous vein conduits for bypass of each of the three major coronary arteries.

The later technique has lowered early mortality rates by reducing postoperative bleeding and operating times. Mayer and associates[13] recently reported a 4.5 year experience with 16 patients with the Marfan or Marfan-like aortic root disease in whom composite replacement of the aortic valve and ascending aorta with implanted native coronary ostia was accomplished. Although 11 of the 16 patients are alive and have minimal or no symptoms of cardiac dysfunction, two developed aneurysms at the site of coronary anastomoses on the aortic graft and a third developed an aneurysm at the anastomosis of the graft to the distal aorta. Despite these late complications, the composite graft method is clearly superior to the older operative procedures.

Dr. Roberts: Most students of cardiovascular diseases are aware that patients with the Marfan syndrome and form fruste varieties of it may have *floppy or prolapsing mitral leaflets.*[2] Our patient had severe mitral regurgitation and yet, at operation, the posterior mitral leaflet was normal, and the anterior leaflet did not protrude enough toward the left atrium to be considered "a prolapsed leaflet." Both grossly and histologically, the anterior leaflet was thickened by fibrous tissue and the amount of acid mucopolysaccharide material in it was not increased. Our patient indicates

127

that there are causes of mitral regurgitation in these patients other than a prolapsing or floppy leaflet. Another major cause is *dilatation of the mitral anulus*. The anulus in the present patient, however, was 12.5 cm in circumference, which is not enough to produce severe mitral regurgitation.[14] Another cause of mitral regurgitation in these patients is *mitral anular calcific deposits*, but none occurred in the present patient.[15] A fourth cause of mitral regurgitation in these patients is *marked dilatation of the left ventricle from associated aortic regurgitation*. The present patient, however, had no aortic regurgitation during his last 12 years, and his left ventricle was not very dilated at necropsy. Thus, it appears that the mitral regurgitation in our patient resulted mainly from the fibrous contracture of the anterior mitral leaflet, possibly a process initiated by *infective endocarditis* which healed.[16] The leaflet thickening, however, could be the *anatomic equivalent of the "Austin-Flint" murmur* from the previously severe aortic regurgitation.

A final unusual finding in our patient was the *origin of the left main coronary artery as the first branch of the right coronary artery*. The left main passed behind the ascending aorta and between the wall of aorta and anterior wall of left atrium. Consequently, only one ostium of a coronary artery was present in the aorta. Dr. Waller, is there any specific danger of replacing both mitral and the aortic valves in a patient in whom either the left main or the left circumflex coronary arteries course behind the aorta in between the mitral and aortic valve "rings"?

Dr. Waller: In this laboratory, we have studied two patients who had anomalous origin of the left circumflex coronary artery as the first branch of the right coronary artery and in whom either the mitral or both the mitral and aortic valves were replaced with rigid-frame prostheses.[17] The anomalous coronary artery had not been diagnosed preoperatively or at operation in either patient. In the patient with two prostheses, the lumen of the anomalous left circumflex coronary artery was compressed between the two prosthetic-valve rings causing severe narrowing with resulting lateral wall myocardial infarction. Thus, in the present patient, the danger could have been even greater, since not only was the left circumflex potentially compressed, but the entire left system could have been compressed by the rigid frames of the porcine mitral and that of the caged-ball aortic prosthesis.

Dr. Roberts: A final word regarding nomenclature. The lesion in the aorta in patients with the Marfan syndrome or the form fruste varieties of it has been called "medial cystic necrosis." This term, however, is poor because "cysts" are relatively infrequent, and "necrosis" is extremely difficult to be sure of when examining histologic sections of ascending aorta. This term "medial cystic necrosis" was introduced by Gsell in 1928[18] and further used by Erdheim in 1929.[19] These authors had access only to hematoxylin eosin stains at that time, and these stains are simply not adequate to study the configuration of the elastic fibers in the media of aorta. Use of superb elastic tissue stains during the past 25 years has indicated that the dominant histologic finding in the ascending aorta in patients with the Marfan syndrome or in its form fruste varieties is *massive degeneration of elastic fibers* which occurred in the present patient. We estimated that less than 10 percent of the expected number of elastic fibers were present in the media of the wall of the aneurysm in the present patient. Massive elastic-fiber degeneration is the *sine qua non* of the Marfan type aorta. The strength of the aorta is due to the integrity of its elastic fibers, collagen fibrils, and smooth muscle cells. There is no evidence that the smooth muscle cells are abnormal in the aorta in these patients, but there is some ultrastructural evidence that the collagen fibers are abnormal. By simple histologic examination, however, the major and dominant histologic feature is massive degeneration of elastic fibers, and, therefore, the term "medial cystic necrosis" might best be avoided.

REFERENCES

1. Murdoch JL, Walker BA, Halpern BL: Life expectancy and causes of death in the Marfan syndrome. N Engl J Med 1972; 286:804–808

2. Roberts WC: Congenital cardiovascular abnormalities usually "silent" until adulthood: morphologic features of the floppy mitral valve, valvular aortic stenosis, hypertrophic cardiomyopathy, sinus of Valsalva aneurysm, and the Marfan syndrome. In: Roberts WC, ed. Congenital heart disease in adults. Philadelphia: FA Davis Co, 1979; 407–453 (Cardiovascular Clinics 10 [#11: 1–574, 1979)

3. Brown OR, DeMots, Kloster FE, Roberts A, Menashe VD, Beals RK: Aortic root dilatation and mitral valve prolapse in Marian's syndrome: an echocardiographic study. Circulation 1975; 52:652–802

4. Payvandi MN, Kerber RE, Phelps CD, Judisch GF, El-Khoury G, Schrott HG: Cardiac, skeletal and ophthalmologic abnormalities in relatives of patients with the Marfan syndrome. Circulation 1977; 55:797–802

5. Johnson ML, Paton BC, Holmes JH: Ultrasonic evaluation of prosthetic valve motion. Circulation 1970; 42 (Suppl 2):5–15

6. Siggers DC, Srwongse SA, Deuchar D: Analysis of dynamics of mitral Starr-Edwards valve prosthesis using reflected ultrasound. Br Heart J 1971; 33:401–406

7. Bahnson HT, Nelson AR: Cystic medial necrosis as a cause of localized aortic aneurysms amenable to surgical treatment. Ann Surg 1956; 144:519–529

8. Cooley DA, DeBakey ME: Resection of entire ascending aorta in fusiform aneurysm using cardiac bypass. JAMA 1956; 162:1158

9. Wheat MW, Wilson JR, Bartley TD: Successful replacement of the entire ascending aorta and aortic valve. JAMA 1964; 188:717–719

10. Bloodwell RB, Hallman GL, Cooley DA: Aneurysm of the ascending aorta with aortic valvular insufficiency. Arch Surg 1966; 92:588–599

11. Ferlic RM, Goot B, Edwards JE, Lillehei CW: Aortic valvular insufficiency associated with cystic medial necrosis. Ann Surg 1967; 165:1–9

12. Bentall H, DeBono A: A technique for complete replacement of the entire ascending aorta. Thorax 1968; 3:338–339

13. Mayer JE, Lindsay WG, Wang Y, Jorgensen CR, Nicoloff DM: Composite replacement of the aortic valve and ascending aorta. J Thorac Cardiovasc Surg 1978; 76:816–823

14. Bulkley BH, Roberts WC: Dilatation of the mitral anulus: a rare cause of mitral regurgitation. Am J Med 1975; 59:457–463

15. Roberts WC, Perloff JC: Mitral valvular disease: a clinicopathologic survey of the conditions causing the mitral valve to function abnormally. Ann Intern Med 1972; 77:936–975

16. Roberts WC, Buchbinder NA: Healed left-sided infective endocarditis: a clinicopathologic study of 59 patients. Am J Cardiol 1977; 40:878–888

17. Roberts WC, Morrow AG: Compression of anomalous left circumflex coronary arteries by prosthetic valve fixation rings. J Thorac Cardiovasc Surg 1969; 57:834–838

18. Gsell O: Wandnekrosen der Aorta als Selbstandige Erkrankung und ihre Beziehung zur Spontanruptur. Virchows Arch Path Anat Physiol 1928; 270:1–9

19. Erdheim J: Medionecrosis aortae idiopathica. Virchow's Arch Path Anat Physiol 1929; 273:454–463

Case 402 Disseminated *Petriellidium Boydii* and Pacemaker Endocarditis

William A. Davis, MD, Jeffrey M. Isner, MD*, Arthur W. Bracey, MD,
William C. Roberts, MD and Vincent F. Garagusi, MD
Washington, D.C. and Bethesda, Maryland

Clinical and morphologic findings are described in a 62 year old woman with "mixed connective tissue disease" who received corticosteroid therapy, and in whom disseminated and fatal Petriellidium boydii infection with right-sided endocarditis developed. The patient was a gardener. The organism is ubiquitous in soil in many parts of the United States; therefore, it is likely that the infection was introduced by this means. Endocarditis due to P. boydii has not been reported previously. In the patient described, massive vegetations nearly obliterated the tricuspid valve orifice, encasing a pacemaker catheter which had been inserted eight years earlier. Although never previously isolated from blood cultures, P. boydii was isolated from 11 consecutive blood cultures. P. boydii is a true fungus and has only recently been appreciated as an opportunistic pathogen in a compromised host.

Infection is one of the major factors limiting survival of a compromised host. Many microorganisms previously considered benign have been recognized more recently to be pathogens in patients whose immunologic status has been compromised. P. boydii (previously Allescheria boydii), a true fungus found in soil, for years was believed to have its pathogenicity primarily limited to maduromycosis of the foot.[1] Recently, this organism has gained increasing recognition as an opportunistic pathogen.[2,3] This report describes previously unreported findings in a patient with widely disseminated, fatal P. boydii infection.

CASE REPORT

A 62 year old black woman, who died August 19, 1977, was first seen at Georgetown University Hospital when she was 41 years old (21 years before death) because of arthralgias, proximal muscle weakness and dermal "tightness," especially of the skin over the face. Upper gastrointestinal tract films at that time suggested changes of scleroderma, and a deltoid muscle biopsy specimen was consistent with polymyositis. The patient was considered to have a mixed collagen vascular syndrome, with elements of both scleroderma and polymyositis. Therapy with prednisone (20 mg per day) resulted in symptomatic improvement.

Subsequent medical problems included chronic anemia (hemoglobin 7.0 g/dl), intermittent mild renal insufficiency (creatinine 1.2–2.0 mg/dl), and congestive

From the Infectious Disease Division, Department of Medicine, and the Department of Pathology, Georgetown University Hospital, Washington, D.C., and the Pathology Branch, National Heart, Lung, and Blood Institute, National Institutes of Health, Bethesda, Maryland. Requests for reprints should be addressed to Dr. William A. Davis, Georgetown University Hospital, 3800 Reservoir Road, Washington, D.C. 20007. Manuscript accepted February 4, 1980.
* Present address: Department of Medicine, Tufts University Medical Center, Boston, MA 02111.

DOI: 10.1201/9781003409281-21

heart failure requiring therapy with digoxin and diuretics. Raynaud's phenomenon began at age 46, and the dose of prednisone was increased to 30 mg/day and continued as such until one year before death (age 61) when the dose was reduced to 20 mg/day. In addition, therapy with chloroquine, 500 mg/day was begun and continued for the patient's remaining 16 years. At age 54, syncope occurred, complete heart block was found, and a permanent pacemaker was implanted. The patient encountered no additional problems until age 62 at which time she planted a garden for the first time in several years. After working daily in the garden for one month, she noted the onset of dyspnea, right pleuritic chest pain and right upper quadrant pain; she was hospitalized two months before death. A chest film demonstrated an infiltrate in the lower lobe of the right lung and a bloody effusion in the right pleural cavity. Smears and cultures of sputum, blood, pleural fluid and fluid aspirated from the pacemaker generator site showed no abnormalities. An etiology was never established and the pulmonary process resolved incompletely after therapy with cefazolin and tobramycin. The patient was discharged after two weeks at the family's request. During the next seven weeks, she complained of anorexia and lost 9 kg in weight. Because of increasing lethargy, somnolence and left eye pain, associated with decreased visual acuity of one day's duration, she was rehospitalized seven days before death. On admission, she was cachectic and somnolent. The rectal temperature was 38.6°C. The skin over the face and hands was taut, and there were contractures around the mouth. The left periorbital tissues were swollen, the left eyeball was tender, and the left eye visual acuity was reduced to light perception. A panuveitis was diagnosed. The subcutaneous pacemaker pocket was in the right infraclavicular area. A grade 3/6 holosystolic murmur without respiratory variation was heard at the lower left sternal border. The hemoglobin level was 5.4 g/dl; white blood cell count, 17,000/mm^3 (69 polymorphonuclear cells, 18 band forms, 10 lymphocytes, 3 monocytes); platelet count 16,000/mm^3 and reticulocyte count 8 percent. The erythrocyte sedimentation rate was 45 mm in one hour. Coagulation studies were consistent with disseminated intravascular coagulation. Chest film disclosed an enlarged cardiac silhouette and patchy interstitial infiltrates in the lower lobe of the right lung. Electrocardiogram showed sinus tachycardia at a rate of 120 beats/min. In each QRS complex there was pacemaker artifact from an R-wave triggered pacemaker. An echocardiogram (Figure 1) showed abnormal echoes around the expected echoes from a transvenous pacemaker in the right ventricle. The cerebrospinal fluid pressure was 18 cm of water and the fluid contained glucose 19 mg/dl (serum 82 mg/dl), protein 95 mg/dl, erythrocytes 24/mm^3 and leukocytes 130/mm^3 (80 lymphocytes, 20 polymorphonuclear leukocytes). Smears and culture specimens of the cerebrospinal fluid, blood and urine were negative for growth at 36 hours. Sputum cultures grew "normal flora." On the day of death, the heart and respiratory rates increased, chest pain was apparent, and an electrocardiogram showed that the pacemaker was failing to sense and capture. Cardiopulmonary arrest ensued.

The day following the patient's death, growth was observed on the surface of the broth (Columbia Broth (Pfizer Diagnostic Division) of several (antemortem) blood cultures. Within one week, all 11 antemortem cultures (both aerobic and anaerobic) had a whitish, floating mass of growth on the surface of the broth, but no growth in the media or at the bottom of the culture bottles. Fluid aspirated from the pacemaker generator pocket eventually was positive on fungal media as were postmortem cultures of the vitreous fluid from the left eye. Studies of the organism on subculture revealed a rapidly growing, cotton-like mass which later became darker in color. Positive identification of the fungus as P. boydii was established by the Center for Disease Control in Atlanta.

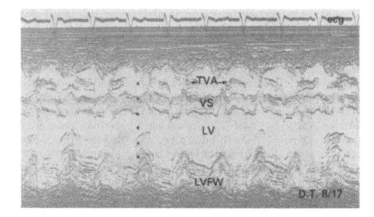

Figure 1 Echocardiogram recorded one day before death. Adventitious echoes are seen in the right ventricular cavity due to the pacemaker and associated tricuspid valve vegetation (TVA). VS = ventricular septum; LV = left ventricle; LVFW = left ventricular free wall; ECG = electrocardiogram.

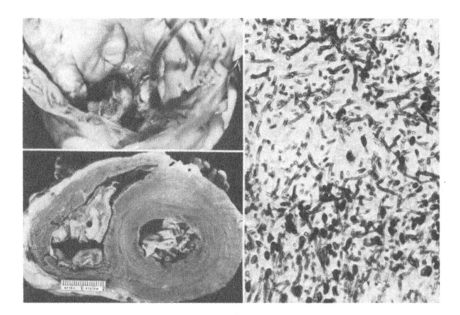

Figure 2 Tricuspid valve vegetation. **Top left**, view of the vegetation and pacemaker wire from the right atrium. **Bottom left**, vegetation in the tricuspid valve orifice and right ventricle as viewed from the ventricular aspect. The hole in the center of the anterior portion of the vegetation was formerly occupied by the pacemaker electrode. **Right**, photomicrograph of histologic section of a portion of the vegetation showing septated hyphal fungi with single terminal conidia, consistent with P. boydii. Gomori methenamine silver stain; magnification × 350, reduced by 65 percent.

At necropsy (GT #77A-130), the patient had a taut face and hands. The pacemaker pocket in the right side of the chest contained a tan-white exudate. The pericardial sac contained 370 ml of serosanguineous fluid, but neither the parietal nor visceral pericardium was scarred or thickened. The heart weighed 410 g. A pacemaker wire was fixed in the right atrium to the atrial septum by fibrous tissue; at the level of the tricuspid valve orifice, it was encased by a vegetation (Figure 2), measuring about 4 by 3 by 2 cm, which occupied most of the valve orifice, and pressed the anterior and posterior leaflets against the right ventricular mural endocardium. Distally, the pacemaker wire was encased by collagen; the pacemaker tip made firm contact with the right ventricular apical endocardium. The generator function of the pacemaker was intact with an output of 2.2 milliampere and a postmortem film showed the pacemaker electrode to be intact. Sections of the vegetation (Figure 2) disclosed septated hyphal fungi with single terminal conidia, consistent with P. boydii, with extensive fibrin deposits and inflammatory cells. There was a 2 by 3 cm transmural scar in the posterior wall of the left ventricle, but all portions of the right, left main, left anterior descending and left circumflex coronary arteries were narrowed less than 75 percent in cross-sectional area by atherosclerotic plaque. There were multiple fresh and organizing pulmonary emboli with a recent infarct in the lower lobe of the right lung but histologically no microorganisms were present. The distal third of the esophagus was fibrotic and ulcerated. The liver (weight 1,000 g) had a nutmeg appearance. The adrenal glands together weighed 5.1 g and their cortices was atrophic. The kidneys weighed 145 and 130 g, respectively, and were within normal limits. The meninges and brain showed no abnormalities; histologically, no microorganisms were found. Postmortem serum for extractable nuclear antigen was positive at a dilution of 1:1,000 and ribo-nuclease sensitive, consistent with the diagnosis of "mixed connective tissue disease."

COMMENTS

The patient described is most unusual for several reasons. (1) Fatal P. boydii endocarditis with massive vegetations in the tricuspid valve orifice occurred; (2) fungemia was present (11 positive blood cultures); (3) fungal infection of any type of a permanent pacemaker is rare, and P. boydii infection of a permanent pacemaker has not been reported previously. As in several previously described patients with disseminated P. boydii infections, our patient incurred infection of the eye and probably also of the central nervous system. Fewer than 10 patients with disseminated P. boydii infection have been described previously.[3]

P. boydii exists in asexual (Monosporium apispermum) or sexual forms (A. boydii); it is similar morphologically to Aspergillus species; grows rapidly in culture and changes in color as it ages; is ubiquitous in soil in many parts of the United States, and causes infection by direct innoculation or by inhalation of ascospores, which are aerosolized when soil, containing the organism, is disturbed.[4,5] Our patient planted and regularly maintained a garden for several weeks before evidence of infection developed.

P. boydii infections may be external or internal or both. Noninvasive localized mycetomas occur on the conjunctivas, lacrimal glands and eyelids, and excisional biopsy is usually required for diagnosis and cure. Pulmonary mycetomas occur in patients with previously normal or abnormal lungs,[6] and signs and symptoms of infection may be minimal, or cough and hemoptysis may occur. The mycetomas might require excision. P. boydii was cultured in drainage from purulent sphenoidal sinusitis in a recently reported, presumably normal host.[7] Therapy with intravenous miconazole (41 g) resulted in clearing of the purulent drainage.

Invasive P. boydii infections may be localized, disseminated or both. Local infections may result from direct tissue inoculation and produce a chronic destructive process with abcess and granuloma formation. Maduromycosis of the foot is the most notable of such infections and in the United States is most commonly caused by P. boydii. Both normal and compromised hosts may be infected. Corneal ulceration, endophthalmitis, necrotizing pneumonia, pulmonary abscess, meningoencephalitis and prostatitis have been reported.[2,3,5] Disseminated infection is rare,[3] but when present the central nervous system usually is involved,[3,8–10] and occasionally the thyroid gland, bone and soft tissues.

Treatment of invasive P. boydii infections is often unsuccessful, especially when it is disseminated. When feasible, surgical resection is preferred for localized disease. Chemotherapy with amphotericin B, and 2-hydroxy-stibamidine, griseofulvin and chloramphenicol has been attempted, but success has been limited.[11] Miconazole is a more recently used agent.

The pacemaker-related vegetation that essentially obstructed the tricuspid valve orifice in our patient is remarkable for several reasons. First, infections involving permanently implanted endocardial pacemakers are uncommon; the reported frequency is less than 6 percent of all units implanted.[12–20] When such infections do occur, they most often are limited to the subcutaneous pocket housing the pacemaker pulse generator. Nearly all of these infections occur soon after implantation and are due to contamination of the operative wound. Local signs of sepsis at the site of the pulse-generator pocket allow early diagnosis and initiation of antibiotic therapy. Such conservative management generally prevents extension of the infective process. As a result, pacemaker infections involving the pacing electrode and tricuspid valve, such as occurred in our patient, account for few pacemaker infections. Second, the etiologic agent of the vast majority of pacemaker infections is Staphylococcus species. Pacemaker-related endocarditis of the tricuspid valve due to a fungus is decidedly rare[21] and, to our knowledge, has never resulted from P. boydii. Third, although the vegetations in patients with fungal endocarditis are generally larger than bacterial endocarditis,[22] transorifice vegetations, as occurred in our patient, are unusual. The presence of a foreign body (pacing wire) in the tricuspid valve orifice likely contributed to the size of the vegetations in our patient. The size of the vegetations was almost certainly the factor that allowed echocardiographic identification of the pacemaker-related valvular endocarditis.

REFERENCES

1. Conant NF, Smith DT, Baker RD, et al.: Manual of clinical mycology, 3rd ed. Philadelphia: W.B. Saunders Co., 1971:458.
2. Lutwick LI, Galgiani JN, Johnson RH, et al.: Visceral fungal infections due to Petrillidium boydii. Am J Med 1976; 61:632.
3. Winston D], Jordan MC, Rhodes J: Allescheria boydii infections in the immuno-suppressed host. Am J Med 1977; 63:830.
4. Emmons CW, Binford CH, Utz JP: Medical mycology, 3rd ed. Philadelphia: Lea & Febiger, 1977:389–418.
5. Arnett JC, Hatch HB: Pulmonary allescheriasis. Arch Intern Med 1975; 135:1250.
6. Hainer JW, Ostrow JH, Mackenzie DW: Pulmonary monosporosis: report of a case with precipitating antibody. Chest 1974; 66:601.
7. Mader JT, Ream SR, Heath PW: Petriellidium boydii (Allescheria boydii) sphe-noidal sinusitis. JAMA 1978; 239:2368.
8. Forno LS, Billingham ME: Allescheria boydii infection of the brain. J Pathol 1972; 106:195.
9. Rosen F, Deck JH, Remeastle NB: Allescheria boydii unique systemic dissemina-tion to thyroid and brain. Can Med Assoc J 1965; 93:1125.
10. Selby R: Pachymeningitis secondary to allescheria boydii. J Neurosurg 1972; 36:225.

11. Utz JP: Mycetoma *In:* Hoeprich PD, ed. Infectious diseases. New York: Harper & Row, 1978.
12. Imparato AM, Kim GE: Electrode complications in patients with permanent cardiac pacemakers. Ten years' experience. Arch Surg 1972; 105:705.
13. Lìnschoten H, Meijne NG, Mellink HM, et al.: Pacemaker implantation and infection. J Cardiovasc Surg 1973; 14:126.
14. Yarnoz MD, Attai LA, Furman S: Infection of pacemaker electrode and removal with cardiopulmonary bypass. J Thorac Cardiovasc Surg 1974; 86:43.
15. Kennelly BM, Piller LW: Management of infected transvenous permanent pacemakers. Br Heart J 1974; 36:1133.
16. Conklin EF, Giannelli S Jr, Nealon TF Jr: Four hundred consecutive patients with permanent transvenous pacemakers. J Thorac Cardiovasc Surg 1975; 69:1.
17. Grögler FM, Frank G, Greven G, et al.: Complications of permanent transvenous cardiac pacing. J Thorac Cardiovasc Surg 1975; 69:895.
18. Chavcez CM, Conn JH: Septicemia secondary to impacted infected pacemaker wire. Successful treatment by removal with cardiopulmonary bypass. J Thorac Cardiovasc Surg 1977; 73:796.
19. Morgan G, Ginks W, Siddons H, et al.: Septicemia in patients with an endocardial pacemaker. Am J Cardiol 1979; 44:221.
20. Jara FM, Toledo-Pereyra L, Lewis JW, et al.: The infected pacemaker pocket. J Thorac Cardiovasc Surg 1979; 78:298.
21. Davis JM, Moss AF, Schenk EA: Tricuspid Candida endocarditis complicating a permanently implanted transvenous pacemaker. Am Heart J 1969; 77:818.
22. Andriole VT, Kravetz HM, Roberts WC, et al.: Candida endocarditis. Clinical and pathologic studies. Am J Med 1962; 32:251.

Case 413 Calcific Deposits Developing in a Bovine Pericardial Bioprosthetic Valve 3 Days After Implantation

Tokuhiro Ishihara, MD, Victor J. Ferrans, MD, PhD, Michael Jones, MD, Henry S. Cabin, MD, and William C. Roberts, MD

SUMMARY Calcific deposits, localized in a thin layer of thrombus covering the cuspal surfaces, were present 3 days after implantation in a valved pulmonic conduit that contained an Ionescu-Shiley bovine pericardial valve and was placed in a 29-year-old man with double outlet right ventricle, valvular and infundibular pulmonic stenosis, and ventricular septal defect. Factors that may have contributed to such a rapid calcification were the relatively young age of the patient, the development of acute renal insufficiency postoperatively, and the administration of large amounts of calcium chloride intravenously during blood transfusions and during episodes of cardiac arrest.

CALCIFICATION of bioprosthetic cardiac valves can lead to prosthetic stenosis, regurgitation or both.[1-10] Calcific deposits usually produce valvular dysfunction only after the bioprostheses have been in place for several years.[1] In some patients, however, calcific deposits have developed within a few months after implantation.[1-6,10] In one exceptional patient,[4] a porcine bioprosthetic valve had to be removed because of calcification only 19 days after implantation. In this communication we describe anatomic findings in a pericardial bioprosthesis that developed calcific deposits within 3 days of implantation. Such rapid calcification of a valvular bioprosthesis has not been described previously.

CASE REPORT

S. H. (CC. # 12-81-67-7), a 29-year old man, had double outlet right ventricle, valvular and infundibular pulmonic stenosis, ventricular septal defect and patent foramen ovale. At 4 years of age, he had had a left-sided Blalock-Taussig subclavian-pulmonary arterial anastomosis. At age 27 years (1978), this shunt was occluded. The blood hematocrit was 78%; studies of renal function and blood coagulation gave normal results, and the serum uric acid and bilirubin were slightly elevated. The peak systolic pressure gradient between the body of the right ventricle and the pulmonary trunk was 95 mm Hg. The systemic arterial oxygen saturation was 88%. A right-sided Blalock-Taussig subclavian-pulmonary arterial shunt was performed in October 1978. In November 1979, because he did not improve despite a functioning shunt, he underwent closure of the ventricular septal defect and patent foramen ovale, and insertion of a valved conduit containing a size 22 Ionescu-Shiley bovine pericardial valve between the right ventricle and the pulmonary trunk. After operation, the patient was reexplored because of extensive bleeding.

From the Pathology and Surgery Branches, National Heart, Lung, and Blood Institute, National Institutes of Health, Bethesda, Maryland.

Address for correspondence: Victor J. Ferrans, M.D., Ph.D., Building 10, Room 7N208, National Institutes of Health, Bethesda, Maryland 20205.

Received May 8, 1980; revision accepted June 30, 1980.

Circulation 63, No. 3, 1981.

DOI: 10.1201/9781003409281-22

He had multiple areas of oozing, without a large source of bleeding and without a specific coagulation defect. He then developed a low cardiac output state, with a marked decrease in renal function and blood urea nitrogen and creatinine values of 54 and 5.2 mg/dl, respectively. Serum calcium was 4.2 mg/dl. Peritoneal dialysis was instituted. Hemodynamic evaluation revealed persistent right ventricular hypertension (104/4 mm Hg) and a pressure gradient of 80 mm Hg at the distal anastomosis between the conduit and the pulmonary artery. On the third day after operation, a revision of the distal anastomosis of the conduit was performed, but the patient died several hours later.

During the entire postoperative period, the serum calcium was never elevated. Because of bleeding, the patient received 65 units of whole blood, 18 units of fresh-frozen plasma and 39 units of platelets. He also received a total of 20 g of calcium chloride during the 3-day postoperative period, in association with the transfusions and during resuscitative efforts.

At necropsy, the pericardial tissue leaflets in the valved conduit were covered with a very thin layer of thrombus that did not interfere with leaflet mobility. Histologic study of right and left ventricular myocardium disclosed focal areas of necrosis, infiltration by polymorphonuclear leukocytes, and calcific deposits within necrotic myocardial cells.

MATERIALS AND METHODS

Histologic and scanning and transmission electron microscopic studies were made of the pericardial tissue leaflets of the bioprosthesis implanted in the pulmonic conduit. For purposes of comparison, similar studies were made of three uflimplanted Ionescu-Shiley valves obtained through courtesy of Ionescu-Shiley Laboratories, Inc., Irvine, California.

For histologic study, the tissues were fixed with buffered formalin, embedded in glycolmethacrylate plastic medium, sectioned at a thickness of 1 μ and stained using the hematoxylin-eosin, alkaline toluidine blue and von Kossa methods. For scanning electron microscopy, the tissues were fixed with phosphate-buffered glutaraldehyde, dehydrated, dried according to the critical point method, coated with gold-palladium, and examined with a JEOL-35C scanning electron microscope at an accelerating voltage of 20 kV.[11] For transmission electron microscopy, tissues were fixed with phosphate-buffered glutaraldehyde and prepared as described previously.[11]

RESULTS

Histologic Observations

On histologic study, the pericardial connective tissue in the leaflets of the implanted valve appeared structurally comparable to that in unimplanted pericardial bioprostheses (Figures 1A and 1B). However, both the inflow and outflow surfaces and the free edge (tip) of each leaflet were covered by a continuous layer of thrombotic material that was 20–180 μ thick (Figures 1B–1D). These surface thrombi were composed of fibrin, erythrocytes and platelets. The thrombi showed basophilic staining in preparations stained with hematoxylin-eosin (Figure 1D) and gave a strongly positive reaction with the von Kossa method (Figure 1C). Pericardial mesothelial cells were not identified in any of the leaflets of the implanted valve or of the unimplanted valves. Small numbers of macrophages were present on the valvular surfaces. Giant cells were not found. A few strongly birefringent fibers that were about 15 μ in diameter were found on the valvular surfaces (Figures 1C–1E), where they had been incorporated into thrombi. These fibers were considered to be cotton fibers.

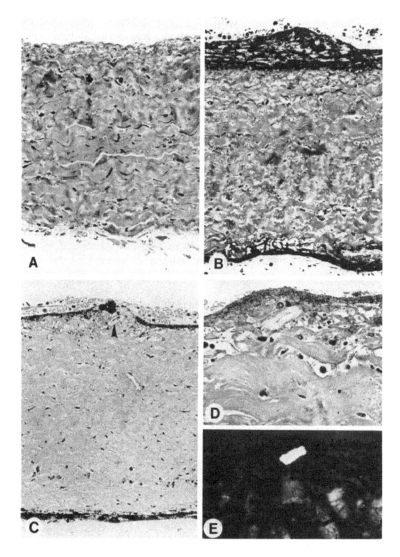

Figure 1 Histologic sections of pericardial tissue leaflets of unimplanted (A) and implanted (B–E) Ionescu-Shiley valves. (A) Leaflet of unimplanted valve, showing outflow surface (top), which appears smooth in contour, and inflow surface, which is rough and is composed of coarse bundles of collagen. Alkaline toluidine blue stain; original magnification × 160. (B) Valve recovered after having been in place for 3 days, showing layer of thrombus covering both the outflow (top) and inflow (bottom) surfaces. Alkaline toluidine blue stain; original magnification × 160. (C) As in (B) but stained by the von Kossa method, to demonstrate calcific deposits (darkly stained) in layer of thrombus. A cotton fiber (arrowhead) is present in thrombus in outflow surface; original magnification × 160. (D) Higher magnification view of area similar to that in (C). The calcific deposits in the thrombus appear as small, dark granules (compare with figure 3A). Hematoxylin-eosin stain; original magnification × 400. (E) Polarization micrograph of area in (D), showing birefringence of cotton fiber; original magnification × 270.

Scanning Electron Microscopic Observations

The outflow surfaces of the leaflets of unimplanted Ionescu-Shiley valves showed straight or curved grooves 10–20 μ wide (Figure 2A). The inflow surfaces of the same leaflets appeared much rougher in texture than the outflow surfaces, but did not

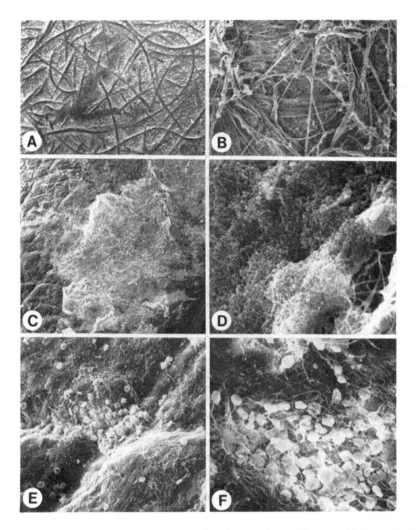

Figure 2 Scanning electron micrographs of unimplanted Ionescu-Shiley valve (A and B) and of valve implanted for 3 days (C–F). (A) Outflow surface of unimplanted valve has numerous grooves that follow straight or curved paths. Magnification × 55. (B) Inflow surface of same leaflet as in (A) is composed of coarse bundles of collagen. No grooves are evident on this surface. Magnification × 55. (C) A thin layer of thrombotic material is present on outflow surface of implanted valve. Magnification × 55. (D) High-magnification view (× 2700) showing finely granular material in calcified thrombus. (E) Erythrocytes are located in two intersecting grooves (one groove runs from bottom left to upper right, and the other from mid-left to mid-right) in outflow surface of the valve. Magnification × 460. (F) High-magnification view (× 920) of small thrombus composed of erythrocytes enmeshed in fibrin.

139

show grooves (Figure 2B). Both the inflow and outflow surfaces of the leaflets of the valve that had been implanted in the patient were covered with thrombi that were directly superimposed on the most superficial layers of valvular collagen (Figures 2C–2F). Some of the grooves in the outflow surfaces of the explanted valve contained platelets, fibrin strands and erythrocytes (Figure 2E), even in areas where the surface adjacent to the grooves was free of thrombus. In areas of calcification of surface thrombi (Figure 2D), the fibrin strands were covered by clumps of finely granular material.

Transmission Electron Microscopic Observations

Observations on ultrathin sections examined by transmission electron microscopy revealed that the calcific deposits consisted of irregularly shaped masses (Figure 3A), usually 0.25–$2.2\,\mu$ in diameter, composed of very fine needles or plate-like crystals of high electron density (Figure 3B). These crystals averaged 70 Å in thickness. These calcific masses were located between fibrin strands, which were not calcified. The calcific masses often appeared to be superimposed upon remnants of cells, which were identified as platelets, macrophages and leukocytes (Figure 3C). Most of these cells showed extensive degenerative and autolytic changes. The larger calcific masses were extremely dense, and structures associated with these masses were not discernible. A few calcific deposits were associated with the most superficial layers of valvular collagen (Figure 3D). Elastic fibers were not calcified, and there was no evidence of collagen degeneration. Deposits of fibrin were interspersed with the most superficial layers of collagen.

DISCUSSION

Ionescu-Shiley pericardial valves have been used for several years with good clinical results;[12] however, anatomic studies have been made of limited numbers of valves of this type which have been removed after being implanted in patients,[12] and little information is available on the occurrence of calcific deposits in these valves. Calcific deposits are known to develop in other types of bioprostheses,[1] but the time of onset and the rate of deposition of calcium in bioprostheses are not known.

The host factors and tissue factors that cause calcification of bioprostheses are poorly understood. It is not known to what extent conclusions derived from studies of porcine bioprostheses will be applicable to pericardial bioprostheses. Porcine bioprostheses calcify more frequently and to a greater extent in patients who have one or more of the following predisposing conditions: younger than 35 years of age,[1,3,4,7–10,13–16] chronic renal disease,[1,2,10] and infection of the bioprosthesis.[1,17,18] Morphologic studies of Ionescu-Shiley valves have been too limited to determine the importance of these factors in predisposing to calcification of this type of bioprosthesis. Our patient was young and did have acute renal insufficiency, but had no evidence of infection in the bioprosthesis.

Ultrastructural studies have demonstrated that the two main anatomic sites of calcification of porcine valvular bioprostheses are collagen fibrils in the leaflets and surface thrombi and vegetations.[1] Evidence has been presented indicating that the initial deposits of calcium phosphate in thrombi and vegetations are localized in mitochondria of blood cells and platelets trapped in the fibrin mesh.[1] In the present study, calcific deposits were demonstrated in collagen and in surface thrombi, but almost all of the deposits were localized in thrombotic material. These deposits were structurally similar to those observed in porcine bioprostheses.[1] Studies in experimental animals have shown that a thin layer of fibrin is deposited on the leaflets of porcine bioprostheses within a few minutes after implantation.[19] In humans, such a layer of fibrin was observed in two Hancock bioprostheses that had been in place for only 2 and 3 days, respectively, but neither contained calcific deposits.[11] Thus, the changes

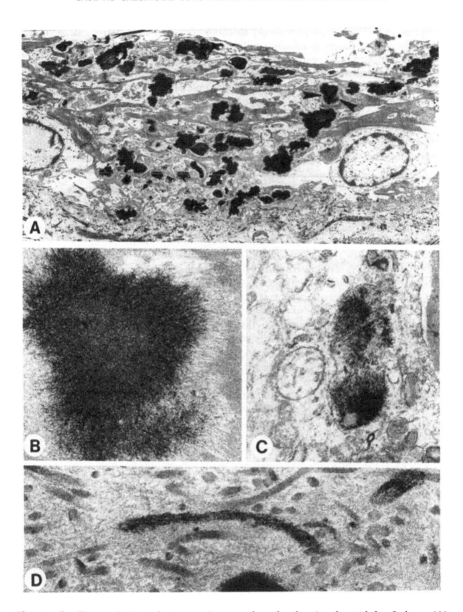

Figure 3 Transmission electron micrographs of valve implanted for 3 days. (A) Low-magnification view of area near free edge of leaflet, showing calcific deposits, which appear black, and mononuclear cells within the mesh of fibrin in thrombus overlying the collagen at the leaflet surface. Arrowheads indicate calcific deposit shown at high magnification in (B). Magnification × 7000. (B) Calcific deposit in thrombus is composed of very fine needle-like crystals. Magnification × 58,500. (C) Calcific deposits are localized within cytoplasm of mononuclear cell. Magnification × 33,500. (D) Calcific deposits (black) overlie collagen fibrils in area near leaflet surface. Magnification × 56,250.

we report apparently represent a very unusual phenomenon of early calcification of this surface layer. These calcific deposits probably would have become the cause of clinically significant bioprosthetic stenosis if our patient had survived longer.

Several factors may have contributed to the early calcification of the bioprosthesis in our patient: the low cardiac output syndrome, which led to renal insufficiency requiring peritoneal dialysis, and the large amounts of calcium chloride given intravenously because of the multiple blood transfusions and at times of resuscitative efforts. Another factor is the presence of proteins in the blood, which function in the coagulation process and which contain γ-carboxyglutamic acid, an unusual amino acid capable of avidly binding calcium.[20,21] This amino acid has been extracted from calcified (but not from noncalcified) porcine bioprostheses.[20] Its association with calcification of pericardial bioprostheses has not been investigated.

Uptake of calcium by mitochondria of hypoxic or ischemic cells is known to occur not only in myocardium but also in other tissues,[22] and the availability of large amounts of calcium to blood cells incorporated into thrombi may have resulted in significant accumulation of calcium in these cells (thus initiating bioprosthetic calcification) under conditions of hypoxia associated with the low cardiac output state in our patient. The finding of calcific deposits in necrotic myocardial cells as in our patient is not unusual; it is frequently observed in patients who have the low cardiac output syndrome postoperatively.[23]

The cotton fibers on the surfaces of the cusps of the bioprosthesis may have been derived from the packing material in the valve container. Such fibers were not found in pulmonary or myocardial vessels. A fatal coronary embolus was produced by fragments of packing material in a porcine bioprosthesis.[24]

The morphologic observations on the unimplanted Ionescu-Shiley valves reveal marked asymmetry in the texture of the inflow and outflow surfaces of the pericardial tissue leaflets. The inflow surface is very rough and corresponds to the pericardial surface that faces the sternum. In contrast, the outflow surface is much smoother; it contains grooves that appear to have been made by a mechanical process and corresponds to the pericardial surface that faces the heart. These differences, which were consistently observed in the three unimplanted valves examined, provide a basis for the identification of the surfaces of Ionescu-Shiley valves; however, in animal experiments (unpublished observations) we found that the grooves tend to be obscured (as was the case in the valve from our patient) by the deposition of fibrin on the surfaces after the valves are implanted.

REFERENCES

1. Ferrans VJ, Boyce SW, Billingham ME, Jones M, Ishihara T, Roberts WC: Calcific deposits in porcine bioprostheses: structure and pathogenesis. Am J Cardiol **46**: 721, 1980

2. Hetzer R, Hill JD, Kerth WJ, Wilson AJ, Adappa MG, Gerbode F: Thrombosis and degeneration of Hancock valves: clinical and pathological findings. Ann Thorac Surg **26**: 317, 1978

3. Rose AG, Forman R, Bowen RM: Calcification of glutaraldehyde-fixed porcine xenograft. Thorax **33**: 111, 1978

4. Forfar JC, Cotter L, Morritt GN: Severe and early stenosis of porcine heterograft mitral valve. Br Heart J **40**: 1184, 1978

5. Albert HM, Bryant LR, Schechter FG: Seven year experience with mounted porcine valves. Ann Surg **185**: 717, 1977

6. Bachet J, Bical O, Goudot B, Menu P, Richard T, Barbagelatta M, Guilmet D: Early structural failure of porcine xenografts in young patients. *In* Bioprosthetic Cardiac Valves, edited by Sebening F, Klövekorn WP, Meisner H, Struck E. München, Deutsches Herzzentrum, 1979, pp. 341–349

7. Thandroyen FT, Whitton IN, Pirie D, Rogers MA, Mitha AS: Severe calcification of glutaraldehyde-preserved porcine xenografts in children. Am J Cardiol **45**: 690, 1980

8. Silver MM, Pollock J, Silver MD, Williams WG, Trusler GA: Calcification in porcine xenograft valves in children. Am J Cardiol **45**: 685, 1980

9. Sanders SP, Freed MD, Norwood WI, Castaneda A, Nadas AS: Early failure of porcine valves implanted in children, (abstr) Am J Cardiol **45**: 449, 1980

10. Fishbein MC, Gissen SA, Collins JJ Jr, Barsamian EM, Cohn LH: Pathologic findings after cardiac valve replacement with glutaraldehyde-fixed porcine valves. Am J Cardiol **40**: 331, 1977

11. Ferrans VJ, Spray TL, Billingham ME, Roberts WC: Structural changes in glutaraldehyde-treated porcine heterografts used as substitute cardiac valves. Transmission and scanning electron microscopic observations in 12 patients. Am J Cardiol **41**: 1159, 1978

12. Ionescu MI, Tandon AP, Mary DAS, Abid A: Heart valve replacement with the Ionescu-Shiley pericardial xenograft. J Thorac Cardiovasc Surg **73**: 31, 1977

13. Kutsche LM, Oyer P, Shumway N, Baum D: An important complication of Hancock mitral valve replacement in children. Circulation **60** (suppl I): 1–98, 1978

14. Brown JW, Dunn JM, Spooner E, Kirsh MM: Late spontaneous disruption of a porcine xenograft mitral valve. Clinical, hemodynamic, echocardiographic, and pathological findings. J Thorac Cardiovasc Surg **75**: 606, 1978

15. Geha AS, Stansel HC Jr, Cornhill JF, Kilman JW, Buckley MJ, Roberts WC: Late failure of porcine valve heterografts in children. J Thorac Cardiovasc Surg **78**: 351, 1979

16. Magilligan DJ Jr, Lewis JW Jr, Jara FM, Stein PD, Riddle JM, Lee MW: Spontaneous degeneration of porcine bioprosthetic valves. Ann Thorac Surg **30**: 259, 1980

17. Zuhdi N: The porcine aortic valve bioprosthesis: a significant alternative. Ann Thorac Surg **21**: 573, 1976

18. Magilligan DJ Jr, Quinn EL, Davila JC: Bacteremia, endocarditis, and the Hancock valve. Ann Thorac Surg **24**: 508, 1977

19. Geroulanos S, Gossler W, Walpoth B, Turina M, Senning A: Frühe rasterelektronenoptische Oberflächenveränderungen nach orthotoper Pulmonalklappen-Xenotransplantation durch glutaraldehyd-konditionierte Schweineklappen. Eine experimentelle Studie an Hunden. Helv Chir Acta **46**: 91, 1979

20. Levy RJ, Lian JB: Studies on the etiology of calcific aortic valve disease: the role of the calcium binding amino acid, y-carboxyglutamic acid, (abstr) Circulation **58** (suppl II): 11–54, 1978

21. Levy RJ, Zenker JA, Lian JB: Vitamin K-dependent calcium binding proteins in aortic valve calcification. J Clin Invest **65**: 563, 1980

22. Trump BF, Berezesky IK, Laiho KU, Osomio AR, Mergner WJ, Smith MW: The role of calcium in cell injury. A review. Scan Electron Microsc, **2**: 437–492, 1980

23. Reichenbach DD, Benditt EP: Catecholamines and cardiomyopathy: the pathogenesis and potential importance of myofibrillar degeneration. Hum Pathol **1**: 125, 1970

24. Tubbs RR, Picha GC, Levin HS, Groves L, Barenberg S: Cotton emboli (cellulose II polymorph, "rayon") of the coronary arteries. Hum Pathol **11**: 76, 1980

Case 458 Inward Stent-Post Bending of a Porcine Bioprosthesis in the Mitral Position

Cause of Bioprosthetic Dysfunction

A. Michael Borkon, MD, Charles L. McIntosh, MD, PhD, Michael Jones, MD, William C. Roberts, MD, and Andrew G. Morrow, MD
Bethesda, MD

Certain clinical and morphologic features are described in a patient with severe bioprosthetic obstruction 9 years after mitral valve replacement. At reoperation, severe inward bending of the stent-posts was found without significant bioprosthetic cuspal abnormalities. "Polymer creep" is considered responsible for the stent-post deformity.

The morphologic features of late bioprosthetic valve failure have been well described.[1-5] In most patients, bioprosthetic failure was the result of cuspal calcification and collagen disruption. Deterioration of the other components of the bioprosthesis infrequently has been responsible for failure. Recently, permanent inward stent-post deformity producing secondary valvular orifice obstruction and valvular failure has been reported after aortic valve replacement with Hancock bioprostheses and is believed to have resulted from stent-post compression from a narrow aortic root.[6,7] Experimental studies have shown that stent-post deformity may result also from "polymer creep," an aging characteristic of polypropylene.[8] Stent-post deformity has not been described previously in the mitral position. Such was the case, however, in the case described herein.

CASE REPORT

A 50-year-old white woman underwent closed mitral commissurotomy in September, 1960, and was well thereafter until November, 1969, when congestive heart failure reappeared and repeat cardiac catheterization was performed (Table 1). On Nov. 3, 1970, she underwent aortic valve replacement with a No. 8 Starr-Edwards Model 2310 prosthesis and mitral replacement with a No. 29 Hancock bioprosthesis. The postoperative course was uncomplicated, and she was discharged receiving warfarin sodium. Cardiac catheterization (Table 1), 7 months after operation, disclosed a residual mean gradient across the Hancock mitral bioprosthesis of 7 mm Hg and a calculated mitral valve orifice area of 2.4 cm². She was symptomatically improved (New York Heart Association Functional Class II). In September, 1979, she began to have increasing symptoms of congestive heart failure. A Grade 2/6 systolic ejection murmur was heard at the right upper sternal border and a Grade 2/6 holosystolic murmur at the apex and axilla. These murmurs were unchanged from prior examinations. No diastolic murmur was heard. Repeat cardiac catheterization

From the Clinic of Surgery and the Pathology Branch, National Heart, Lung and Blood Institute, Bethesda, Md.

Received for publication March 2, 1981.

Accepted for publication May 19, 1981.

Address for reprints: Andrew G. Morrow, M.D., National Heart, Lung and Blood Institute, Bethesda, Md. 20205.

DOI: 10.1201/9781003409281-23

Table 1: Hemodynamic data

	Immediately preoperatively	Months preoperatively	
		7	106
Rhythm	Atrial fibrillation	Sinus	Atrial fibrillation
Pressures (mm Hg):			
Right atrium (mean)	5	2	11
Right ventricle (s/d)*	53/5	38/6	108/10
Pulmonary artery (s/d)	53/25	38/18	108/10
Pulmonary artery	m = 26	m = 15	m = 32
wedge (PAW)	v = 36	a = 16	v = 46
		v = 22	
Left ventricle (LV) (s/d)	170/8	170/12	190/14
Aorta (s/d)	160/80	155/77	190/86
PAW/LV mdg = mean	8	7	11
diastolic gradient			
Cardiac output (L/min)	3.4	5.4	3.3
Mitral valve area (cm²)	—	2.4	1.0

*s/d = systolic/diastolic.

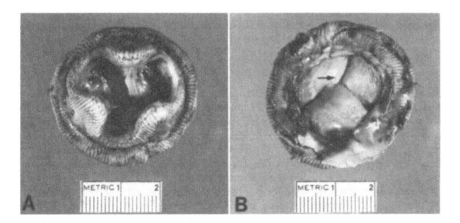

Figure 1 Mitral bioprostheses removed from the patient 107 months after implantation. *A*, Ventricular aspect. The stent-posts are bent inward, producing secondary valve orifice obstruction. Valve leaflets are thin and pliable. *B*, Atrial aspect. There is a pinhole leaflet perforation *(arrow)*.

(Table 1) on Sept. 19, 1979, demonstrated severe stenosis of the bioprosthetic mitral valve (mean mitral gradient 11 mm Hg and calculated orifice area 1.0 cm²). The mitral Hancock bioprosthesis was replaced with a Starr-Edwards valve. The postoperative course was uneventful, and she remains well.

    The cusps of the bioprosthesis removed at operation were thin and delicate and a small tear was present adjacent to one commissure. The stent-posts were indented inward and appeared to result in bioprosthetic obstruction (Figure 1).

COMMENTS

The flexible stent was developed in 1970 by Reis and associates[9] to improve Hancock valve durability by diminishing stress on the bioprosthetic cusps. In most instances

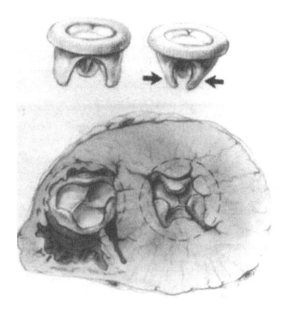

Figure 2 Mechanism of stent-post deformity due to left ventricular compression from bioprosthesis-ventricular disproportion.

leaflet calcification and collagen disruption result in bioprosthetic dysfunction. Deterioration of the Stellite ring, polypropylene stent, or Dacron cloth covering has seldom been implicated as a primary mechanism of bioprosthetic valve failure. In two recently reported cases there was permanent inward stent-post deformity causing significant valve orifice obstruction after aortic valve replacement with Hancock bioprostheses. In both cases, the bioprosthesis was compressed by a small aortic root and was associated with bioprosthetic thrombosis[6] or severe hemolysis.[7]

Stent-post deformity producing obstruction and requiring reoperation has not previously been reported after mitral valve replacement. Spray and Roberts[1] observed stent-post deformity associated with bioprosthetic failure due to leaflet degeneration, but they did not discuss its significance. Pohlner et al[8] demonstrated that polypropylene may be subject to "polymer creep" from persistent cyclic fatigue, producing permanent inward stent-post migration and bioprosthetic failure. Possibly, "polymer creep" may have been responsible for the secondary valve orifice obstruction in our patients, as cardiac catheterization documented worsening of the bioprosthetic stenosis and no cuspal abnormalities were identified that could account for this degree of obstruction.

Left ventricular compression may also result in stent-post deformity owing to bioprosthesis-ventricular disproportion if proper care is not taken in sizing not only the mitral valve anulus, but also the ventricular cavity, as demonstrated in Figure 2. It is unlikely that this was the mechanism of stent-post deformity in the patient presented because obstruction developed late and the ventricular cavity at both operations was of adequate size.

REFERENCES

1. Spray TL, Roberts WC: Structural changes in porcine xenografts. Am J Cardiol **40**:319–330, 1977

2. Ferrans VJ, Spray TL, Billingham ME, Roberts WC: Structural changes in glutaraldehyde-treated porcine heterografts used as substitute cardiac valves. AM J CARDIOL **41**:1159–1184, 1978

3. Ferrans VJ, Spray TL, Billingham ME, Roberts WC: Ultrastructure of Hancock porcine valvular heterografts. Pre-and postimplantation changes. CIRCULATION 58:Suppl 1:10–18, 1978

4. Hezter R, Hill JD, Kerth WJ, Wilson AJ, Adappa MG, Gerbode F: Thrombosis and degeneration of Hancock valve. Clinical and pathological findings. ANN THORAC SURG **26**:317–322, 1978

5. Fishbein MC, Gissen SA, Collin JT, Barsamian EM, Cohn LH: Pathologic findings after cardiac valve replacement with glutaraldehyde-fixed porcine valves. AM J CARDIOL **40**:331–337, 1977

6. Salomon NW, Copeland JG, Goldman S, Larson DF: Unusual complication of the Hancock porcine heterograft. Strut compression in the aortic root. J THORAC CARDIOVASC SURG **77**:294–296, 1979

7. Magilligan DJ, Fisher E, Alam M: Hemolytic anemia with porcine xenograft aortic and mitral valves. J THORAC CARDIOVASC SURG **79**:628–631, 1980

8. Pohlner PG, Thompson FJ, Hjelm E, Barratt-Boyes BG: Experimental evaluation of aortic hemograft valves mounted on flexible support frames and comparison with glutaraldehyde-treated porcine valves. J THORAC CARDIOVASC SURG **77**:287–293, 1979

9. Reis RL, Hancock WD, Yarbrough JW, Glancy DL, Morrow AG: The flexible stent. J THORAC CARDIOVASC SURG **62**:683–689, 1971

Case 491 Acquired Cor Triatriatum (Left Ventricular False Aneurysm)

Complication of Active Infective Endocarditis of the Aortic Valve with Ring Abscess Treated by Valve Replacement

Bruce M. McManus, MD, PhD,* Nevin M. Katz, MD, Brian D. Blackbourne, MD, John S. Gottdiener, MD, Robert B. Wallace, MD, and William C. Roberts, MD
Bethesda, MD, and Washington, D.C.

Cor triatriatum is a congenital anomaly in which the left atrium (LA) is essentially partitioned into two chambers with a small orifice between them. The cephalad chamber receives the pulmonary veins and the caudal chamber is connected to the mitral valve. The concept of "cor triatriatum" as an *acquired* condition is new. Recently, however, we studied the heart of a 31-year-old opiate addict who had

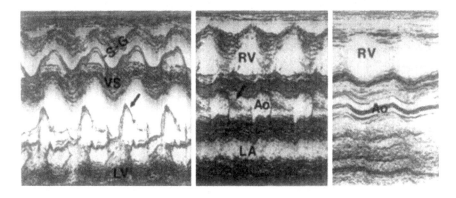

Figure 1 M-mode echocardiograms. *Left*, Preoperative view showing a Swan-Ganz *(S-G)* catheter in the right ventricular outflow tract, a hyperdynamic ventricular septum *(VS)* and left ventricular free wall *(LV)*, and vibratory movement *(arrow)* of the anterior mitral leaflet and ventricular septum. *Middle*, Preoperative view at the level of aortic valve and left atrium revealing "shaggy" thickenings *(arrow)* of the aortic valve cusps and echo-dense zones between right ventricular outflow tract *(RV)* and aorta *(Ao)*, and between Ao and left atrium *(LA)* that are believed to represent aortic valve ring abscess. *Right*, Postoperative view at the level of aortic valve and left atrium showing the bioprosthesis in aorta and increased echo densities behind the aorta. The latter may represent a portion of the false aneurysm.

From the Pathology Branch, National Heart, Lung and Blood Institute, National Institutes of Health; the Departments of Surgery and Medicine, Georgetown University; and the Medical Examiner's Office, Washington, D.C.

Received for publication March 29, 1982; accepted Apr. 20, 1982.

Reprint requests: William C. Roberts, M.D., Pathology Branch, NIH-NHLBI, Bldg. 10A, Room 3E-30, Bethesda, MD 20205.

* Present address: Department of Pathology, University of Nebraska Medical Center, Omaha, NE 68105.

                                                     DOI: 10.1201/9781003409281-24

three chambers at the atrial level rather than two. He had developed *Staphylococcus aureus* endocarditis of the aortic valve resulting in severe aortic regurgitation (AR), causing severe congestive heart failure and associated with hemorrhagic pericardial tamponade. At operation, each of the three aortic valve cusps was virtually destroyed by the active infection. A ring abscess was found at operation and the mouth into it was just caudal to the junction of the left and posterior cusps. The cusps were excised and the mouth into the ring abscess was debrided. A porcine bioprosthesis (23 mm size) was inserted at the level of the "anulus." The patient died of a narcotic overdose 75 days after an otherwise uneventful clinical postoperative course. A murmur of AR was never present postoperatively and he had received antibiotics for 6 weeks after operation. Echocardiograms recorded 2 days before and 18 days after operation are shown in Figure 1.

At necropsy, an opening was found just caudal to the ring of the bioprosthesis that led into a large chamber situated adjacent to both atria (Figures 2 and 3). This

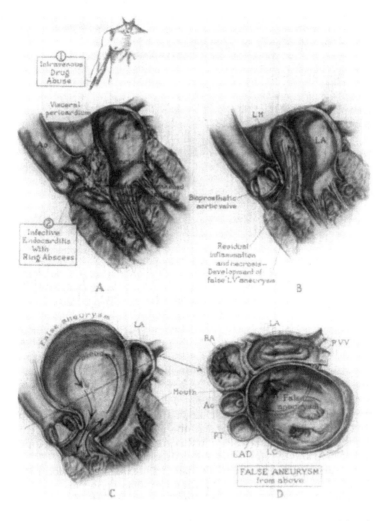

Figure 2 Drawings of the false aneurysm and its likely mechanism of development.

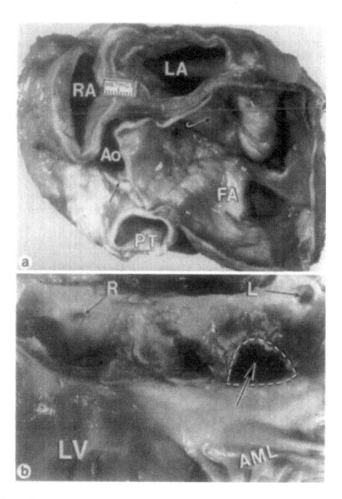

Figure 3 False aneurysm. *a*, Opened false aneurysm *(FA)* viewed from above showing its fibrous wall and site of communication with the left ventricle *(curved arrow)*. The false aneurysm is much larger than either atrium and overlays the aortic root *(Ao)* where a strut of the bioprosthesis is seen *(arrow)*. PT = pulmonary trunk. *b*, Opened aorta and left ventricular *(LV)* outflow tract showing the entry site *(broken-lined area)* into false aneurysm *(large arrow)*. AML = anterior mitral leaflet; L and R = ostium of the left and right coronary arteries *(small arrows)*. (Photos by M.M.M. Moore.)

accessory chamber, which was much larger than either the right atrium or the compressed LA, ended in a blind pouch, the wall of which consisted entirely of dense fibrous tissue. No residual infection was present in the heart. The bioprosthetic cusps were normal and the ring was securely in place.

Thus, the above described patient had active infective endocarditis on a previously anatomically normal aortic valve and an adjacent ring abscess.[1] The mouth into the abscess was incompletely closed at the time of aortic valve replacement. In retrospect, however, it may have been advisable to have obliterated completely the mouth of the abscess by sutures buttressed with prosthetic material or by a prosthetic patch.[2] Residual infection just caudal to the bioprosthetic valve ring at the aorto-LA angle plus the likely occurrence of a small gradient postoperatively between left ventricle (LV) and aorta are circumstances allowing entrance of blood into the ring abscess. The resulting accessory chamber, which was not present at operation, presumably progressively enlarged postoperatively due to its receiving blood under LV systolic pressure. The aneurysm of the ring abscess represents a false LV aneurysm, although situated at the atrial level, because its wall was not previously myocardium.

The development of a false aneurysm of LV after aortic valve replacement at the site of a ring abscess secondary to infective endocarditis of the aortic valve has not been described previously to our knowledge. Despite the impressive size of the false aneurysm, it apparently caused no symptoms or signs of cardiac dysfunction.

REFERENCES

1. Arnett EN, Roberts WC: Valve ring abscess in active infective endocarditis: Frequency, location, and clues to clinical diagnosis from the study of 95 necropsy patients. Circulation **54**:140, 1976.
2. Frantz PT, Murray GF, Wilcox BR: Surgical management of left ventricular-aortic discontinuity complicating bacterial endocarditis. Ann Thorac Surg **29**:1, 1980.

Case 497 Severe Aortic Regurgitation from Systemic Hypertension

Bruce F. Waller, MD, F.C.C.P.; Joan C. Kishel, MD; and William C. Roberts, MD, F.C.C.P.

Although about 10 percent of patients with systemic hypertension have a basal diastolic blowing murmur indicating aortic regurgitation (AR) (Figure 1),[1-7] the degree of aortic regurgitation is usually minimal or mild. The occurrence of severe aortic regurgitation from systemic hypertension unassociated with aortic dissection is rare,[8] but herein we describe such a patient who had aortic regurgitation severe enough to require aortic valve replacement.

CASE REPORT

A 64-year-old woman, who died on August 3, 1981, had systemic arterial hypertension noted for the first time at age 36 years (1953). At age 40, she began antihypertensive treatment (reserpine). At age 50 (1967), a grade 2/6 diastolic blowing murmur of aortic regurgitation was noted and the blood pressure was 240/120 mm Hg (Figure 2). During the next seven years, the blood pressure remained elevated despite administration of diuretics, reserpine and alpha-methyldopa. At age 55 years (1973), angina pectoris appeared and thereafter it progressed. On examination at age 56, the intensity of the aortic regurgitation murmur was grade 3/6. The ECG (Figure 3) showed sinus bradycardia and left ventricular hypertrophy, and the chest radiograph (Figure 4), an enlarged cardiac silhouette. On M-mode echocardiogram (Figure 5), the left ventricular free wall and ventricular septum were of similar thickness and the ascending aorta was dilated. The results of the cardiac catheterization are summarized in Table 1. She underwent aortic valve replacement with a tilting-disc prosthesis and had two aortocoronary bypass conduits placed to the left anterior descending coronary system. The aortic valve was three-cuspid; each cusp was freely mobile, but mildly thickened by fibrous tissue without calcific deposits, and no commissure was fused.

The blood pressure in the first six weeks postoperation was reduced compared to the preoperation and late postoperation values (Figure 2). Later she was treated with beta-blocking and vasodilating agents. A murmur of aortic regurgitation was absent postoperatively. At age 62 (1980), angina pectoris and exertional dyspnea reappeared. The blood pressure was 210/100 mm Hg. She took warfarin only intermittently, and in July, 1981 she developed acute pulmonary edema without audible prosthetic aortic valve sounds, and died several days later.

At necropsy, the heart weighed 530 g. The orifice of the aortic-valve prosthesis was severely narrowed by thrombus which made the occluder immobile. A healed transmural left ventricular infarct was present (Figure 6) and the left main, left anterior descending, and right coronary arteries were each narrowed >75 percent in cross-sectional area by atherosclerotic plaques.

From the Pathology Branch, National Heart, Lung and Blood Institute, National Institutes of Health, Bethesda.

Reprint requests: Dr. Roberts, Bldg 10A, Rm 3E30, NHLBI, National Institutes of Health, Bethesda 20205

DOI: 10.1201/9781003409281-25

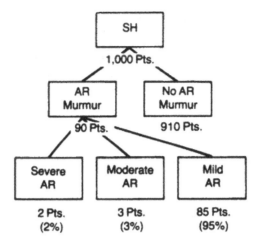

Figure 1 Frequency and severity of aortic regurgitation (AR) in patients (pts) with systemic hypertension (SH) based on previously reported data.[1-7]

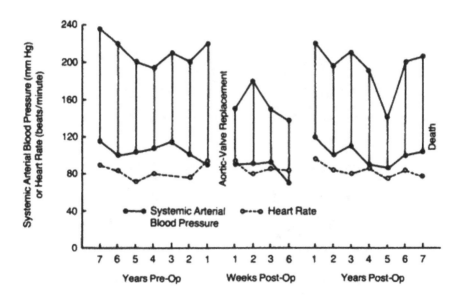

Figure 2 Systolic and diastolic systemic arterial pressures before and after aortic-valve replacement.

COMMENTS

The patient described above had systemic hypertension and aortic regurgitation severe enough to warrant aortic-valve replacement without clinical or morphologic explanation for the aortic regurgitation other than systemic hypertension. Recently, we reported four other patients, all men aged 43–59 years (mean 50), with severe systemic hypertension, chronic congestive heart failure, and aortic regurgitation severe enough to warrant aortic-valve replacement.[8] The hypertension had been present from 1–30 years (mean 13). In each of the four previous patients and in the

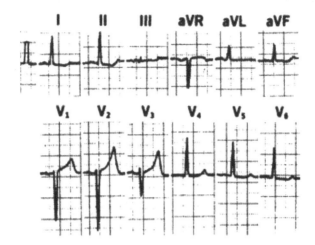

Figure 3 Electrocardiogram in patient at age 56 years (eight years before death) showing left ventricular hypertrophy and nonspecific ST segment and T wave changes. The total QRS amplitude is 195 mm.

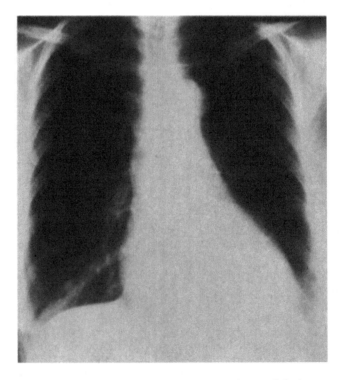

Figure 4 Posteroanterior chest roentgenogram obtained before aortic valve replacement eight years before death showing an enlarged cardiac silhouette.

154

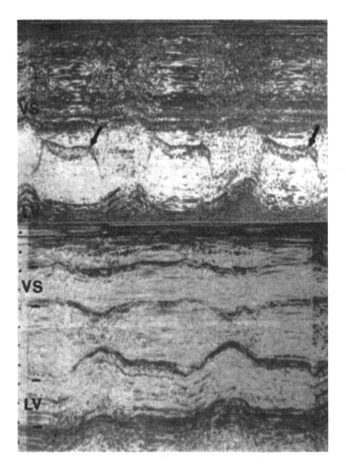

Figure 5 M-mode echocardiograms recorded just before aortic valve replacement. The anterior mitral valve leaflet flutters *(arrow), (upper)*. The ventricular septum (VS) and left ventricular free wall (LV) are of similar thickness *(lower)*.

present patient, the aortic valve was three-cuspid; each cusp was free of calcific deposits and freely mobile.

Until these five patients were encountered, we had not observed severe aortic regurgitation from systemic hypertension alone and are unaware of any reports describing aortic valve replacement for aortic regurgitation in such patients. At least 79 patients with systemic hypertension and aortic regurgitation (by auscultation), however, were reported between 1940 and 1971, but none had aortic valve replacement.[7] Of the 79 patients, the aortic regurgitation was severe in 17 (22 percent) and mild or moderate in 62 (78 percent). Each of the 17 patients with severe aortic regurgitation had fatal congestive heart failure, but another definite, probable or possible cause of the failure other than aortic regurgitation appears to have been present in six. Of the remaining 11 patients, necropsy information was available in seven. The aortic valve and ascending aorta were reported to be normal in all seven. The aortic valve "ring" was dilated in only one (7–12 cm [mean 9]), the left ventricle

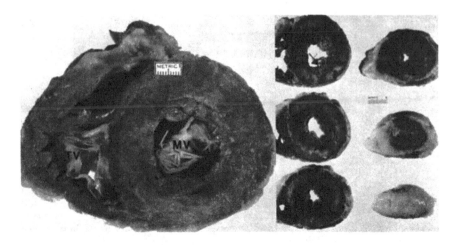

Figure 6 *Left:* Basal portion of the cardiac ventricles. MV=mitral valve leaflets and TV=tricuspid valve leaflets. *Right:* Transverse sections of both cardiac ventricles from base-to-apex showing nondilated cavities, thickened ventricular walls and a healed myocardial infarct.

Table 1: Hemodynamic data (pressures in mm Hg)

Left ventricle (LV) (s/d)	160/11
Femoral artery (FA) (s/d)	160/60
Pulmonary arterial wedge (mean)	7
Right ventricle (s/d)	20/5
Right atrium (mean)	3
Cardiac index (L/min/M2)	1.6
AR by aortogram (1 +-4+)	3 +
Coronary arterial narrowing	
(% diameter reduction)	
Left main	70
Left anterior descending	50
Left circumflex	50
Right	0

s/d = peak systole/end diastole

was dilated in only three patients, but the heart weight was increased in all seven (460–700 g [mean 565 g]).

Certain factors increase the possibility of developing aortic regurgitation in patients with systemic hypertension.[1-7] 1) *Magnitude of systemic arterial pressure.* The higher the pressure, the greater the chance of aortic regurgitation. 2) *Age of patient.* Of patients with similar levels of systemic arterial pressure, *older patients* have a higher frequency of aortic regurgitation than do younger patients. 3) *Duration of systemic hypertension.* Of patients of similar age and similar pressure, those with systemic hypertension of longer duration have a higher frequency of aortic regurgitation than do those of shorter duration. The mechanism by which severe aortic regurgitation develops in some patients with systemic hypertension is unclear.

REFERENCES

1. Barlow J, Kincaid-Smith P. The auscultatory findings in hypertension. Br Heart J 1960; 22:505–514
2. Garvin CF. Functional aortic insufficiency. Am J Med 1940; 13:1799–1704
3. Gouley BA, Sickel EM. Aortic regurgitation caused by dilatation of the aortic orifice and associated with a characteristic valvular lesion. Am Heart J 1943; 26:24–38
4. Hammon L. Diagnostic implications of aortic insufficiency. Cincinnati J Med 1944: 25:95–125
5. Fenichel NM. Arteriosclerotic aortic insufficiency. Am Heart J 1950; 40:117–124
6. Puchner TC, Huston JH, Hellmuth GA. Aortic valve insufficiency in arterial hypertension. Am J Cardiol 1960; 5:758–760
7. Matalon R, Moussalli ARJ, Nidus BD, Katz LA, Eisinger RP. Functional aortic insufficiency—a feature of renal failure. N Engl J Med 1971; 285:1522–1523
8. Waller BF, Zoltick JM, Rosen JH, Katz NM, Gomes MN, Fletcher RD, et al. Severe aortic regurgitation from systemic hypertension without aortic dissection requiring aortic valve replacement Analysis of 4 patients. Am J Cardiol 1982; 49:473–477

Case 523 Aortic Valve Stenosis and Left Ventricular Apical Aneurysm and/or Rupture

Real or Potential Complications of Persistent Left Ventricular Systolic Hypertension After Acute Myocardial Infarction

William C. Roberts, MD, Ernest N. Arnett, MD, Seena C. Aisner, MD, and Paul Techlenberg, MD
Bethesda and Baltimore, MD

When acute myocardial infarction (MI) occurs in patients with systemic hypertension, the systemic arterial and left ventricular (LV) pressure generally returns to or toward normal if the MI was fairly large. When acute MI occurs in patients with significant aortic valve stenosis (AS), however, the LV systolic pressure remains elevated and the continuation of this pressure elevation increases the likelihood of LV rupture or aneurysmal formation, particularly when the MI involves the LV apical wall which normally is several times thinner than the LV basal wall.[1,2] Such was the case in a 67-year-old man, who died of progressive congestive heart failure after healing of more than one (by history) acute MI in the previous 5 years. At necropsy he had a severely stenotic congenitally bicuspid aortic valve and a large apical aneurysm at the site of a healed LV MI (Figure 1). The heart weighed 630 gm. Both the left anterior descending and left circumflex coronary arteries were narrowed 76% to 100% in cross-sectional area by atherosclerotic plaques. The occurrence of LV free wall rupture and/or aneurysmal formation has not been reported previously in a patient with severe AS. This fact is surprising in view of the elderly age of many patients with AS.

REFERENCES

1. Roberts WC, Ronan JA Jr, Harvey WP: Rupture of the left ventricular free wall (LVFW) or the ventricular septum (VS) secondary to acute myocardial infarction (AMI): An occurrence virtually limited to the first transmural AMI in the hypertensive individual (abstr). Am J Cardiol **35**:166, 1975.
2. Cabin HS, Roberts WC: True left ventricular aneurysm and healed myocardial infarction. Clinical and necropsy observations including quantification of degrees of coronary arterial narrowing. Am J Cardiol **46**:754, 1980.

From the Pathology Branch, National Heart, Lung and Blood Institute, National Institutes of Health; and the Departments of Cardiology and Pathology, Franklin Square Hospital.

Received for publication July 8, 1982; accepted July 27, 1982.

Reprint requests: William C. Roberts, M.D., National Institutes of Health, Bldg. 10A, Room 3E-30, Bethesda, MD 20205.

DOI: 10.1201/9781003409281-26

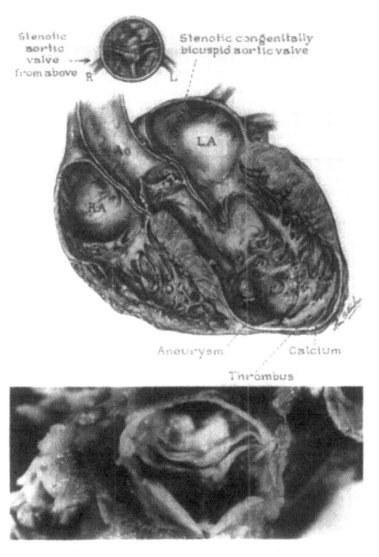

Figure 1 Drawing of heart *(upper panel)* showing the healed left ventricular apical aneurysm and the congenitally bicuspid, stenotic aortic valve; and a photograph of the valve *(lower panel)*.

Case 531 Cholesteryl Ester Crystals in a Porcine Aortic Valvular Bioprosthesis Implanted for Eight Years

Victor J. Ferrans, MD, PhD; Bruce McManus, MD, PhD; and William C. Roberts, MD, F.C.C.P.

Masses of crystals, which were largely composed of cholesteryl esters, were found in a porcine aortic valvular bioprosthesis removed eight years after implantation in the mitral position in a patient with rheumatic mitral valvular stenosis. Histologic sections of grossly raised and nonraised yellow lesions in the three cusps of this bioprosthesis revealed large clefts, which on frozen section contained lipid-positive, birefringent crystals. These crystals gave a positive reaction with the Schultz test for cholesterol. Biochemical analyses of isolated nodules revealed a cholesterol content of 40 nmole/mg of wet tissue. Of this cholesterol, 88 percent was esterified, and the remaining 12 percent was free cholesterol. These cholesterol deposits are most likely derived from blood lipids; however, they were not related to hyperlipidemia, since the patient had normal blood levels of cholesterol and triglycerides.

Small lipid droplets are found relatively frequently in connective tissue of the leaflets of implanted cardiac valvular bioprostheses, as documented by previous electron microscopic observations from this laboratory;[1] however, crystalline deposits of cholesterol have not been reported previously in implanted bioprostheses. Such a finding forms the basis of the present report.

CASE REPORT

A 76-year-old woman with a history of rheumatic mitral valvular stenosis, previous closed mitral commissurotomy (1966), and replacement of the mitral valve with a Hancock porcine aortic valvular bioprosthesis (1973) died in December 1981 in intractable chronic congestive heart failure. She had marked pulmonary arterial hypertension (100/10 mm Hg before mitral replacement and 75/15 mm Hg six months after operation) and elevation of left ventricular end-diastolic pressure (20 mm Hg in 1974); her systemic arterial blood pressure ranged up to 170/90 mm Hg. The bioprosthetic heart valve was considered to have functioned normally until the patient's death. Blood lipids had been within normal limits; cholesterol was 189 ± 36 mg/dl (mean $\pm$ SD of nine values), and triglycerides were 107 mg/dl (mean of three values).

Anatomic Findings

At autopsy, the heart weighed 820 g. The coronary arteries were free of atherosclerotic plaques. Atherosclerotic changes in aorta, cerebral vessels, and peripheral systematic arteries were mild. The left atrium was markedly dilated and contained a small mural thrombus. Both ventricles were hypertrophied, and the left was dilated. Focal fibrous intimal thickening was present in the main left and right pulmonary arteries. The mitral prosthesis was well-secured, without perivalvular leaks. The atrial and ventricular aspects of the prosthetic valve ring were covered by fibrous tissue; this

From the Pathology Branch, National Heart, Lung, and Blood Institute, National Institutes of Health, Bethesda, Maryland.

Reprint requests: Dr. Ferrans, National Institutes of Health, Bldg 10, Rm 7N208, Bethesda 20205

DOI: 10.1201/9781003409281-27

tissue, however, did not impinge on the bioprosthetic cusps. No tears or perforations were present in the cusps. Tiny, elevated, yellow nodules, up to 2 mm in diameter, were evident grossly in each of the cusps, particularly on their outflow surfaces (Figures 1A and B). Calcific deposits were not found on roentgenographic examination of the bioprosthesis (Figure 1C). Study of histologic sections revealed that the yellow nodules on the leaflets were composed of masses of crystals embedded in a coarsely granular, eosinophilic matrix (Figure 2 to 5). In sections of plastic-embedded tissues these crystals appeared as empty, rectangular clefts that measured up to several hundred μ in length. No cellular reaction (macrophages, foam cells, giant cells, or

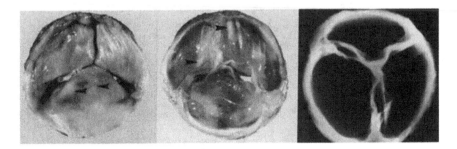

Figure 1   Views of the porcine bioprosthesis after removal from the mitral position and detachment from the stents. A, *left:* Inflow surface, showing light areas (*arrowheads*) corresponding to large crystalline deposits. The cusps appear otherwise normal. B, *center:* Outflow (left ventricular) surface, showing raised crystalline deposits (arrowheads). C, *right:* Radiograph of the bioprosthesis, confirming the absence of calcific deposits in the cusps.

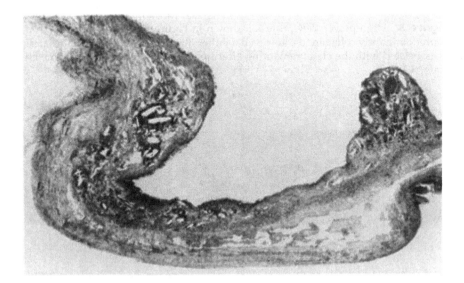

Figure 2   Section of cusp, showing numerous, large clefts within the connective tissue matrix of the cusp and nodular excrescence on the outflow surface. Areas of delamination of cuspal connective tissue are also noted. Alkaline toluidine blue stain, ×50.

161

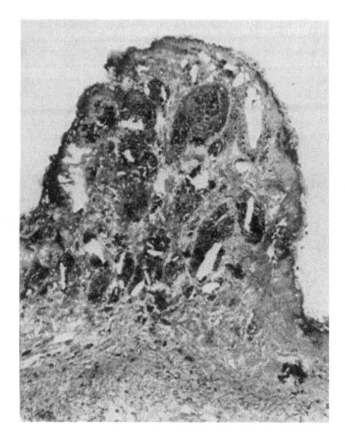

Figure 3 High-power view of lesion shown in Figure 2. Tlie supporting stroma is predominantly collagenous; however, a rather deeply staining, granular material is associated with the clefts remaining after lipid removal. Alkaline toluidine blue stain, × 160.

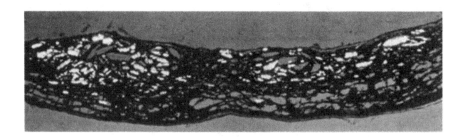

Figure 4 Polarized light micrograph of portion of a cusp, showing diffuse infiltration of the cuspal tissue by birefringent crystals, which tend to be localized on the outflow side of the cusp. Additional clefts without birefringent material represent areas of extensive delamination of collagen. (Sudan black B stain, × 40).

other inflammatory cells) was associated with these nodules of crystals. Smaller, nonraised masses of crystals were also present within the leaflet connective tissue. Sections stained by the von Kossa method did not show calcific deposits either in association with the crystals or elsewhere in the bioprosthetic tissue. Frozen sections stained with oil red O or with Sudan black B revealed multiple, small, nonbirefringent, darkly stained lipid droplets; the crystals described above were much less intensely stained than the lipid droplets. The crystals were markedly birefringent (Figures 4 and 5) and gave a positive reaction with the Schultz method for the histochemical demonstration of cholesterol.

In addition to the lipid infiltration described above, the connective tissue in the bioprosthetic leaflets showed moderate degrees of delamination (separation of the connective tissue layers) and degeneration, with the formation of many empty spaces within the substance of the leaflets. Fibrous sheaths or thrombi were not present over the cusps, and few cells (mostly macrophages) were present on the cuspal surfaces.

In order to further investigate the composition of the crystalline material, two nodules were excised from the leaflets with the aid of a dissecting microscope and submitted for biochemical analysis. The results, expressed in nanomoles per mg of wet tissue weight (mean± SE of quadruplicate determinations), were as follows: total cholesterol, 40.25 ± 2.72, of which 5.18 ± 0.75 was in the form of free cholesterol and 34.07 ±2.82 in the form of cholesteryl esters.

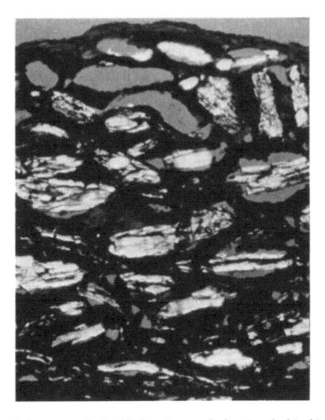

Figure 5 High-power polarized light micrograph showing the birefringent crystals in cuspal tissue. Sudan black B stain, × 400.

DISCUSSION

The observations in the present study document the presence of crystals, composed mainly of cholesteryl esters, in a bioprosthesis which had been implanted in the mitral position for eight years, during which time it had functioned well. Deposits of lipid droplets, presumed to be composed of triglycerides, have been observed in other bioprostheses,[1] but such large, crystalline masses have not been reported previously, to our knowledge, in implanted bioprostheses. Various types of lipid deposits are known to occur in native cardiac valves in a number of metabolic disorders. Most notable among the latter is homozygous type 2 hyperlipoproteinemia, in which the aortic valve is the site of formation of large intracellular (foam cells) and extracellular deposits of cholesteryl esters; other valves are involved to a much lesser extent.[2-6] Other diseases in which lipid deposits have been found in cardiac valves include Fabry's disease,[7,8] Farber's disease,[9] generalized GM_1 gangliosidosis,[10,11] and Sandhoff's disease,[12] in which glycolipids are stored in valvular connective tissue cells, and cholesteryl ester storage disease,[13] in which cholesteryl ester deposits have been detected in aortic valve. Lipid deposits also occur in association with the lesions of calcific aortic stenosis and mitral annular calcification.[14,15] The silicone rubber balls in certain mechanical prosthetic valves have been reported[16] to undergo infiltration with lipids derived from plasma lipoproteins; consequent swelling and deformation of the ball may cause mechanical dysfunction of the prosthesis.

The reason for the accumulation of cholesterol in the bioprosthesis from our patient remains unclear. This patient did not have hyperlipidemia, as demonstrated by multiple measurements of serum cholesterol and triglycerides. Thus, these deposits cannot be regarded as consequences of hypercholesterolemia. The deposits in the bioprosthesis from our patient were localized mainly on the outflow (ventricular) surface of the bioprosthesis, the site receiving the highest ventricular pressure. It was surprising to find that these deposits were not in association with a foreign body reaction or any other type of inflammatory infiltrate, such as occurs with cholesterol deposits in other areas of the body. This lack of inflammatory reaction probably was due to the fact that the cholesterol crystals were localized within the glutaraldehyde-fixed porcine valvular tissue, which usually is not invaded by inflammatory cells.[1] These deposits probably are derived from circulating plasma lipoproteins, since there were no cells identified in adjacent areas of valvular tissue which could have synthesized these large amounts of cholesterol *in situ*. Morphologic observations on valvular bioprostheses implanted for eight years or longer have been few, and it remains to be determined how prevalent this change is in these bioprostheses. This is difficult to judge from review of gross anatomic and histologic observations. On gross anatomic study, these deposits can resemble calcific deposits, which also appear as pale nodules. It is possible that mild degrees of this alteration are relatively frequent, but are not detected by study of routine histologic sections, from which the cholesterol is removed during tissue processing. Polarized light microscopy of frozen sections is the method of choice for the demonstration of these cholesterol deposits.

ACKNOWLEDGMENT: We are grateful to Dr. Jeffrey M. Hoeg of the Molecular Disease Branch, National Heart, Lung, and Blood Institute, for performing the cholesterol analyses.

REFERENCES

1. Ferrans VJ, Spray TL, Billingham ME, Roberts WC. Structural changes in glutaraldehyde-treated porcine heterografts used as substitute cardiac valves: Transmission and scanning electron microscopic observations in 12 patients. Am J Cardiol 1978; 41:1159–1184

2. Stanley P, Chartrand C, Davignon A. Acquired aortic stenosis in a twelve-year-old girl with xanthomatosis. N Engl J Med 1965; 273:1378–1380

3. Rothbard S, Hagstrom JWC, Smith JP. Aortic stenosis and myocardial infarction in hypercholesterolemic xanthomatosis. Am Heart J 1967; 73:687–692

4. Wennevold A, Jacobsen JG. Acquired supravalvular aortic stenosis in familial hypercholesterolemia: a hemodynamic and angiographic study. Am J Med 1971; 50:823–827

5. Barr DP, Rothbard S, Eder HA. Atherosclerosis and aortic stenosis in hypercholesteremic xanthomatosis. JAMA 1954; 156:943–947

6. McCleary JE, Brunsting LA, Kennedy RLJ. Primary xanthoma tuberosum in children; with classification of xanthomas. Pediatrics 1959; 23:67–75

7. Desnick RJ, Blieden LC, Sharp HL, Hofschire PJ, Moller JH. Cardiac valvular anomalies in Fabry disease: clinical, morphologic, and biochemical studies. Circulation 1976; 54:818–825

8. Ferrans VJ, Hibbs RG, Burda CD. The heart in Fabry's disease: a histochemical and electron microscopic study. Am J Cardiol 1969; 24:95–110

9. Farber S, Cohen J, Uzman LL. Lipogranulomatosis. A new lipoglycoprotein "storage" disease. Mt Sinai J Med (NY) 1957; 24:816–837

10. Gonatas NK, Gonatas J. Ultrastructural and biochemical observations on a case of systemic late infantile lipidosis and its relationship to Tay-Sachs disease and gargoylism. J Neuropathol Exp Neurol 1965; 24:318–340

11. Hadley RN, Hagstrom JWC. Cardiac lesions in a patient with familial neurovisceral lipidosis (generalized gangliosidosis). Am J Clin Pathol 1971; 55:237–240

12. Blieden LC, Desnick RJ, Carter JB, Krivit W, Moller JH, Sharp HL. Cardiac involvement in Sandhoffs disease: inborn error of glycosphingolipid metabolism. Am J Cardiol 1974; 34:83–88

13. Fredrickson DS, Ferrans VJ. Acid cholesteryl ester hydrolase deficiency. (Wolmans disease and cholesteryl ester storage disease). In: Stanbury JB, et al, eds. The metabolic basis of inherited disease, 4th ed. New York: McGraw-Hill, 1978:670–687

14. Kim KM, Valigorsky JM, Mergner WJ, et al. Aging changes in the human aortic valve in relation to dystrophic calcification. Hum Pathol 1976; 7:47–60

15. Roberts WC, Perloff JK. Mitral valvular disease: a clinicopathologic survey of the conditions causing the mitral valve to function abnormally. Ann Intern Med 1972; 77:939–975

16. Carmen R, Mutha SC. Lipid absorption by silicone rubber heart valve poppets—in vivo and in vitro results. J Biomed Material Res 1972; 6:327–346

Case 543 Severe Mitral Regurgitation Immediately After Mitral Valve Replacement with a Parietal Pericardial Bovine Bioprosthesis

Marc A. Silver, MD, Philip R. Orenburg, MD and William C. Roberts, MD

The occurrence of severe mitral regurgitation (MR) immediately after mitral valve replacement (MVR) is exceedingly rare. One cause is interference with closure of a prosthetic occluder by the left ventricular wall, calcific deposits, or residual unexcised mitral leaflet or chordae tendineae.[1] Another cause is incomplete obliteration by suture of the space between the prosthetic or bioprosthetic ring and the native anulus, resulting in a paraanular communication.[1] A third and hitherto unreported cause of severe MR immediately after MVR by a bioprosthesis is described in the patient below.

A 64-year-old man who had had a precordial systolic murmur for many years had been asymptomatic until 25 days before MVR, when signs of active infective endocarditis appeared; severe congestive heart failure followed shortly thereafter. Group B beta hemolytic streptococcus was grown on blood cultures. A grade 3/6 precordial apical systolic blowing murmur consistent with MR was audible. The pulmonary arterial wedge mean pressure was 35, V-wave 50, and pulmonary arterial pressure 57/20 mm Hg. At MVR, a vegetation was present on the posterior mitral leaflet to which several chordae had ruptured; the leaflet appeared to prolapse toward left atrium. The purely regurgitant valve was replaced with a 25-mm Ionescu-Shiley bioprosthesis. The patient's early postoperative course was characterized by systemic hypotension and coma. A murmur consistent with MR was heard on precordial examination 2 days after operation. He died 8 days after operation, never having regained consciousness. At necropsy, the heart weighed 690 g. Sutures surrounded 2 of the 3 stents of the mitral bioprosthesis, causing a straight-line stretching of the margins of the bioprosthetic cusps between the 3 commissures. The result was a triangular-shaped severely incompetent bioprosthetic orifice (Figure 1).

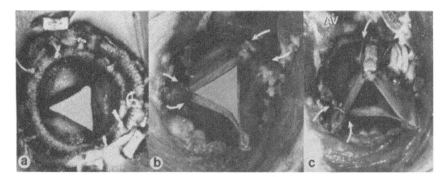

Figure 1 Mitral bioprosthesis in the patient described. **a**, view from left atrium showing a triangular orifice. **b and c**, 2 views from the left ventricular aspect. The arrows point to the 2 sutures which encircled the stents, causing tautness of the cusps and preventing them from coapting during ventricular systole.

From the Pathology Branch, National Heart, Lung, and Blood Institute, National Institutes of Health, Bethesda, Maryland. Manuscript received and accepted April 5, 1983.

DOI: 10.1201/9781003409281-28

Thus, sutures encircling 2 of the 3 bioprosthetic stents tautened the cusps, producing severe MR. The left atrium should not be closed after MVR until it is clear that the cusps of a tissue valve or the occluder of a mechanical valve[2] are freely mobile.

REFERENCES

1. **Roberts WC.** Complications of cardiac valve replacement: characteristic abnormalities of prostheses pertaining to any or specific site. Am Heart J 1982;103:113–122.
2. **Jones AA, Oils JB, Fletcher GF, Roberts WC.** A hitherto undescribed cause of prosthetic mitral valve obstruction. J Thorac Cardiovasc Surg 1977;74:116–117.

Case 633 Fatal Bioprosthetic Regurgitation *Immediately After* Mitral and Tricuspid Valve Replacements with Ionescu-Shiley Bioprostheses

Wanda M. Lester, MD and William C. Roberts, MD

Significant cardiac valve regurgitation *immediately after* cardiac valve replacement is rare. Silver et al[1] described a patient who had severe bioprosthetic regurgitation immediately after replacement of the mitral valve with an Ionescu-Shiley bioprosthesis. The regurgitation resulted from inadvertent encircling of 2 of the 3 stents of the bioprosthesis by sutures, which prevented mobility of the cusps and closure of the bioprosthetic orifice. In this report we describe another patient in whom a similar mechanism caused severe bioprosthetic regurgitation in both mitral and tricuspid valve positions. Because this mechanism of development of severe bioprosthetic regurgitation is apparently not well appreciated, we describe this second patient in hopes of preventing this fatal complication in others.

E.R., a 55-year-old woman, died shortly after her fifth cardiac operation. She had had mitral commissurotomies when 26 and 35 years old, aortic (Björk-Shiley) and mitral (Hancock) valve replacements when 46 years old, and tricuspid valve replacement (Hancock) 1 month later. Apart from an intracranial hemorrhage later in the same year (1976), which led to cessation of warfarin therapy and the use öf aspirin and dipyridamole, she did well until about 4 months before death, when exertional dyspnea, easy fatigability, abdominal swelling and leg edema developed. Because of worsening symptoms and signs, she was hospitalized 2 months later. The neck veins were distended while she was sitting up and v waves were visible. Rales were present over both lower lung fields. The liver was large and pulsatile. Electrocardiogram showed atrial fibrillation and right bundle branch block. At cardiac catheterization, the pressures (in mm Hg) were: right atrial mean 14, v wave 18; right ventricle, 70/16; pulmonary artery, 70/25 (mean 35); pulmonary arterial wedge mean 13, v wave 16; left ventricle, 110/12, and aorta, 110/60. The mean diastolic gradient between pulmonary artery wedge position and left ventricle was 5 mm Hg and the mean gradient between right atrium and right ventricle was 2 mm Hg. On left ventricular angiogram, the bioprosthesis in the mitral position was competent. The ejection fraction was 44%. Selective coronary angiograms showed no abnormalities. Aortogram disclosed 1+/4+ aortic regurgitation. The cardiac index was 2.1 liters/min/m². Pulmonary function tests were consistent with moderate to severe pulmonary obstructive disease.

The Hancock bioprosthesis in the mitral position was replaced with a size 27 and the Hancock bioprosthesis in the tricuspid position was replaced with a size 29 Ionescu-Shiley bioprosthesis. Poor cardiac output with some excessive bleeding was evident immediately after discontinuing bypass. The patient died about 8 hours after beginning the operation. Each cusp of the excised Hancock bioprostheses was intact and both valve orifices were competent. At necropsy, 1 stent of the bioprosthesis in the tricuspid valve position had burrowed into the right ventricular myocardium, and 1 stent of this bioprosthesis was surrounded by a suture (Figures 1 and 2). The consequence of these 2 misadventures was a straightening of the free margins of 2 of the 3 cusps so that this bioprosthetic orifice was fixed in

From the Pathology Branch, National Heart, Lung, and Blood Institute, National Institutes of Health, Bethesda, Maryland 20205. Dr. Lester had a fellowship from the Canadian Heart Foundation. Manuscript received and accepted November 5, 1984.

DOI: 10.1201/9781003409281-29

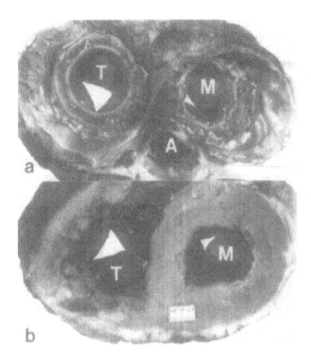

Figure 1   **a**, heart after removal of the atrial walls showing the bioprostheses in the tricuspid (T) and mitral (M) valve positions. The orifices of both bioprostheses are open and triangular in shape. The Björk-Shiley mechanical prosthesis in the aortic (A) valve position appeared to have functioned well. **b**, view from the ventricular aspect.

an open triangular-shaped position. One suture used to insert the bioprosthesis in the mitral position crossed 2 of the 3 bioprosthetic cusps, making each immobile and preventing closure of the bioprosthetic orifices (Figures 1 and 2). The occluder of the Björk-Shiley prosthesis in the aortic valve position moved normally.

The fifth and last operation in the patient was done because of distended neck veins, subcutaneous edema and ascites, findings believed to have resulted from regurgitation of the bioprosthetic valve in the tricuspid valve position. The presence or absence of regurgitation was not confirmed by right ventricular angiography. At operation, no peribasilar bioprosthetic communications were present, each of the 3 cusps of both bioprostheses was intact, and both orifices appeared to close satisfactorily. After replacement of the bioprostheses in both tricuspid and mitral valve positions with "new"—and larger—bioprostheses, the patient had evidence of severe low cardiac output. Necropsy disclosed that at least 2 of the 3 cusps of each of the 2 newly inserted bioprostheses were immobile because either inadvertent suture on the ventricular aspects of the bioprosthetic orifices or burrowing of a stent into the myocardial wall had caused straightening of the distal margins of the bioprosthetic cusps and prevented cuspal movements so that the bioprosthetic orifices could not close during ventricular systole. Had smaller bioprostheses been used in this 81-pound, 61-inch-tall woman, possibly inadvertent anchoring of the sutures over the margins of the cusps and the burrowing of 1 stent into a myocardial wall would have been prevented. It is, of course, unwise to close an atriotomy incision until the

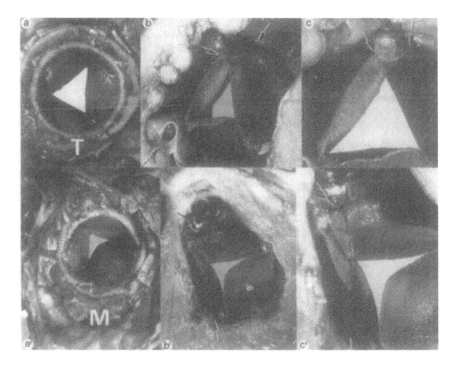

Figure 2 Close-up views of the Ionescu-Shiley bioprostheses in the tricuspid (T) and mitral (M) valve positions. **a** and **a′**, from the atrial aspects, the orifices of each are fixed in a triangular shape. **b**, 1 stent (**dashed arrow**) has burrowed into thê right ventricular free wall. One stent is encircled by a suture (**curved solid arrows**). **b′**, 1 suture (**arrows**) crosses 2 bioprosthetic cusps holding each rigidly in place. The Björk-Shiley prosthesis is visible at the **upper left. c**, another view of the suture encircling the stent. **c′**, close-up of the suture inadvertently holding down 2 biopros- thetic cusps. (Photographs by M.M.M. Moore.)

operator has satisfactorily shown that each cusp of the bioprosthesis is freely mobile, a requirement to prevent bioprosthetic regurgitation.

REFERENCE

1. **Silver MA, Orenburg PR, Roberts WC.** Severe mitral regurgitation after mitral valve replacement with a parietal pericardial bovine bioprosthesis. Am J Cardiol 1983;52:218–219.

Case 724 Extensive Calcification of a Bioprosthesis in the Tricuspid Valve Position and Minimal Calcification of a Simultaneously Implanted Bioprosthesis in the Mitral Valve Position

Deborah J. Barbour, MD, Charles L. Mcintosh, MD, PhD, and William C. Roberts, MD

Previous reports describing results of simultaneously implanted and explanted porcine bioprostheses in the mitral and aortic valve positions[1,2] and mitral and tricuspid valve positions[3] have shown greater degeneration in those bioprostheses in the mitral position than in either aortic or tricuspid valve positions. The reasons for the more rapid degeneration of the bioprostheses in the mitral position than in either the aortic or tricuspid valve positions are not clear, but probably are related to the higher closing pressure on the bioprosthetic cusps in the mitral position. In contrast to previous observations, a patient who had recently undergone study had much heavier calcific deposits on the cusps of the bioprosthesis in the tricuspid valve position than on those of the bioprosthesis in the mitral position. A brief description of this patient follows.

T.H., a 38-year-old Greek woman, had a mitral valve commissurotomy at age 19 years. By age 29, anasarca prompted cardiac catheterization (Table 1) and then simultaneous tricuspid and mitral valve replacements with 31- and 27-mm Hancock porcine bioprostheses for pure tricuspid valve regurgitation and mitral valve stenosis. She did well for 7 years, and then peripheral edema, dyspnea, anasarca and dizziness occurred. Catheterization (Table 1) at age 37 revealed severe stenosis of the bioprosthesis in the tricuspid valve position and moderate stenosis of the bioprosthesis in the mitral valve position, and 105 months after their initial simultaneous implantation, both bioprostheses were replaced, a 29-mm Hancock porcine bioprosthesis in the tricuspid position and a Starr-Edwards mechanical prosthesis in the mitral position. At operation, thrombus was removed from both atria. The bioprosthesis explanted from the tricuspid valve position had far heavier calcific deposits than did the one explanted from the mitral position (Figure 1).

The cause of the greater degree of calcium on the bioprosthetic cusps in the tricuspid valve position than on the bioprosthetic cusps in the mitral valve position

Table 1: Hemodynamic data

Age (yr)	PA (S/d)	RV (s/d)	RA (m)	RA-RV mdg	LV (s/d)	SA (s/d)	PAW (m)	PAW-LV mdg	CI
29	115/60	115/18	18	0	105/12	105/65	25	17	1.8
38	32/19	32/4	16	13	95/4	100/60	12	11	2.4

Pressures are in mm Hg.
CI = cardiac index in liters/min/m²; LV = left ventricle; m = mean; mdg = mean diastolic gradient; PA = pulmonary artery; PAW = pulmonary artery wedge; RA = right atrium; RV = right ventricle; SA = systemic artery; s/d = peak systole/end diastole.

From the Pathology and Surgery Branches, National Heart, Lung, and Blood Institutes, National Institutes of Health, Bethesda, Maryland 20892. Manuscript received and accepted July 1, 1986.

DOI: 10.1201/9781003409281-30

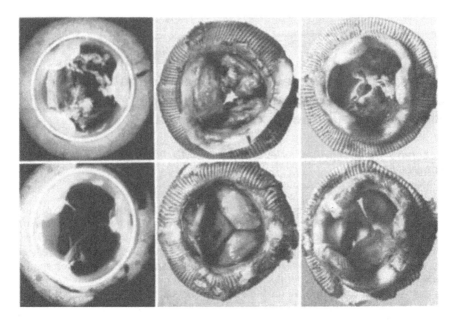

Figure 1 Explanted bioprostheses. *Upper panel*, radiograph *(left)* and photographs *(center* and *right)* of the bioprosthesis explanted from the tricuspid valve position; *lower panel*, radiograph *(left)* and photographs *(center* and *right)* of the bioprosthesis explanted from the mitral position. The photographs in the *center* are the atrial aspect of the bioprosthesis and those at the *right*, the ventricular aspect.

was not determined. The closing pressure on the bioprosthesis in the tricuspid valve position was only one-third of that on the bioprosthetic cusps in the mitral position (32 vs 95 mm Hg).

REFERENCES

1. Warnes CA, Scott ML, Silver GM, Smith CW, Ferrans VJ, Roberts WC. Comparison of late degenerative changes in porcine bioprostheses in the mitral and aortic valve position in the same patient. *Am J Cardiol* 1983;51:965–968.
2. Cipriano PR, Billingham ME, Miller DC. Calcification of aortic versus mitral porcine bioprosthetic heart valves; a radiographic study comparing amounts of calcific deposits in valves explanted from the same patient. *Am J Cardiol* 1984;54:1030–1032.
3. Cohen SR, Silver MA, McIntosh CL, Roberts WC. Comparison of late (62 to 140 months) degenerative changes in simultaneously implanted and explanted porcine (Hancock) bioprostheses in the tricuspid and mitral valve positions in six patients. *Am J Cardiol* 1984;53;1599–1602.

Case 788 Bioprostheses in Tricuspid and Mitral Valve Positions for 100 Months with Heavier Calcific Deposits on the Left-Sided Valve Followed by New Bioprostheses in Both Positions for 95 Months with Heavier Calcific Deposits on the Right-Sided Valve

Benjamin N. Potkin, MD Charles L. Mcintosh, MD, PhD, Richard O. Cannon III, MD, William C. Roberts, MD

Previous reports describing results of simultaneously implanted and explanted bioprostheses in the mitral and aortic valve positions and in the mitral and tricuspid positions usually, but not always, have shown greater degeneration of the bioprostheses in the mitral position than in either the aortic or tricuspid valve position, presumably because of the higher closing pressure on the bioprosthetic cusps in the mitral position.[1-4] Herein, we describe a patient who had simultaneous bioprosthetic replacement of both mitral and tricuspid valves. Later replacement of both bioprostheses revealed heavier calcific deposits on the bioprosthesis in the mitral position after the first bioprosthetic replacement and heavier calcific deposits on the bioprosthesis in the tricuspid valve position after the second bioprosthetic replacement.

E.V., a 62-year-old white woman with systemic hypertension and diabetes mellitus, had 4 cardiac valve operations (Table 1). Congestive heart failure developed during her second pregnancy and 1 year later, at age 35, she underwent closed mitral commissurotomy for mitral stenosis. She was nearly asymptomatic for 2 years thereafter and then congestive heart failure and atrial fibrillation developed. Because of worsening congestive heart failure, at age 46 she had simultaneous replacement of both native mitral and tricuspid valves with Hancock no. 29 and 31 glutaraldehype processed bioprostheses, respectively. She was asymptomatic for the next 8 years when congestive heart failure reappeared at age 54. Left ventricular cineangiogram now demonstrated 4+/4+ mitral regurgitation and a 22 mm Hg mean diastolic pressure gradient across the bioprosthesis in the mitral position. At age 54, the 2 bioprostheses, each of which had been in place for 100 months, were excised along with the diffusely thickened, purely regurgitant aortic valve and all 3 were replaced with Hancock bioprostheses. The excised bioprosthesis in the mitral position had heavier calcific deposits than did the bioprosthesis in the tricuspid valve position (Figure 1). Postoperatively, she again was asymptomatic. Catheterization, 7 months later, disclosed a 11 mm Hg mean diastolic pressure gradient across the bioprosthesis in the mitral position. Pulmonary hypertension persisted. Congestive heart failure recurred at age 61 years, 86 months after the last operation. Nine months later or 3 days before death the 3 bioprosthetic valves were replaced because of refractory congestive heart failure. The bioprosthesis that had been in the tricuspid valve position had heavier calcific deposits than that present on the bioprostheses that had been in either the mitral or aortic valve position (Figure 2).

This patient is unique in that 2 prostheses had each been in place for 100 months and 3 other bioprostheses had each been in place for 95 months. When the initially inserted 2 bioprostheses were explanted, heavier calcific deposits were present in the bioprosthesis that had been in the mitral valve position compared with the one that

From the Pathology, Surgery and Cardiology Branches, National Heart, Lung, and Blood Institute, National Institues of Health, Bethesda, Maryland 20892. Manuscript received October 15, 1987; revised manuscript received and accepted November 13, 1987.

DOI: 10.1201/9781003409281-31

173

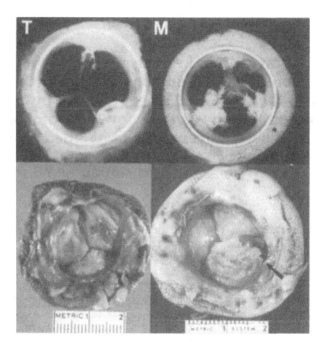

Figure 1 Radiographs (*top*) and photographs (*bottom*) of bioprostheses that had been in place in the tricuspid (T) and mitral (M) valve positions for 100 months. Heavier calcific deposits are present in the prosthesis that had been in the mitral valve position. Additionally, 1 cusp of the prosthesis in the mitral position was torn (*arrow*) and this bioprosthesis was severely regurgitant.

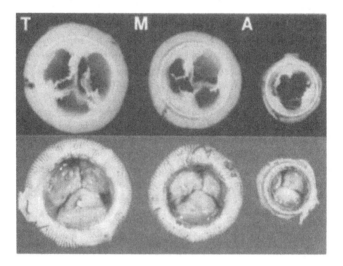

Figure 2 Radiographs (*top*) and photographs (*bottom*) of bioprostheses explanted 3 days before death and which had been in place in the tricuspid (T), mitral (M) and aortic (A) valve positions for 95 months. Heavier calcific deposits are present in the bioprosthesis in the tricuspid valve position than in the bioprosthesis in either the mitral or aortic valve positions.

had been in the tricuspid valve position. When these malfunctioning bioprostheses were excised and replaced with other bioprostheses that were in place for nearly the same amount of time, namely 95 months, heavier calcific deposits developed in the bioprosthesis that had been in the tricuspid valve position compared with that occurring in either bioprosthesis located on the left side of the heart.

The explanation for the reversal of the heavier calcific deposits in the tricuspid and mitral valve positions during the 2 time frames (100 months with the initially inserted bioprostheses and 95 months with the replaced bioprostheses) is unclear. It is likely that during much of the postoperative period after the initial double valve replacement the right ventricular systolic pressure, which represents the closing pressure on the bioprosthesis in the tricuspid valve position, was only mildly elevated (37 mm Hg). In contrast, after the bioprostheses in the tricuspid and mitral valve positions were replaced, the right ventricular systolic pressure remained elevated (65 mm Hg), probably during the entire 95-month period. During this latter 95-month period of high right ventricular systolic pressures, heavier calcific deposits developed on the cusps of the bioprosthesis in the tricuspid valve position than on the cusps of the bioprosthesis in the mitral valve position. The closing pressure, i.e., the left ventricular systolic pressure, on the bioprosthesis in the mitral position, however, was always considerably higher than was the closing pressure on the bioprosthesis in the tricuspid valve position: 160 vs 37 mm Hg after the first valve replacements and 210 vs 65 mm Hg after the bioprosthetic replacements. Thus, factors other than bioprosthetic closing pressures must have played a role in determining which bioprosthesis in the atrioventricular valve positions contained the heavier calcific deposits.

Table 1: Patient's hemodynamic data

Month/year	5/1970	8/1971	6/1979	1/1980	8/1986
Age (yr)	45	46	54	55	61
NYHA FC	III	I	III	I	III
SA (s/d)	160/95	150/90	112/70	205/90	137/76
RA V (mean)	25 (18)	14 (10)	26 (22)	16 (13)	22 (20)
RV (s/d)	60/9	37/7	75/16	65/7	67/20
PA (s/d)	60/30	37/20	80/40	65/28	68/28
PAW V (mean)	34 (25)	26 (20)	47 (38)	40 (28)	34 (25)
LV (s/d)	155/16	160/12	117/16	210/25	158/17
CO/CI	5.4/3.1	6.3/3.8	2.2/1.4	5.2/3.3	4.0/2.5
LV-SA psg	0	10	0	5	21
PAW-LV mdg	13	8	22	11	10
RA-RV mdg	6	7	8	7	6
MVA/MVI	*0.8/0.5	2.8/1.7	†	2.1/1.3	1.3/0.8
TVA/TVI	—	2.2/1.3	1.4/0.9	1.4/0.9	1.4/0.9
AR by AA cine (0 to 4+)	0	0	2+/4+	0	1+/4+
MR by LV cine (0 to 4+)	1+/4+	0	4+/4+	0	0

All pressures are in mm Hg. All valve replacements were with Hancock bioprosthesis (size in parenthesis): mitral commissurotomy, 1959; MVR (29) and TVR (31), 2/1971; MVR (27), TVR (31) and AVR (19), 6/1979.
* Calculated valve area underestimated because of mild mitral regurgitation.
† Not possible to calculate valve area because of severe mitral regurgitation.
AA = ascending aorta; AR = aortic regurgitation; AVR = aortic valve replacement; CI = cardiac index (liters/min/m²); Cine = cineangiography; CO = cardiac output (liters/min); LV = left ventricular; mdg = mean diastolic gradient; MR = mitral regurgitation; MVA = mitral valve area; MVI = mitral valve index; MVR = mitral valve replacement; NYHA FC = New York Heart Association functional class; PA = pulmonary artery; PAW = pulmonary artery wedge pressure; psg = peak systolic gradient; RA = right arterial; RV = right ventricular; SA = systemic artery; s/d = systolic/diastolic; TVA = tricuspid valve area; TVI = tricuspid valve index; TVR = tricuspid valve replacement.

REFERENCES

1. Warnes CA, Scott ML, Silver GM, Smith CW, Ferrans VJ, Roberts WC. Comparison of late degenerative changes in porcine bioprostheses in the mitral and aortic valve position in the same patient. *Am J Cardiol* 1983;51:965–968.
2. Cipriano PR, Billingham ME, Miller DC. Calcification of aortic versus mitral porcine bioprosthetic heart valves: a radiographic study comparing amounts of calcific deposits in valves explanted from the same patient. *Am J Cardiol* 1984;54:1030–1032.
3. Cohen SR, Silver MA, McIntosh CL, Roberts WC. Comparison of late (62 to 140 months) degenerative changes in simultaneously implanted and explanted porcine (Hancock) bioprostheses in the tricuspid and mitral valve positions in six patients. *Am J Cardiol* 1984;53:1599–1602.
4. Barbour DJ, McIntosh CL, Roberts WC. Extensive calcification of a bioprosthesis in the tricuspid valve position and minimal calcification of a simultaneously implanted bioprosthesis in the mitral valve position. *Am J Cardiol* 1987;59:179–180.

Case 806 "Quadricuspidization" of a Previously Three-Cusp Aortic Valve

Jessica M. Mann, MD, and William C. Roberts, MD
Bethesda, MD

Quadricuspid aortic valves have always been described as congenital in origin.[1-4] Surgical manipulation of a previously normal tri-cuspid aortic valve may transform the latter into a quadricuspid valve. Such was the case in the patient described below.

R.B., a 39-year-old man, was found at age 13 years to have discrete subaortic stenosis with a left ventricular (230/8 mm Hg)-to-aortic (96/60 mm Hg) peak systolic pressure gradient of 134 mm Hg. The cardiac index was 3.6 L/min/m². When he was 13 years old he underwent resection of a subaortic "membrane" by Dr. Andrew G. Morrow. At operation, the aortic valve was described as tri-cuspid and each cusp was normal. The patient was asymptomatic after operation. At age 16, no peak systolic pressure gradient between the left ventricle and the aortic valve was present, but an aortic angiogram disclosed 2+/4+ aortic regurgitation. At age 30, he had several dizzy spells and a Holter monitor disclosed multifocal ventricular premature complexes and runs of ventricular tachycardia. Serial echocardiograms showed anterior mitral leaflet flutter and progressive left ventricular dilatation,

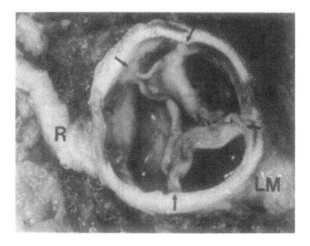

Figure 1 View of the acquired quadricuspid aortic valve from the aorta. The four cusps are thickened by fibrous tissue and some degree of commissural fusion is present. *Arrows* point out the four commissures. The accessory cusp is posterior and smaller than the "true" posterior cusp. *LM* = left main coronary artery; *R* = right coronary artery.

From the Pathology Branch, National Heart, Lung, and Blood Institute, National Institutes of Health.

Reprint requests: Pathology Branch, NHLBI-NIH, Bldg. 10, Room 2N-258, Bethesda, MD 20892.

DOI: 10.1201/9781003409281-32

with a left ventricular diastolic dimension increasing from 66 to 80 mm and the systolic dimension increasing from 38 to 58 mm. He died suddenly at home at age 39. At necropsy, the heart weighed 560 gm. The left ventricular outflow tract was not narrowed. No foci of myocardial fibrosis or necrosis were present. The aortic valve was quadri-cuspid with two posterior cusps of unequal size (Figure 1). The coronary arterial system was right-dominant, and all three coronary arteries had wide-open lumens.

Although there are no photographs to document the appearance of the aortic valve at operation 26 years before death, the surgeon, Andrew G. Morrow, was an excellent describer of both normal and abnormal cardiovascular findings at operation, and consequently there can be little doubt that the aortic valve consisted of three normal cusps at that time. Aortic regurgitation was noted for the first time 2 years after operation, and it persisted for the remaining 24 years of life. Thus operative manipulation of the aortic valve during operative resection of discrete subaortic stenosis can lead to transformation of a tricuspid into a quadricuspid aortic valve.

REFERENCES

1. Simonds JP. Congenital malformations of the aortic and pulmonary valves. *Am J Med Sci* 1923;166:584–595.
2. Robicsek F, Sanger PW, Daugherty HK, Montgomery CC. Congenital quadri-cuspid aortic valve with displacement of the left coronary orifice. *Am J Cardiol* 1969;23:288–290.
3. Luisi VS, Pasque A, Vernelli F, Aliboni M, Urbano V, Reginato E. Quadricuspid aortic valve. *J Cardiovasc Surg* 1984;25:252–254.
4. Matsumoto M, Miki S, Kusuhara K, Ueda Y, Ohkita Y, Tahata T, Komeda M. Quadricuspid aortic valve associated with severe aortic regurgitation. *Jpn Circ J* 1984;49:190–191.

Case 811 Development of Severe Stenosis in a Previously Purely Regurgitant, Congenitally Bicuspid Aortic Valve

Jay M. Kalan, MD, Charles L. McIntosh, MD, PhD, Robert O. Bonow, MD, and William C. Roberts, MD

A congenitally bicuspid aortic valve may function normally, it may be stenotic with or without associated regurgitation or it may be purely regurgitant (no associated stenosis).[1,2] Such a valve may function normally for many years and then it may become stenotic (as calcific deposits build up) or it may become purely regurgitant (because of superimposed infective endocarditis or because of reasons unclear). Once a bicuspid valve develops some degree of stenosis, its course thereafter is one of gradually worsening stenosis; once a bicuspid valve develops some degree of pure regurgitation (without associated stenosis), its course thereafter is one of gradually worsening regurgitation. Recently, we encountered a man who 8 years earlier had evidence of severe pure aortic regurgitation (no element of stenosis) and thereafter he went on to develop severe aortic valve stenosis with virtual loss of the regurgitation. To our knowledge, conversion from pure aortic regurgitation to severe aortic stenosis has not been reported. This report records such an occurrence.

A.H., a 70-year-old white man, had a precordial murmur when inducted into the armed forces at about age 25. At age 60, two transient episodes of paroxysmal nocturnal dyspnea occurred and digoxin therapy was started. He remained without symptoms of cardiac dysfunction, able to swim and play tennis, until age 70, when aortic valve replacement was done. At age 62 (1979) his blood pressure was 160/ 70 mm Hg. Peripheral signs of aortic regurgitation were present, including a rapid carotid artery upstroke, water-hammer pulse and Quincke's sign. A grade 3/6 precordial systolic ejection murmur radiated to the neck, and a grade 3/6 diastolic blow was present and loudest at the left sternal border. Echocardiographic and catheterization data are shown in Table 1 and Figure 1. Ejection fraction by radionuclide angiography was 63% at rest and 52% with exercise. Exercise capacity by exercise stress test was good. He remained asymptomatic but gradually developed left ventricular hypertrophy without dilatation (Table 1). At age 70, transient second-degree heart block was seen on electrocardiogram. The systemic blood pressure was 130/90 mm Hg and the carotid upstroke was delayed. A harsh, grade 4/6 systolic precordial murmur that radiated to the neck was present. No precordial diastolic murmur was heard. Cardiac catheterization (Table 1) now showed a 75-mm Hg peak systolic pressure gradient across the aortic valve (Figure 1). The aortic valve was replaced (August 1987) with a 23-mm Hancock porcine bioprosthesis. Seven months postoperatively, he is asymptomatic and active, with an ejection fraction by radionuclide angiography of 70% at rest.

The excised native aortic valve consisted of 2 cusps weighing together 5.9 g (Figure 2). The posterior cusp was mobile but thickened by fibrous tissue; it contained a single small deposit of calcium. The anterior cusp, in contrast, was immobile and contained heavy calcific deposits.

From the Pathology, Surgery and Cardiology Branches, National Heart, Lung, and Blood Institute, National Institutes of Health, Bethesda, Maryland 20892. Manuscript received May 19, 1988; revised manuscript received and accepted June 19, 1988.

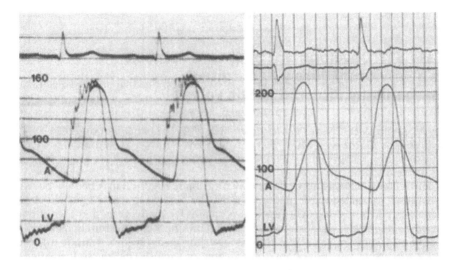

Figure 1 Simultaneous pressure tracings from the aorta (A) and left ventricle (LV) at catheterization at age 62 (*left*) and at age 70 *(right)*. The left tracing shows no pressure gradient at peak systole across the aortic valve and the right tracing shows a 75-mm Hg peak systolic pressure gradient across the aortic valve.

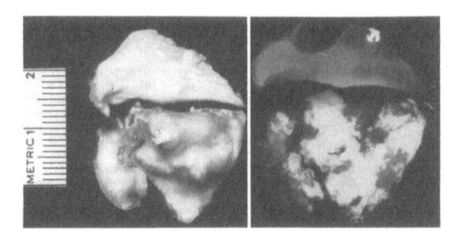

Figure 2 Photograph and roentgenogram of the excised aortic valve showing heavy calcific deposits in the anterior cusp and a single small deposit in the posterior cusp.

When calcium is deposited on a congenitally bicuspid valve, it usually is distributed relatively evenly on each of the 2 cusps.[1] In the aforementioned patient, 1 cusp contained heavy deposits and the second was nearly devoid of calcific deposits. The reason for this uneven distribution of the calcific deposits is unclear. There was never clinical evidence of infective endocarditis. The cause of the valvular stenosis was the deposition on one of the cusps of extremely heavy calcific deposits that made this cusp, which was larger than the other cusp, completely immobile. The

Table 1: Echocardiographic and catheterization data

	Age 62	Age 70
Dimensions		
Left ventricular wall (mm)	12	18
Left ventricular cavity (ed/ps) (mm)	60/35	53/35
Fractional shortening (%)	42	34
Pressures (mm Hg)		
Right atrium (mean)	7	7
Right ventricle (ps/ed)	30/10	32/8
Pulmonary artery (ps/ed)	28/12	28/15
Pulmonary artery wedge (mean)	12	10
Left atrium (mean)	12	10
Left ventricle (ps/ed)	155/13	210/17
Aorta (ps/ed)	155/60	135/70
Aorta to left ventricle peak systolic gradient	0	75
Cineangiogram		
Aortic regurgitation	3+/4	trace
Aortic valve calcium	0	3+/4+
Cardiac output (liter/min)	5.7	6.5
Cardiac index (liter/min/m2)	2.8	3.1

Ed/ps = end-diastole/peak systole.

explanation for the deposition of heavy deposits of calcium on a previously purely regurgitant aortic valve is unclear, but such a documentation has not been recorded previously.

REFERENCES

1. Roberts WC. The congenitally bicuspid aortic valve. A study of 85 autopsy cases. *Am J Cardiol* 1970;26:72–83.
2. Roberts WC, Morrow AG, McIntosh CL, Jones M, Epstein SE. Congenitally bicuspid aortic valve causing severe, pure aortic regurgitation without superimposed infective endocarditis. Analysis of 13 patients requiring aortic valve replacement. *Am J Cardiol* 1981;47:206–209.

Case 840 Extensive Multifocal Myocardial Infarcts from Cloth Emboli After Replacement of Mitral and Aortic Valves with Cloth-Covered, Caged-Ball Prostheses

Allen L. Dollar, MD, Marie-Lydie Pierre-Louis, MD, Charles L. McIntosh, MD, PhD, and William C. Roberts, MD

The early Starr-Edwards prosthetic heart valve models (series 1000, 1200 and 1260) contained no cloth on the inner aspects of the ring or on the struts. In an attempt to reduce the frequency of thrombus on the prostheses, a cloth covering was later added to cover the inside portion of the ring and the struts. Almost simultaneously, a stellite poppet was substituted for the silicone rubber poppet in many prostheses. Although these modifications did reduce the frequency of embolic events, a new problem was introduced, namely cloth wear. Cloth wear led in some patients to dysfunction of prostheses, hemolytic anemia and systemic emboli.[1-7] As the cloth on these prosthetic valves wore, cloth occasionally embolized to 1 or more systemic organs. Such resulting organ infarcts were usually not visible on gross inspection.

We recently studied a patient at necropsy who had multiple ventricular scars from cloth emboli from caged-ball prostheses. Such myocardial scars from this etiology have not been described previously.

A 58-year-old man underwent replacements of his stenotic mitral and aortic valves on January 23, 1970, and he died on November 1, 1988. Cloth-covered Starr-Edwards prostheses with metallic poppets, models 2310 and 6310, were implanted. Unilateral occlusion of a central retinal artery occurred at age 53 (13 years postoperatively); it resolved spontaneously and sight returned. A ventricular demand pacemaker was implanted at age 54 because of symptomatic bradycardia. Cardiac catheterization at that time disclosed a 10 mm Hg mean diastolic gradient between the pulmonary artery wedge and left ventricle, and no peak systolic gradient between the left ventricle (140/11 mm Hg) and aorta (140/85 mm Hg). The coronary arteries were normal by angiogram. On echocardiogram, the diameter of the left ventricular cavity was 55 mm in end-diastole and 38 mm in peak systole. Left ventricular fractional shortening was 31%. On evaluation 8 months before death, he was asymptomatic. Death resulted from injuries sustained when, as a pedestrian, he was struck by a truck traveling at a high speed.

Thirteen electrocardiograms recorded from July 16, 1969, to March 16, 1988, were reviewed. Each of the 3 recorded before double valve replacement showed atrial fibrillation, Q waves in leads V_1 through V_3 and total 12-lead QRS amplitudes of 234, 240 and 216 mm (10 mm = 1 mV).[8] The first 8 electrocardiograms recorded from 5 days to 14 years after the double valve replacement also showed Q waves in leads V_1 through V_3 and total 12-lead QRS amplitudes ranging from 129 to 179 mm (mean 164); atrial fibrillation was present in 5 and sinus rhythm in 3 of these 8 electrocardiograms. Two electrocardiograms recorded after the pacemaker was inserted showed total 12-lead QRS amplitudes of 199 and 213 mm, respectively.

From the Pathology and Surgery Branches, National Heart, Lung, and Blood Institute, National Institutes of Health, Bethesda, Maryland 20892, and the District of Columbia Medical Examiner's Office, District of Columbia, Washington, DC. Manuscript received April 19, 1989; revised manuscript received and accepted May 11, 1989.

DOI: 10.1201/9781003409281-34

At necropsy, the heart weighed 545 g. The epicardial coronary arteries were virtually devoid of atherosclerotic plaques. Cloth wear on both struts and rings was severe on both prostheses (Figure 1). There were numerous focal scars measuring 1 to 10 mm in the myocardial walls of both ventricles (Figure 2). Histologic examination revealed focal fibrosis and scattered basophilic staining, slightly refractile, foreign body material occluding

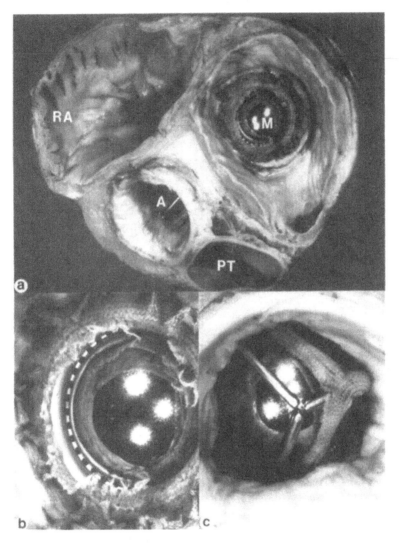

Figure 1 Photographs of the heart in the patient described. *a*, view of atria and great arteries from above showing the cloth-covered Starr-Edwards prostheses in the mitral (M) and aortic (A) valve positions. The cloth on the mitral prosthetic ring is frayed. PT = pulmonary trunk; RA = right atrium. *b*, close-up view of the mitral valve prosthesis from the left atrium with the torn cloth pulled away from the metallic ring. *c*, close-up view of the aortic valve prosthesis viewed from the aorta showing detachment of the cloth covering from each of the 3 struts due to wear of the cloth on the inside of the cage.

183

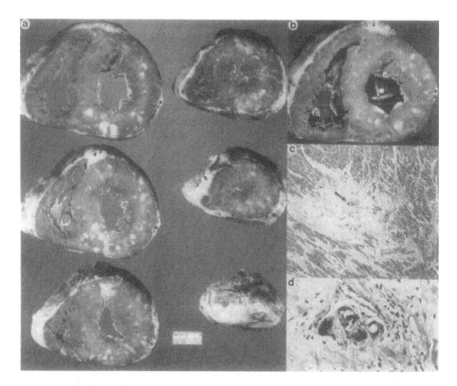

Figure 2 Ventricular myocardium in the patient described. *a*, views of the cardiac ventricles after transverse cutting showing numerous focal scars *(white)* in the walls of both ventricles. *b*, the most basal section showing the Starr-Edwards prosthetic valve in the mitral position. The cloth covering the struts of this valve is intact. *c*, photomicrograph of a portion of left ventricular myocardium showing a focal scar, in the center of which is basophilic staining, foreign body material *(arrow)* surrounded by multinucleated giant cells. *d*, higher power magnification of the embolized foreign-body material and associated giant cells seen in *c*. Hematoxylin and eosin stains, × 32 (*c*), × 250 (*d*).

small intramyocardial arteries, often surrounded by multinucleated giant cells (Figure 2). By polarized light this basophilic material was anisotropic and typical of cloth fragment. Histologic examination of the kidneys and brain disclosed similar foreign body material associated with multinucleated giant cells. The foreign body emboli in these organs was not associated with gross or microscopic scars. No foreign body material was found in lung, liver, spleen, pancreas or thyroid gland.

The extensive focal right and left ventricular wall scarring in this patient is presumed to have resulted from multiple cloth emboli dislodged from the cardiac valve prostheses. Despite these multiple emboli, there were no clinical or electrocardiographic consequences.

REFERENCES

1. Niles NR, Sandilands JR. Pathology of heart valve replacement surgery: autopsies of 62 patients with Starr-Edwards prostheses. *Dis Chest* 1969;56:373–382.
2. Niles NR. Teflon embolism from Starr-Edwards valves. *J Thorac Cardiovasc Surg* 1970;59:794–799.

3. Boruchow IB, Ramsey HW, Wheat MW Jr. Complications following destruction of the cloth covering of a Starr-Edwards aortic valve prosthesis. *J Thorac Cardiovasc Surg* 1971;62:290–293.

4. Thomas CS Jr, Killen DA, Alford WC Jr, Burrus GR, Stoney WS. Cloth disruption in the Starr-Edwards composite mitral valve prosthesis. *Ann Thorac Surg* 1973;15:434–438.

5. Crawford FA, Sethi GK, Scott SM, Takaro T. Systemic emboli due to cloth wear in a Starr-Edwards Model 2320 aortic prosthesis. *Ann Thorac Surg* 1973;16:614–619.

6. Shah A, Dolgin M, Tice DA, Trehan N. Complications due to cloth wear in cloth-covered Starr-Edwards aortic and mitral valve prostheses and their management. *Am Heart J* 1978;96:407–414.

7. Huber S, Burckhardt D, Raeder EA, Follath F, Hasse J, Gradel E. Complications in patients with cloth-covered Starr-Edwards prostheses. *J Cardiovasc Surg* 1980;21:19–24.

8. Siegel RJ, Roberts WC. Electrocardiographic observations in severe aortic valve stenosis: correlative necropsy study to clinical, hemodynamic, and ECG variables demonstrating relation of 12-lead QRS amplitude to peak systolic transaortic pressure gradient. *Am Heart J* 1982;103:210–221.

Case 876 Huge, Unattached Left Atrial Thrombus in Mitral Stenosis

C. S. Roberts, MD, W. C. Roberts, MD

INTRODUCTION

While thrombus isolated to the appendage of the left atrium is common, its presence in the body of the left atrium is infrequent, occurring nearly always in association with mitral stenosis. When thrombus is located in the body of the left atrium and attached to its mural endocardium, similar attached thrombus is virtually always present in the appendage. Nonadherent thrombus in the body of the left atrium is rare, and when it occurs, thrombus is usually absent in the appendage. Wood,[1] in 1814, observed at necropsy an unattached, spherical thrombus in the left atrial body of a 15-year-old girl with mitral stenosis. Abramson,[2] in 1924, found 19 reported necropsy cases aged 15 to 49 years (mean 36) of unattached left atrial thrombus and all 19 patients had associated mitral stenosis. In the last 35 years, only 3 cases of unattached left atrial body thrombus observed at necropsy have been reported. In 1955, Read and associates[3] described a 62-year-old man with a spherical 5 cm left atrial thrombus without associated mitral stenosis. In 1976, Lie and Entman[4] described an 83-year-old woman with a 3.8 cm spherical left atrial thrombus with associated mitral stenosis. In 1981, Söogaard[5] reported a 76-year-old woman with a 4.5 cm left atrial thrombus without associated mitral stenosis. The rarity of unattached left atrial body thrombus prompted the present report.

CASE REPORT

LC, a 75-year-old white woman, who had acute rheumatic fever at age 20 years, was well until age 60 when atrial fibrillation and systemic hypertension were detected. Soon thereafter she had a stroke, resulting in permanent right hemiplegia. At age 75 she had acute onset of aphasia. On examination the next day, she was obese and semiconscious (responded only to painful stimuli). Blood pressure was 140/90 mmHg and arterial pulse was 100 beats/min. A grade 1/6 systolic precordial murmur was recorded. No diastolic precordial murmur was described. The patient's legs were cool and pale and no femoral, popliteal, dorsalis pedal, or posterior tibial arterial pulses were palpated. The electrocardiogram showed atrial flutter with 2:1 atrioventricular block, left anterior hemiblock, and nonspecific ST-segment changes. Translumbar aortogram showed near complete occlusion of the aorta at the level of the renal arteries and distally. She was anuric and acidotic. Bilateral femoral endarterectomy was performed and peritoneal dialysis started, but she died 6 days later.

Surgery and Pathology Branches, National Heart, Lung, and Blood Institute, National Institutes of Health, Bethesda, Maryland, USA

Address for reprints:
Charles Stewart Roberts, M.D.
Surgery Branch
National Heart, Lung and Blood Institute
National Institutes of Health
Bethesda, MD 20892, USA
Received: November 7, 1989
Accepted with revision: January 2, 1990

                                   DOI: 10.1201/9781003409281-35

At necropsy, the heart weighted 500 g. Both atria were dilated. The myocardium was free of grossly visible foci of necrosis or fibrosis. The tricuspid, pulmonic, and aortic valves were normal. The mitral leaflets and chordae tendineae were diffusely fibrotic and the mitral orifice was severely stenotic (Figures 1, 2). The body of the left atrium contained a nonadherent, smooth-surfaced, spherical thrombus weighing 53 g and measuring 4.6 cm in diameter. The abdominal aorta was severely atherosclerotic and aneurysmal, and its lumen was filled with thrombus which obstructed the ostia of both renal arteries, the inferior mesenteric artery, and both common iliac arteries (Figure 3). Both kidneys had multiple cortical infarcts. An old infarct was found in the left cerebral hemisphere. (It is likely that the thrombi in these various systemic arteries were not embolic in nature.)

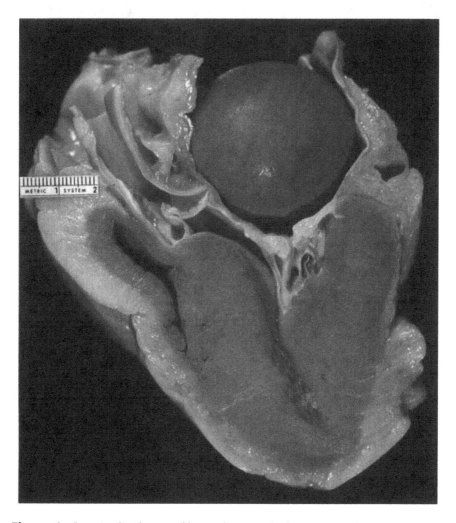

Figure 1 Longitudinal view of heart showing the large unattached, smooth-sur-faced thrombus in the left atrial chamber and a stenotic mitral valve. The left ventricular cavity is not dilated but its wall is thicker than normal.

187

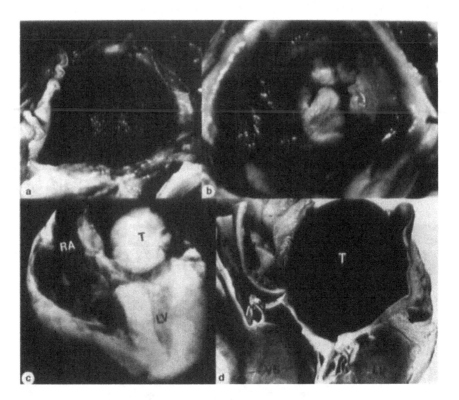

Figure 2 (A) View of thrombus from above after incising the wall from a right pulmonary vein to a left pulmonary vein. (B) View of opened left atrium from above after removing the thrombus. The valve is stenotic and the mural endocardium is smooth. (C) Radiograph of the heart at necropsy showing the four chambers and the left atrial thrombus. RA = right atrial cavity; RV = right ventricular cavity; T = thrombus. (D) Longitudinal view of left side of the heart after cutting the thrombus in half. The thrombus histologically consisted virtually entirely of fibrin. Ao = aorta; LV = left ventricular wall; VS = ventricular septum.

DISCUSSION

The most unusual features of the aforementioned patient are the huge size of the left atrial thrombus and its nonadherence to left atrial endocardium. There were no left atrial endocardial lesions to suggest that the thrombus had at one time been attached. We have never observed thrombus in the body of left atrium, in contrast to that in appendage only, without associated mitral stenosis, but most thrombi in this chamber, of course, are attached to its mural endocardium. How the left atrial thrombus in the present patient could have developed to such a large size without its ever having become attached is unknown.

REFERENCES

1. Wood W: Letter enclosing the history and dissection of a case in which a foreign body was found within the heart. *Edinburgh Med Surg J* 10, 50 (1814)
2. Abramson JL: Ball thrombi of the heart. *Ann Clin Med* 3, 327 (1924)

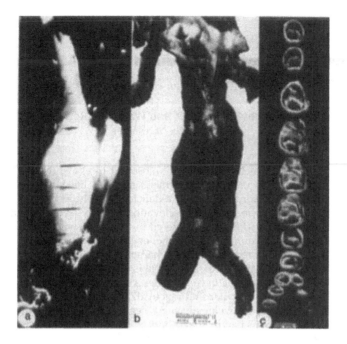

Figure 3 Abdominal aorta. (A) Radiograph of the abdominal aorta showing an aneurysm, intraaneurysmal thrombus-narrowed lumen, and calcific deposits. (B) Abdominal aorta itself. (C) Transverse sections of the abdominal aorta showing the narrowed lumen due entirely to thrombus.

3. Read JL, Porter RR, Russi S, Kriz JR: Occlusive avricular thrombi. *Circulation* 12, 250 (1955)
4. Lie JT, Entman ML: "Hole-in-one" sudden death: Mitral stenosis and left atrial ball thrombus. *Am Heart J* 91, 798 (1976)
5. Söogaard PE: Free ball thrombus of the left atrium. *Eur J Cardiol* 12, 177 (1981)

Case 898 Cardiovascular Findings in Alkaptonuric Ochronosis

Amy H. Kragel, MD, Joyce A. Lapa, MD, and William C. Roberts, MD
Bethesda, MD

Hereditary alkaptonuric ochronosis is an autosomal recessive metabolic disorder that affects about one in one million persons and has been shown to exist for over 3500 years.[1,2] The disorder is due to a deficiency of the enzyme homogentisic acid oxidase and the deficiency leads to elevation of body levels of homogentistic acid. The homogentisic acid is either excreted in the urine, where it oxidizes in an alkaline pH causing darkening of the urine, or (after polymerization) deposits in the connective tissues of the body causing characteristic pigmentation.[1,2] While the most debilitating complication of alkaptonuria is ochronotic arthropathy, a variety of cardiovascular abnormalities have been described in ochronosis. In this report we describe typical cardiovascular findings in alkaptonuric ochronosis.

R.B., a 72-year-old man, developed severe degenerative arthritis during his 30s and was diagnosed then as having alkaptonuria. His arthritis was progressive and severely limited his activity. At age 54, angina pectoris appeared and at age 55 he had an uncomplicated acute myocardial infarction. Subsequently, he had angina pectoris with moderate exertion, but his activity was limited primarily by the arthritis. Other medical problems included systemic hypertension, Raynaud's phenomenon, severe chronic obstructive pulmonary disease, chronic urinary obstruction with a nonfunctioning right kidney, orchiectomy for a benign teratoma, and an abdominal aortic aneurysm. He was admitted to the hospital 19 days before death because of severe respiratory distress. The blood pressure was 160/80 mm Hg; the pulse was 109 beats/min and irregular, and the respiratory rate was 28 breaths/min. He had diffuse pulmonary wheezes. He had a grade 2/6 systolic ejection murmur over both base and apex and a third heart sound. The electrocardiogram showed multifocal atrial tachycardia and Q waves were present in leads II, III, AVF, V_5 and V_6. Shortly before death, he developed electrocardiographic changes consistent with an anterior wall acute myocardial infarction. He died of severe respiratory failure.

Necropsy (NNMC No. A88–41) findings included severe degenerative bone disease with extensive black pigmentation of his skeleton, emphysema, generalized atherosclerosis, obstruction of the right ureter with a black pigmented stone, and an adjacent papillary transitional cell carcinoma of the ureter. Multiple pigmented stones also were present in the prostate gland. The heart weighed 645 gm. Large deposits of dark pigment were present on the aortic and mitral valve cusps and in atherosclerotic plaques of the coronary arteries (Figure 1). Calcific deposits were present in the mitral valve anulus and on the aortic aspects of the aortic valve cusps. Neither the mitral nor aortic valves were stenotic. The lumens of the left anterior descending, left circumflex, and right coronary arteries were narrowed >75% in cross-sectional area by calcified, pigmented plaque. A healed, focally pigmented,

From the Pathology Branch, National Heart, Lung, and Blood Institute, National Institutes of Health, and the Department of Laboratory Medicine, National Naval Medical Center.

Reprint requests: William C. Roberts, MD, NHLBI-NIH, Building 10, Room 2N258, 9000 Rockville Pike, Bethesda, MD 20892.

DOI: 10.1201/9781003409281-36

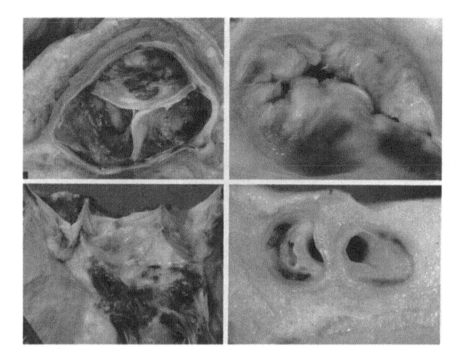

Figure 1 Pigmented heart. **Top left**, Aortic valve viewed from above. **Top right**, Mitral valve from left atrium. **Bottom right**, Cross-sections of the proximal left anterior descending and first diagonal coronary arteries. The blue-black pigment represents ochronotic deposits. Pigment deposition is heaviest in areas associated with calcific deposits, that is, the aortic aspect of the aortic valve, the ventricular aspect of the mitral valve, and calcified atherosclerotic plaque in epicardial coronary arteries.

transmural infarct was present in the posterior left ventricular wall (Figure 2). The posteromedial papillary muscle was atrophied, focally pigmented, and focally calcified. The aorta was extensively calcified, ulcerated, and pigmented (Figure 3). The abdominal aorta was aneurysmal (4 cm wide). Hematoxylin and eosin stained sections of the transmural left ventricular scar showed black pigment within areas of fibrosis. Similar pigment was seen within plaque in the epicardial coronary arteries. This pigment stained with the Nile blue stain.

Alkaptonuric ochronosis has been associated with pigmentation of various cardiovascular structures including the aortic, pulmonic, and mitral valves, mitral anulus, mural endocardium, areas of replacement myocardial fibrosis, and in atherosclerotic plaques of aorta and epicardial coronary arteries.[3–12] Pigment is deposited both intracellularly and extracellularly. It may be seen within macrophages and fibrocytes of endocardial and valvular tissue.[12] Pigment may be seen in all three layers (intima, media, and adventitia) of the arterial wall, in atherosclerotic plaque, and in the smooth muscle cells of media.[11,12]

Both fatal and symptomatic atherosclerotic coronary artery disease and aortic stenosis have been described in association with alkaptonuric ochronosis.[4,6–11] O'Brien et al.[1] found no increase in the frequency of either aortic stenosis or coronary artery disease in a large series of patients. Others, however, have suggested that the frequency of aortic stenosis may be increased[8,11] and that ochronotic pigment in the aortic valve may lead to acceleration of degenerative changes in that structure.[11]

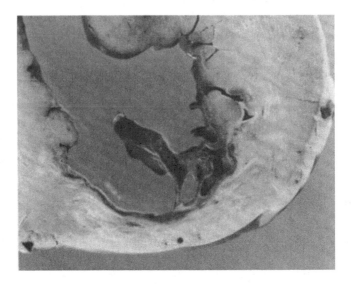

Figure 2 Transverse section of posterolateral left ventricular free wall showing a healed transmural infarct. The posterior free wall and adjacent papillary muscle are thin and fibrotic. Ochronotic pigment is present within some of the scarred tissues.

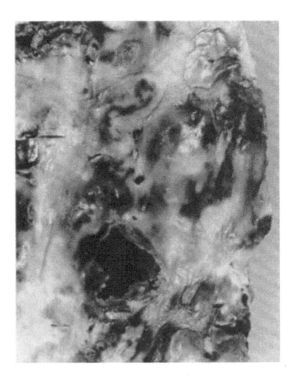

Figure 3 Portion of opened descending thoracic aorta showing pigmented, calcified, and ulcerated atherosclerotic plaques.

Although the aortic valve in our patient was focally thickened by fibrous tissue, calcium, and ochronotic pigment, it was not stenotic.

REFERENCES

1. O'Brien WM, LaDu BN, Bunim JJ. Biochemical, pathologic and clinical aspects of alcaptonuria, ochronosis and ochronotic arthropathy. Review of world literature (1584–1962). *Am J Med* 1963;34:813–838.
2. Lee SL, Stenn FF. Characterization of mummy bone ochronotic pigment. *JAMA* 1978;240:136–138.
3. Skinsnes OK. Generalized ochronosis. Report of an instance in which it was misdiagnosed as melanosarcoma, with resultant enucleation of an eye. *JAMA* 1942;120:552–558.
4. Lichtenstein L, Kaplan L. Hereditary ochronosis. Pathologic changes observed in two necropsied cases. *Am J Pathol* 1954;30:99–119.
5. Nishimori I, Itoh J, Hakuno T. An autopsy case of alkaptonuria with ochronosis. *Acta Pathol Jpn* 1970;20:505–512.
6. Reginato A, Riera M, Martinez V, et al. Alcaptonuria, artropatia ochronotica y estenosis aortica. *Rev Med Chil* 1972;100:529–533.
7. Gould L, Reddy CVR, DePalma D, et al. Cardiac manifestations of ochronosis. *J Thorac Cardiovasc Surg* 1976;72:788–791.
8. Levine HD, Parisi AF, Holdsworth DE, et al. Aortic valve replacement for ochronosis of the aortic valve. *Chest* 1978;74:466–467.
9. Ptacin M, Sebastian J, Bamrah VS. Ochronotic cardiovascular disease. *Clin Cardiol* 1985;8:441–445.
10. Vlay SC, Hartman AR, Culliford AT. Alkaptonuria and aortic stenosis [Abstract]. *Ann Intern Med* 1986;104:446.
11. Gaines JJ, Pai GM. Cardiovascular ochronosis. *Arch Pathol Lab Med* 1987;111:991–994.
12. Gaines JJ. The pathology of alkaptonuric ochronosis. *Hum Pathol* 1989;20:40–46.

Case 903 Extreme Obstruction to Left Ventricular Outflow by a Bioprosthesis in the Mitral Valve Position

William C. Roberts, MD, and Allen L. Dollar, MD
Bethesda, MD

Obstruction to left ventricular outflow is a recognized potential or real complication of mitral valve replacement.[1-13] It usually results from the use of a large-sized prosthesis or bioprosthesis in patients with relatively small-sized left ventricular cavities. As surgeons gained more experience in cardiac valve replacement and particularly when the use of smaller-framed prostheses became commonplace, left venticular outflow obstruction after mitral replacement became uncommon and is now rare. Recently we studied the heart of a patient who had extreme obstruction to left ventricular outflow after mitral replacement. Because this complication may be fatal and because it is preventable, a brief description of this patient is presented as a reminder of this unfortunate complication.

A 72-year-old woman, who was known for several years to have a precordial murmur, at age 70 developed atrial fibrillation and symptoms of congestive heart failure. Left ventricular angiography disclosed severe mitral valve prolapse, moderately severe mitral regurgitation, normal left ventricular systolic function, a normal-sized left ventricular cavity, and an enlarged left atrial cavity. She was electrically cardioverted to sinus rhythm and was treated with medication and her symptoms improved. At age 72, 6 months before death, exertional dyspnea worsened and nocturnal dyspnea appeared. Shortly before mitral replacement she was evaluated. She was 65 inches (163 cm) tall and weighed 110 pounds (50 kg). The blood pressure was 120/60 mm Hg, and the cardiac ventricular rate was 74 beats/min. A grade 3/6 holosystolic precordial murmur consistent with mitral regurgitation was present. The electrocardiogram showed atrial fibrillation and evidence of left ventricular hypertrophy. The chest radiograph showed an enlarged cardiac silhouette and evidence of chronic obstructive lung disease. At surgery, mitral valve repair was considered, but the valve leaflets were believed to be so abnormal that valve replacement was performed. The floppy mitral valve was excised and was replaced with a 29 mm Carpentier-Edwards bioprosthesis. The excised mitral valve was typical of mitral valve prolapse. The patient was weaned from cardiopulmonary bypass without difficulty; however, upon arrival in the recovery room, she was severely hypotensive and vasopressors were given. Nevertheless, the hypotension worsened, and 3 hours postoperatively, fatal cardiac arrest occurred. Initially, closed-chest cardiac massage was performed. When it was unsuccessful, the chest was opened, and the posterior wall of the left ventricle was found to have ruptured. The tear was repaired. The left ventricular cavity was distended and was difficult to empty by manual compression. (The ventricle likely ruptured as a result of external chest compressions on the distended, non-emptying left ventricle.) Further resuscitative efforts were unsuccessful. The heart weighed 425 gm. A 2.5 cm transverse tear in the posterior wall of the left ventricle had been closed with sutures. The ventricular cavities were of normal size. The bioprosthesis nearly occluded left ventricular outflow (Figure 1).

From the Pathology Branch, National, Heart, Lung, and Blood Institute, National Institutes of Health.

DOI: 10.1201/9781003409281-37

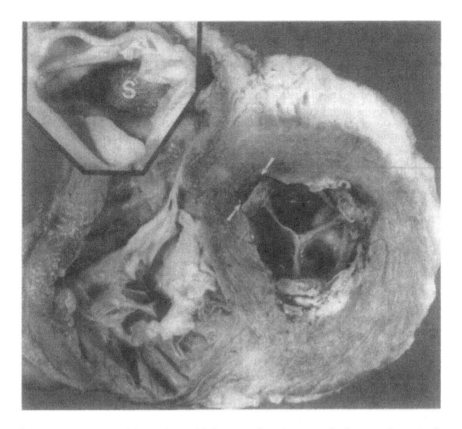

Figure 1 Interior of the right and left ventricles, showing the bioprosthesis in the mitral valve position. Each of the three stents contacts left ventricular endocardium. *Arrows* indicate the minute area for left ventricular outflow. The insert *(upper left)* is a view of the obstructing stent(s) of the bioprosthesis in the mitral valve position from the aorta after the three aortic valve cusps had been excised.

The three other cardiac valves were normal, no foci of myocardial necrosis or fibrosis were present, and the epicardial coronary arteries were normal.

In the above-described patient, the substitute cardiac valve inserted was too large (or the heart was too small), and the consequence was extreme obstruction to left ventricular outflow. Why was such a large-sized prosthesis inserted in this small-sized person? The hemodynamic mitral lesion before operation was pure regurgitation, i.e., no element of mitral stenosis, a lesion which when chronic usually results in dilatation of the left ventricular cavity. In the described patient, however, the left ventricular cavity was not dilated preoperatively (confirmed by left ventricular angiography). Although the heart was larger (425 gm) than normal in mass, it contained an excessive amount of fat, which probably accounted for the increased weight.

What precautions can a surgeon take to prevent this mechanical complication of mitral valve replacement? (1) He/she should utilize relatively small-sized prostheses in relatively small-sized persons irrespective of the type of hemodynamic lesion produced by the native valve to be replaced. (2) If the left ventricular cavity is of normal or near-normal size, the surgeon should err on the side of smaller-sized rather than larger-sized prostheses or bioprostheses. (3) The surgeon should be

195

aware that any type of prosthesis or bioprosthesis is capable of producing left ventricular outflow obstruction, or specifically that a central flow substitute valve, as was inserted in the aforedescribed patient, does not prevent this complication. (4) If the prosthesis or bioprosthesis fills the entire "floor" of the left atrial cavity, it may be too large for the left ventricle, where the major portion of some substitute valves will reside. (5) Mechanical obstruction to left ventricular outflow (or inflow) may be suspected when a patient has a difficult time being weaned from cardiopulmonary bypass or develops severe hypotension shortly after weaning from bypass. (6) Intraoperatively, echocardiography is useful in diagnosing this complication.[13]

REFERENCES

1. Roberts WC, Morrow AG. Mechanisms of acute left atrial thrombosis after mitral valve replacement. Pathologic findings indicating obstruction to left atrial emptying. *Am J Cardiol* 1966;18:497–503.
2. Roberts WC, Morrow AG. Causes of early postoperative death following cardiac valve replacement. Clinico-pathologic correlation in 64 patients studied at necropsy. *J Thorac Cardiovasc Surg* 1967;54:422–437.
3. Roberts WC, Morrow AG. Anatomic studies of hearts containing caged-ball prosthetic valves. *Johns Hopkins Med J* 1967;121:271–295.
4. Shepard RL, Glancy DL, Stinson EB, Roberts WC. Hemodynamic confirmation of obstruction to left ventricular inflow by a caged-ball prosthetic mitral valve. Case report. *J Thorac Cardiovasc Surg* 1973;65:252–254.
5. Roberts WC, Bulkley BH, Morrow AG. Pathologic anatomy of cardiac valve replacement: a study of 224 necropsy patients. *Prog Cardiovasc Dis* 1973;15:539–587.
6. Seningen RP, Bulkley BH, Roberts WC. Prosthetic aortic stenosis. A method to prevent its occurrence by measurement of aortic size from preoperative aortogram. *Circulation* 1974;49:921–924.
7. Roberts WC, Hammer WJ. Cardiac pathology after valve replacement with a tilting-dics prosthesis (Björk-Shiley type). A study of 46 necropsy patients and 49 Björk-Shiley prostheses. *Am J Cardiol* 1976;37:1024–1032.
8. Roberts WC. Complications of cardiac valve replacement: characteristic abnormalities of prostheses pertaining to any or specific site. *Am Heart J* 1982;103:113–122.
9. Rahimtoola SH. The problem of valve prosthesis-patient mismatch. *Circulation* 1978;58:20–24.
10. Pelikan PCD, Chew PH, Fortuin NJ, Yin FCP. Left ventricular outflow obstruction caused by a Starr-Edwards mitral prosthesis. *Am J Cardiol* 1983;52:552–553.
11. Currie PJ, Seward JB, Lam JB, Gersh BJ, Pluth JR. Left ventricular outflow tract obstruction related to a valve prosthesis: case caused by a low-profile mitral prosthesis. *Mayo Clin Proc* 1985;60:184–187.
12. Mihaileanu S, Marino JP, Chauvaud S, Perier P, Forman J, Vissoat J, Julien J, Dreyfus G, Abastado P, Carpentier A. Left ventricular outflow obstruction after mitral valve repair (Carpentier's technique). *Circulation* 1988;78:78–84.
13. Byrnes TJ, Cuillory WR, Hanley HG. Left ventricular outflow obstruction by a mitral valve prosthesis: Doppler ultrasound and cardiac catheterization findings. *Cathet Cardiovasc Diagn* 1989;17:34–38.

Case 919 Massive Calcification of a Porcine Bioprosthesis in the Aortic Valve Position and the Role of Calcium Supplements

Heinrich G. Klues, MD, Lowell S. Statler, MD, Robert B. Wallace, MD, and William C. Roberts, MD
Washington, D.C., and Bethesda, MD

The development of calcific deposits in porcine aortic valve cusps used in bioprostheses for cardiac valve replacement in humans is well recognized. Often the calcific deposits cause tearing of the porcine aortic valve cusps and the tearing may lead to severe valvular regurgitation. The calcific deposits on occasion may be large enough to decrease the mobility of the cusps and the immobility may lead to varying degrees of dysfunction. Bioprosthetic regurgitation, however, is a more common major complication of bioprosthetic replacement than is stenosis. In this report we describe massive calcific deposits with resulting extreme stenosis unassociated with significant regurgitation in a porcine bioprosthesis in the aortic valve position, and we discuss the possible relation of daily calcium supplements on the amount of bioprosthetic calcific deposits.

A 74-year-old woman had aortic valve replacement for a stenotic (47 mm Hg peak systolic pressure gradient between the left ventricle and the ascending aorta) congenitally bicuspid aortic valve stenosis in September 1978 when she was 64 years old. The native valve was replaced with a porcine bioprosthesis (Hancock 27 mm, Johnson & Johnson Cardiovascular, King of Prussia, Pa.). She was asymptomatic thereafter until January 1989, when while she was on a cruise, she noted dyspnea upon walking up stairs on the ship. Three days later, she was in acute pulmonary edema and was hospitalized. An echocardiogram (Figure 1) disclosed a peak systolic pressure gradient between the left ventricle and the aorta of approximately 140 mm Hg. At cardiac catheterization, the bioprosthesis in the aortic valve position could not be crossed by the catheter despite repeated attempts. Five days after the onset of the dyspnea on the ship, the Hancock bioprosthesis in the aortic valve position was replaced with a Carpentier-Edwards bioprosthesis (29 mm, Baxter Healthcare Corp., Edwards Division, Santa Ana, Calif.). Eighteen months later (August 1990) she was asymptomatic and was working daily in her garden. The operatively excised Hancock bioprosthesis is shown in Figure 2. Each cusp is heavily calcified, virtually immobile, and the deposits are present on both aortic and ventricular aspects of the cusps. No cusp is torn or perforated. Early postoperatively it was learned that this woman had been taking a calcium supplement daily for no specific medical indication for at least 20 years, including each of the 3769 days that the porcine bioprosthesis had been in the aortic valve position. Each Caltrate tablet (Lederle Laboratories, Pearl River, N.Y.) she took contained 1500 mg of calcium carbonate. Thus she took at

From the Division of Cardiology, Department of Medicine, and the Department of Surgery, Georgetown University Medical Center; and the Pathology Branch, National Heart, Lung, and Blood Institute, National Institutes of Health.

Reprint requests: William C. Roberts, MD, Bldg. 10, Room 2N258, NHLBI-NIH, Bethesda, MD 20892.

DOI: 10.1201/9781003409281-38

197

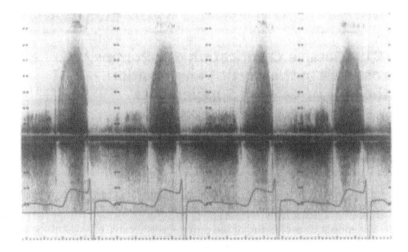

Figure 1 Continuous-wave Doppler tracing obtained from the left ventricular apex demonstrating a 6 m/sec jet across the aortic valve, corresponding to a calculated peak systolic gradient of approximately 140 mm Hg between the left ventricle and aorta. The tracing also shows a mild aortic regurgitation jet.

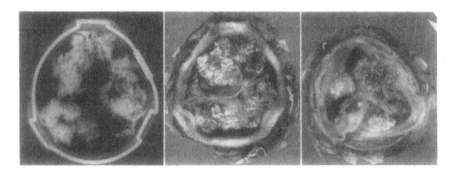

Figure 2 Massively calcified bioprosthetic valve removed from the aortic valve position 126 months after implantation. **Left panel**, Radiograph; **center panel**, view from the aortic aspect; **right panel**, view from the ventricular aspect. It is extremely unusual to have calcific deposits on both ventricular and aortic aspects of the cusps; they are usually only found on the aortic aspects.

least 5654 gm of Caltrate during the 3769 days. Each Caltrate tablet contains 600 mg of elemental calcium; therefore she took 2261 gm of elemental calcium during this 126-month postoperative period. Just before aortic valve replacement the blood urea nitrogen was 18 mg/dl and the creatinine was 1.0 mg/dl.

The unusual features of the patient described herein are the massive quantity of calcific deposits on the cusps of the porcine bioprosthesis, the degree of the pressure gradient across the bioprosthesis, the lack of tearing or perforations in the bioprosthetic cusps despite the huge calcific deposits, and the possibility that the taking of daily calcium supplements played a role in the development of the heavy calcific deposits. Search of reports describing late follow-up of patients having bioprostheses in the aortic valve position did not uncover any reported patients having a peak systolic pressure gradient >100 mm Hg across a bioprosthesis in the aortic valve position. Furthermore, we have not encountered any bioprostheses in any valve position previously having as extensive calcific deposits as were present in the bioprosthesis of the patient described herein. At least one other report has attempted to link heavy calcific deposits in a bioprosthesis to the taking of calcium supplements. Moront and Katz[1] described a 72-year-old woman who developed massive calcific deposits on a bioprosthesis in the mitral valve position in an 18-month period and the mean diastolic pressure gradient across the bioprosthesis was 19 mm Hg. This woman also took calcium carbonate supplements daily. It would appear from the study of the patient by Moront and Katz and from the study of the patient described herein that persons having bioprostheses should not take calcium supplements.

REFERENCE

1. Moront MG, Katz NM. Early degeneration of a porcine aortic valve bioprosthesis in the mitral valve position in an elderly woman and its association with long-term calcium carbonate therapy. *Am J Cardiol* 1987;59:1006–1007.

Case 1167 Congenitally Bicuspid Stenotic Aortic Valves in Octogenarians

Stuart R. Lander, MD; Jeff E. Taylor, MD; William C. Roberts, MD

An 84-year-old white woman was apparently asymptomatic until about 2 months before aortic valve replacement when she went to her physician because of developing exertional dyspnea and chest tightness. A transthoracic echocardiogram showed a normally contracting left ventricle, a normal sized left ventricular cavity, and an estimated aortic valve area of 0.6 cm². The possibility of aortic valve replacement was discussed with the patient but she declined operative intervention.

She was then in her usual state until nearly 2 months later when the dyspnea and chest tightness worsened and she came to the hospital's emergency room. Precordial examination disclosed a grade 3/6 systolic ejection type murmur heard best along the left sternal border with radiation into the neck. No diastolic murmur was heard. Electrocardiogram disclosed sinus rhythm, nonspecific ST, T wave changes, and total 12 lead QRS voltage of 184 mm (10 mm= 1 mV) (normal <175 mm).[1] Chest radiograph disclosed bilateral pleural effusions and mild cardiomegaly; no calcium was seen in either the mitral valve region or in the aortic valve cusps. Cardiac catheterization disclosed the following pressures: left ventricle 173/19 mm Hg; aorta 122/54 mm Hg, yielding a peak systolic pressure gradient of 51; pulmonary artery, 33/14 mm Hg (mean 20), and pulmonary artery wedge mean 12. The aortic valve area was calculated to be 0.51 cm² and the valve area index, 0.3 cm²/body surface area. The patient weighed 145 lbs (68 kg) and was 63 inches tall (160 cm). Coronary angiogram disclosed a dominant right coronary system. The distal left anterior descending coronary artery was narrowed up to 70% in diameter, the left circumflex up to 30%, and the right coronary artery <20%. The left main was normal.

On January 12, 1999, the aortic valve was excised and replaced with a Baxter parietal pericardial 21 mm bioprosthesis. Coronary bypass also was performed. The operatively excised valve was congenitally bicuspid (Figure 1). Early postoperatively the patient was transiently confused, developed atrial fibrillation, and had mild elevation in blood urea nitrogen. She went home the eleventh postoperative day. By that time she was again in sinus rhythm, mentally alert, and had normal renal function. Eight months after operation she was asymptomatic, and cared for herself living alone.

The above case indicates that a congenitally bicuspid aortic valve can be seen in octogenarians and that a stenotic one can be successfully replaced. The oldest reported patient having aortic valve replacement for congenitally stenotic aortic valve was a 92-year-old man.[2] The present patient was asymptomatic until just a few weeks before aortic valve replacement. A recent study from the Mayo Clinic[3] described 527 patients >20 years of age with operative excision of congenitally bicuspid aortic valves including stenotic ones (444 patients), purely regurgitant ones without infection (67 patients), and infected ones (16 patients). Of the 527 patients >20 years of age, 28 (5.3%) were octogenarians. At Baylor University Medical Center since January 1993, 397 patients >20 years of age have undergone

From the Baylor Cardiovascular Institute, Baylor University Medical Center, Dallas, TX

     DOI: 10.1201/9781003409281-39

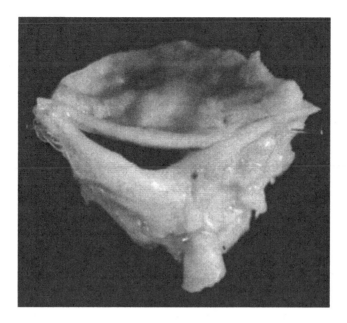

Figure 1 Operatively excised congenitally bicuspid stenotic aortic valve in the 84-year-old patient described herein.

Table 1: Published reports of aortic valve replacement with and without coronary artery bypass in octogenarians

First Author (Year)	Number Of Patients	Age (Mean)	Procedure (Number of Patients)	Operative Mortality	30 Day Mortality (%)	Actuarial Survival (Years)		
						1	3	5
Aranki	188	80–95	AVR (83)	4%	—	—	—	—
(1983)		(-)	AVR + CABG (105)	9%	—	—	—	—
Elayda	152	80–91	AVR (77)	5%				
(1983)		(93)	AVR + CABG (75)	24%	18%	84%	79%	57%
Deiwick	37	80–92	AVR (23)	—				
(1997)		(81)	AVR & CABG (14)	—	8%	88%	79%*	73%
Schmitz	52	>80	AVR (33)	3%	—	—	—	87%
(1998)		(-)	AVR + CABG (19)	22%	—	—	—	59%

* 2 year postoperative follow up; AVR=aortic valve replacement; CABG=coronary bypass grafting.

isolated aortic valve replacement (no replacement of the mitral valve) (115 were described elsewhere[4]): the aortic valve in 169 (43%) was congenitally bicuspid; in 13 (3%) it was unicuspid; in 211 (53%) it was tricuspid; and in 4 (1%) the valve structure was unclear. Of the 169 patients with a congenitally bicuspid aortic valve, 60 (36%) were <65 years of age and 109 (64%) were aged 65 or over including 19 (11%) who were octogenarians.

Only one major coronary artery in the above described patient was narrowed >50% in diameter. As a rule, the cleaner the coronary arteries in older individuals the greater the chance that a stenotic aortic valve will be congenitally bicuspid.[5]

Recent reports of octogenarians undergoing isolated aortic valve replacement with or without coronary artery bypass are reviewed in the Table.[6–9] Operative mortality of combined valve replacement and coronary bypass was relatively high. Of the 52 patients reported by Schmidtz et al,[9] 81% of the early survivors stated that their functional status had improved and 97% stated that the operation was worthwhile.

Finally, as the population continues to age the frequency of aortic valve stenosis will almost certainly increase. Congenital heart disease is not limited to the younger population but indeed may occur in the elderly.

REFERENCES

1. Odom H II, Davis JL, Dinh H, Baker BJ, Roberts WC, Murphy ML. QRS voltage measurements in autopsied men free of cardiopulmonary disease: A basis for evaluating total QRS voltage as an index of left ventricular hypertrophy. *Am J Cardiol.* 1986;58:801–804.
2. Karalis DG, Wahl JM, Mintz GS, Chandrasekaran K. Severe stenosis involving a congenitally bicuspid aortic valve in the tenth decade of life. *Am J Cardiol.* 1990;65:264–265.
3. Sabet HY, Edwards WD, Tazelaar HD, Daly RC. Congenitally bicuspid aortic valves: A surgical pathology study of 542 cases (1991 through 1996) and a literature review of 2,715 additional cases. *Mayo Clin Proc.* 1999;74:14–26.
4. Stephan PJ, Henry III AC, Hebeler Jr RF, Whiddon L, Roberts WC. Comparison of age, gender, number of aortic valve cusps, concomitant coronary artery bypass grafting, and magnitude of left ventricular-systemic arterial peak systolic gradient in adults having aortic valve replacement for isolated aortic valve stenosis. *Am J Cardiol.* 1997;79:166–172.
5. Mautner GC, Mautner SL, Cannon RO III, Hunsberger SA, Roberts WC. Clinical factors useful in predicting aortic valve structure in patients >40 years of age with isolated valvular aortic stenosis. *Am J Cardiol.* 1993;72:194–198.
6. Aranki SF, Rizzo RJ, Couper GS, Adams DH, Collins Jr JJ, Gildea JS, Kinchla NM, Cohn LH. Aortic valve replacement in the elderly. Effect of gender and coronary artery disease on operative mortality. *Circulation.* 1993;88:17–23.
7. Elayda MAA Hall RJ, Reul RM, Alonzo DM, Gillette N, Reul Jr, GJ, Cooley DA. Aortic valve replacement in patients 80 years and older. Operative risks and long-term results. *Circulation.* 1993;88:11–16.
8. Deiwick M, Tandler R, Mollhoff T, Kerber S, Rotker J, Roeder N, Scheld HH. Heart surgery in patients aged eighty years and above: Determinants of morbidity and mortality. *Thorac Cardiovasc Surg.* 1997;45:119–126.
9. Schmitz C, Welz A, Reichart B. Is cardiac surgery justified in patients in the ninth decade of life? *J Card Surg.* 1998;13:113–119.

Case 1306 Severe Late (16 Years) Dysfunction of a Bioprosthesis in the Mitral Valve Position Without Dysfunction of a Bioprosthesis in the Aortic Valve Position

Paul A. Grayburn, MD, Baron L. Hamman, MD, and William C. Roberts, MD

A man who was born in 1939 underwent replacement of both mitral and aortic valves with porcine bioprostheses in 1987 (age 48). Thereafter, he was asymptomatic until 2003 (age 64), when he developed signs and symptoms of heart failure. Cardiac catheterization in late 2003 disclosed the following pressures in mm Hg: pulmonary artery, 70/31; right ventricle, 70/18; right atrial mean, 9; pulmonary artery wedge mean, 30, with v waves averaging 54; left ventricle, 108/25; and aorta, 104/65. Left ventricular angiography disclosed a normal-sized left ventricular cavity and severe mitral regurgitation. Aortic root angiogram disclosed trace aortic regurgitation. The preoperative echocardiogram and the operatively excised (late 2003) bioprosthesis, which had been in the mitral valve position, are shown in the *Figure*. Coronary angiography preoperatively showed insignificant coronary arterial narrowing.

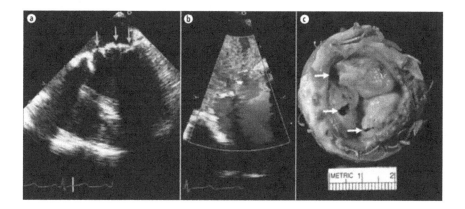

Figure 1 Echocardiographic and gross anatomic images of the bioprosthesis in the mitral valve position for 16 years showing severe bioprosthetic regurgitation. **(a)** A midesophageal 4-chamber view showing 3 distinct defects in the porcine cusps (arrows). **(b)** A magnified image in the same projection showing multiple color flow jets with severe mitral regurgitation through the cusps. There was no perivalvular leak. **(c)** The excised bioprosthesis with 3 perforations in the cusps (arrows). This is a classic example of structural porcine bioprosthetic deterioration.

From the Division of Cardiology, Department of Internal Medicine (Grayburn), Department of Cardiothoracic Surgery (Hamman), and Department of Pathology and the Baylor Heart and Vascular Institute (Roberts), Baylor University Medical Center, Dallas, Texas.

Corresponding author: Paul A. Grayburn, MD, Baylor Hamilton Heart and Vascular Hospital, 621 N. Hall Street, Dallas, Texas 75226 (e-mail: PaulGr@bhcs.com).

This case demonstrates that when bioprostheses are placed in both mitral and aortic valve positions during the same operation, the bioprosthesis in the mitral valve tends to degenerate more rapidly than a similar bioprosthesis in the aortic valve.[1] The likely reason is that the closing pressure exerted on the mitral bioprosthesis is the left ventricular systolic pressure, whereas the closing pressure exerted on the aortic prosthesis is the aorta's diastolic pressure, which in general is about a third lower than the left ventricular peak systolic pressure. In the present patient, the left ventricular peak systolic pressure was 108 mm Hg and the aorta's end-diastolic pressure was 65 mm Hg, a 40% difference.

REFERENCE

1. Warnes CA, Scott ML, Silver GM, Smith CW, Ferrans VJ, Roberts WC. Comparison of late degenerative changes in porcine bioprostheses in the mitral and aortic valve position in the same patient. *Am J Cardiol* 1983;51: 965–968.

Case 1335 Severe Regurgitation Immediately After Replacement of a Dysfunctional Bioprosthesis in the Mitral Valve Position

Hassan Farooq, MD, Paul Grayburn, MD, and William Clifford Roberts, MD

Severe regurgitation immediately after replacement of a cardiac valve with a mechanical prosthesis or a bioprosthesis is a rare occurrence. Such, however, was the case in the patient described. ©2005 by Excerpta Medica Inc.

(Am J Cardiol 2005;95:703–704)

A 74-year-old woman, who was born in September 1929, had her purely regurgitant mitral valve replaced with a bioprosthesis in 1986, when she was 57 years old. Thereafter, she was asymptomatic until age 74, when exertional dyspnea appeared. Four months later, she entered the hospital. She was 57 inches tall and weighed 115 pounds (body mass index 25 kg/m^2). A grade 3/6 holosystolic murmur was heard over the cardiac apex, and it radiated into the left axilla. An echocardiogram disclosed a normal-sized left ventricle, a dilated right ventricle, and severe bioprosthetic regurgitation. At cardiac catheterization, the pressures in mm Hg were as follows: pulmonary artery wedge "a" wave, 33, V wave, 43, and mean, 28; right ventricle, 58/23, simultaneous left ventricle, 166/26, and aorta 162/ 92. Left ventricular angiography disclosed severe (4+/4+) bioprosthetic regurgitation.

• • •

Reoperation on April 14, 2004, disclosed that 1 of the 3 bioprosthetic cusps had prolapsed severely toward the left atrium, despite the absence of calcium in any of the bioprosthetic cusps. The dysfunctional bioprosthesis in the mitral position was replaced with another bioprosthesis (Carpentier-Edwards, 25 mm, Edwards Lifesciences, Irvine, California). At operation, the left atrium was opened by an incision parallel to the atrial septum just anterior to right superior pulmonary vein. After the excision of the initially inserted bioprosthesis and the insertion of the newer bioprosthesis, the patient apparently came off cardiopulmonary bypass, which lasted 68 minutes, without difficulty.

When entering the intensive care unit, the patient's blood pressure was 100/60 mm Hg, and her heart rate was 92 beats/min. Her extremities were cool, and the pedal pulses were barely palpable. Pulmonary artery pressure was 36/18 mm Hg. Later that day, the patient's blood pressure decreased to 60/30 mm Hg, and atrial fibrillation appeared. Sinus rhythm was restored by cardioversion (50 J) but without improvement in hemodynamics. On postoperative day 4, the patient again reverted to atrial fibrillation, but with amiodarone sinus rhythm returned. By day 8, she was still intubated, sinus tachycardia (110 beats/min) persisted, her respirations were rapid (25 breaths/min), and vasopressors were required to maintain adequate systemic

From the Baylor University Medical Center, Baylor Heart & Vascular Institute, Dallas, Texas. Dr. Roberts's address is: Baylor University Medical Center, Baylor Heart & Vascular Institute, 621 North Hall Street, Dallas, Texas 75226. E-mail: wc.roberts@baylorhealth.edu. Manuscript received and accepted October 29, 2004.

DOI: 10.1201/9781003409281-41

arterial pressures. A repeat echocardiogram (Figure 1) showed severe bioprosthetic regurgitation, and a third cardiac operation was performed on postoperative day 9 (April 23, 2004). The left atrium was opened through the previous incision, and the bioprosthesis in the mitral position was excised. The orifice of the bioprosthesis was found to be in a fixed open position because of a single suture that had encircled 1 of the 3 stents, resulting in the tethering down of 2 cusps (Figure 1). After excision of the tethered bioprosthesis and replacement with another bioprosthesis, the patient came off cardiopulmonary bypass easily, and her postoperative course was relatively uneventful. She left the hospital on May 14, 2004.

• • •

In the early days of cardiac valve replacement, certain technical complications occurred fairly commonly simply because the procedure was new, and good techniques had to be developed. In recent years technical complications of cardiac valve replacement have been infrequent. The complication described in the present patient, namely, the tethering down of 2 bioprosthetic cusps by a suture tied down inadvertently on 1 bioprosthetic stent located on the ventricular aspect of the bioprosthesis, was originally described and reported in 1983.[1] The present case indicates that even 21 years later, this complication has not yet been completely eliminated. It is still a good idea before closing the left atrium after mitral

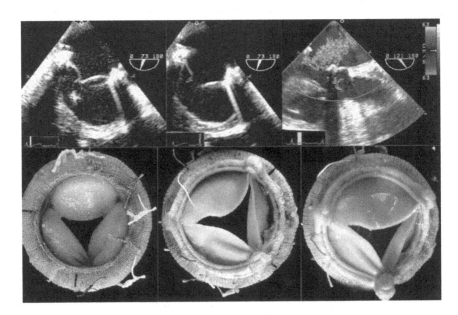

Figure 1 Transesophageal echocardiographic images *(top panels)* obtained in ventricular systole *(top left)* and ventricular diastole *(top middle)* showing marked restriction in the opening of 2 cusps. The *top right* shows mitral regurgitation by color Doppler flow mapping. The vena contracta of the mitral regurgitation jet measured 0.9 cm, a thickness consistent with severe mitral regurgitation. The *bottom panels* show the bioprosthetic valve as seen from the left atrial aspect *(bottom left)* and from the left ventricular aspect *(bottom middle and bottom right)*. A single suture encircled 1 of the 3 stents, tethering down 2 cusps and resulting in an opened, roughly triangular orifice in ventricular systole and diastole.

replacement to ensure that each bioprosthetic cusp is freely mobile. Intraoperative transesophageal echocardiography should be used routinely to evaluate the valve before leaving the operating suite.

REFERENCE

1. Silver MA, Oranburg PR, Roberts WC. Severe mitral regurgitation immediately after mitral valve replacement with a parietal pericardial bovine bioprosthesis. *Am J Cardiol* 1983;52:218–219.

Case 1357 Mitral "Annular" Calcium Forming a Complete Circle "O" Causing Mitral Stenosis in Association with a Stenotic Congenitally Bicuspid Aortic Valve and Severe Coronary Artery Disease

Kevin P. Theleman, MD,[1,3] Paul A. Grayburn, MD,[1,3] William C. Roberts, MD[1,2,3]

Calcific deposits in the epicardial arteries, mitral valve annulus, and aortic valve cusps are common in older persons in the Western world.[1] Recently, we encountered a patient with massive mitral annular calcium causing mitral stenosis in association with a stenotic congenitally bicuspid aortic valve and heavy coronary calcific deposits. The extent of the cardiac calcific deposits is unusual and prompted this report.

A 73-year-old man had an orthotopic liver transplant for alcoholic cirrhosis at age 60, a renal transplant at age 65, a dual-chamber pacemaker inserted for sick sinus syndrome at age 72, and had corticosteroid-induced diabetes mellitus and systemic hypertension. The present examination was prompted by the recent onset of pedal edema. A grade 2/6 systolic ejection murmur that was loudest over the right base of the precordium was present. His body mass index was 22 kg/m^2. Echocardiography disclosed a 6-mm Hg mean diastolic gradient at the mitral orifice and a left ventricular ejection fraction of about 55% (Figure 1). Cardiac catheterization revealed a peak systolic pressure gradient between the left ventricle and aorta of 50 mm Hg (mean gradient, 38 mm Hg) and an aortic valve area of 0.6 cm^2. The left anterior descending artery was narrowed up to 70% in diameter proximally, the second diagonal artery up to 80% proximally, and the ramus intermedius artery up to 80% proximally. The left main coronary artery was widely patent. The dominant left circumflex artery was narrowed up to 50% in diameter and was heavily calcified. The nondominant right coronary artery was free of narrowing.

The aortic valve was replaced with a 21-mm Medtronic Mosaic (Medtronic, Inc., Mineapolis, MN) bioprosthesis. The surgically removed aortic valve was congenitally bicuspid (Figure 2). Aortosaphenous vein grafts were placed to the left anterior descending and the first marginal coronary arteries. An intra-aortic balloon pump was placed intraoperatively. Aortic cross-clamp time was 149 minutes. The postoperative course was complicated by the low cardiac output syndrome, and death occurred 5 days postoperatively.

From the Departments of Medicine (Division of Cardiology)[1] and Pathology[2] and the Baylor Heart and Vascular Institute,[3] Baylor University Medical Center, Dallas, TX

Address for correspondence: William C. Roberts, MD, Baylor Heart and Vascular Institute, Baylor University Medical Center, 621 North Hall Street, Suite H-030, Dallas, TX 75226

E-mail: wcroberts@baylorhealth.edu

DOI: 10.1201/9781003409281-42

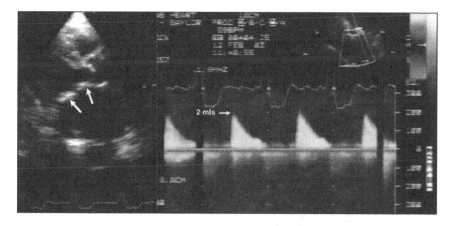

Figure 1 Echocardiogram. Left panel: parasternal long-axis view showing extensive calcification deposits of the mitral annulus (arrows) and aortic valve; right panel: transmitral Doppler inflow showing a peak velocity of 2.0 m/sec and a mean gradient of 6 mm Hg.

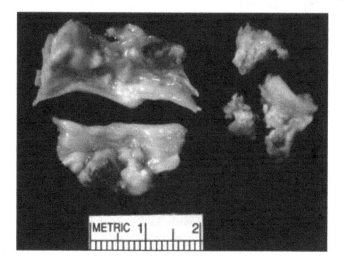

Figure 2 Photograph of the operatively excised focally calcified, stenotic, congenitally bicuspid aortic valve.

At necropsy, the coronary arteries and mitral annular region were massively calcified (Figure 3). The ventricular cavities were not dilated (Figure 4). The bioprosthesis in the aortic valve position appeared to have functioned normally. The venous conduits to the left anterior descending and obtuse marginal arteries were patent.

The most prevalent site of cardiac calcific deposits is the epicardial coronary arteries, followed by the mitral annular area and aortic valve cusps. The apical portions of the left papillary muscles are the fourth most common area of the heart to have calcific deposits.[1] The term "mitral annular calcium" is not accurate in that the calcium deposits are actually located between the ventricular surface

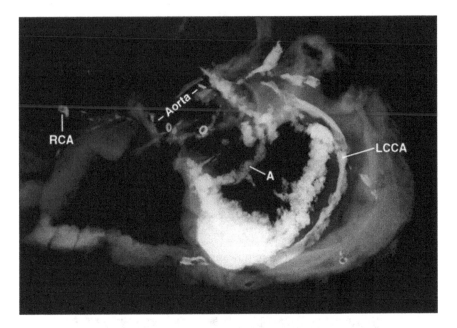

Figure 3 Radiograph of the heart at necropsy. A huge amount of calcium is located beneath the posterior mitral leaflet and extends across the anterior (A) mitral leaflet forming a circle "O." The left circumflex coronary artery (LCCA) is heavily and diffusely calcified (about 50% of patients with a congenitally bicuspid aortic valve have a dominant left circumflex rather than a dominant right coronary artery [RCA], the situation in about 90% of patients with a tricuspid aortic valve). Calcific deposits also are present in the left main and left anterior descending coronary arteries.

of the posterior mitral valve leaflet and the mural endocardium of the left ventricle. When the calcium deposits are extensive, a "C"-shaped or "J"-shaped configuration can appear on radiograph. In rare cases, the calcium extends across the anterior mitral leaflet forming an "O"-shaped configuration.[2] Mitral annular calcium is often associated with mild or moderate mitral regurgitation, but severe regurgitation due to the calcium deposits alone probably does not occur.[2] Significant mitral stenosis due to annular calcium has been reported only in the setting of left ventricular outflow obstruction, as occurred in the present patient.[3]

REFERENCES

1. Roberts WC. The senile cardiac calcification syndrome. *Am J Cardiol* 1986;58:572–574.
2. Roberts WC, Waller BF. Mitral valve "annular" calcium forming a complete circle or "O" configuration: clinical and necropsy observations. *Am Heart J* 1981;101:619–621.
3. Hammer WJ, Roberts WC, deLeon AC. "Mitral stenosis" secondary to combined "massive" mitral annular calcific deposits and small, hypertrophied left ventricles. Hemodynamic documentation in four patients. *Am J Med* 1978;64:371–376.

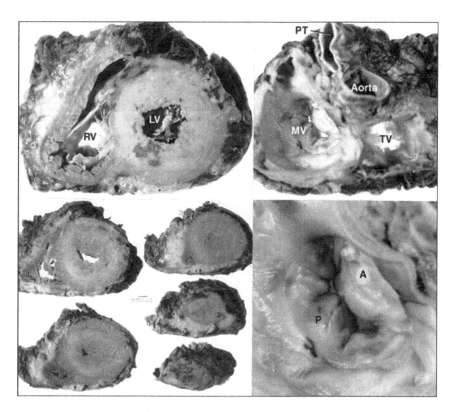

Figure 4   Photographs of the heart at necropsy. Upper left: view of left (LV) and right (RV) ventricles showing normal-sized cavities and a small area of myocardial necrosis in the posterior wall; lower left: transverse sections of the cardiac ventricles showing small cavities and no myocardial lesions; upper right: view of mitral (MV) and tricuspid valve (TV) orifices from the atrial aspects, with pulmonary trunk (PT); lower right: close-up view of the MV from the left atrium showing the anterior (A) and posterior (P) leaflets.

Case 1359 The Heaviest Known Operatively-Excised Aortic Valve

John B. Sims, MD[a,b], Brad J. Roberts, BS, RDCS[a,b], William C. Roberts, MD[a,b], Robert F. Hebeler, Jr., MD[a,c], and Paul A. Grayburn, MD[a,b]*

A 60-year-old man whose operatively excised stenotic and regurgitant aortic valve weighed nearly 15 g, approximately 30 times the normal weight in an adult, is described. To the investigators' knowledge, this is the heaviest aortic valve ever encountered in a human being. © 2006 Elsevier Inc. All rights reserved.
(Am J Cardiol 2006;97:588–589)

The normal tricuspid aortic valve in adults weighs on average 0.5 g.[1] Most stenotic operatively excised aortic valves weigh from 1 to 6 g, and the heaviest, until the present case, seen by 1 of us (WCR) over a 40-year period was just >11 g.[2] In this report, we describe a patient whose operatively excised stenotic aortic valve weighed nearly 15 g.

• • •

A 60-year-old weightlifter born in August 1944 was referred due to a thoracic aortic aneurysm. At age 55, he was told that his heart was "too severely damaged to undergo a cardiac operation." In recent months, he had developed exertional and nocturnal dyspnea, lower leg edema, and a 20-pound increase in weight. His body mass index was 26 kg/m². He was well developed and muscular. A grade 4/6 diastolic blowing murmur was present and best heard over the cardiac apex, and a grade 3/6 systolic ejection murmur was present and best heard over the right upper sternal border. The lungs were clear, and there was no subcutaneous edema. The blood hematocrit was 36%. An electrocardiogram showed sinus bradycardia with left bundle branch block and a QRS width of 160 ms. By transthoracic echocardiography, the diameter of the aorta at or near the sinotubular junction was 6.5 cm, the left ventricular peak systolic diameter was 7.7 cm, and the left ventricular peak diastolic diameter was 8.3 cm. The left ventricular ejection fraction was about 25%. The aortic valve was bicuspid, severely regurgitant, moderately stenotic, and heavily calcified. Calcific deposits were also present in the mitral annular region, and moderate mitral regurgitation was present. During evaluation, the patient developed atrial fibrillation, with a ventricular rate of 120 beats/min, his blood pressure decreased to 90/60 mm Hg, and severe dyspnea ensued. Rapid cardioversion was successfully performed, and the dyspnea lessened. His serum creatinine decreased from 1.8 to 1.4 mg/dl with diuresis.

Cardiac catheterization disclosed normal epicardial coronary arteries and the following pressures: pulmonary artery wedge A wave 35, V wave 42, and mean

[a]Department of Internal Medicine, Division of Cardiology, [b]Heart and Vascular Institute, and [c]Department of Cardiothoracic Surgery, Baylor University Medical Center, Dallas, Texas. Manuscript received August 31, 2005; revised manuscript received and accepted September 2, 2005.
* Corresponding author: Tel: 214-820-7712; fax: 214-820-7533.
E-mail address: paulgr@baylorhealth.edu (P.A. Grayburn).

DOI: 10.1201/9781003409281-43

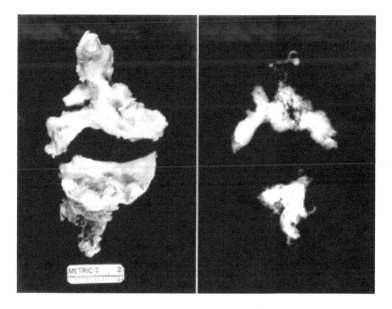

Figure 1 The patient's aortic valve is shown in a photograph *(left)* and an x-ray *(right)*. The valve consists of 2 cusps. One cusp has a raphe, and the length of the raphe from the free margin to its extension of the aorta measures about 3.8 cm. The raphe cusp is heavily calcified and weighs 8.78 g. The nonraphe cusp weighs 5.53 g. The 2 cusps together weigh 14.31 g.

33 mm Hg; pulmonary artery 65/30 mm Hg; right ventricle 63/17 mm Hg; and aorta 90/52 mm Hg (mean 69). The left ventricular cavity was not entered by the catheter. The cardiac index was 2.54 L/min/m².

On December 14, 2004, the ascending aorta was replaced with a 30-mm Hemashield graft (Boston Scientific, Natick, Massachusetts), which included a 29 free style porcine xenograft with implantation of the coronary arteries into the graft. Mitral valvuloplasty was also performed. The aortic valve weighed 14.31 g (Figure 1). Because of early bleeding postoperatively, the patient was taken back to the operating room for reexploration of the mediastinum, where a hematoma was found and evacuated. Because of complete heart block produced at operation, a biventricular pacemaker was inserted 7 days postoperatively. When contacted 7 months after the operation, the patient had no symptoms attributable to heart disease.

• • •

What might be the explanation for the huge mass of this patient's aortic valve? It is now well established that congenitally unicuspid and bicuspid stenotic aortic valves are on average much heavier than stenotic tricuspid aortic valves.[2] The present patient had a congenitally bicuspid aortic valve. Furthermore, it is now well established that men with stenotic aortic valves on average have heavier valves than women with stenotic aortic valves, and the patient described herein was a man.[2] It is also known that patients with significantly elevated serum cholesterol levels have more calcific deposits in their aortic valve cusps, mitral annuli, and epicardial coronary arteries than other subjects of similar ages and the same gender with much lower levels.[3] Patients with homozygous familial hypercholesterolemia, for example, have serum total cholesterol levels >800 mg/dl at birth and by age 10 years may develop considerable calcific aortic stenosis.[4] Unfortunately, the cholesterol numbers in the present patient were uncertain. Larger adult patients with stenotic aortic valves tend to have larger valves than smaller patients of similar ages and the same gender. The present patient, however, weighed only 165 pounds (75 kg) and was 68 inches (173 cm) in height.

The weight of a stenotic aortic valve is determined principally by the quantity of calcium in the valve. Of nearly 2,000 operatively excised stenotic aortic valves in patients >20 years of age examined by 1 of us (WCR), only 2 did not have calcific deposits. The quantity of deposits in the aortic valve in this patient was by far the greatest any of us had seen previously, but the reason for such a large quantity of calcium in the present patient was unclear.

REFERENCES

1. Silver MA, Roberts WC. Detailed anatomy of the normally functioning aortic valve in hearts of normal and increased weight. *Am J Cardiol* 1985;55:454–461.
2. Roberts WC, Ko JM. Weights of operatively-excised stenotic unicuspid, bicuspid, and tricuspid aortic valves and their relation to age, sex, body mass index, and presence or absence of concomitant coronary artery bypass grafting. *Am J Cardiol* 2003;92:1057–1065.
3. Boon A, Cheriex E, Lodder J, Kessels F. Cardiac valve calcification: characteristics of patients with calcification of the mitral annulus or aortic valve. *Heart* 1997;78:472–474.
4. Sprecher DL, Schaefer EJ, Kent KM, Gregg RE, Zech LA, Hoeg JM, McManus B, Roberts WC, Brewer HB Jr. Cardiovascular features of homozygous familial hypercholesterolemia: analysis of 16 patients. *Am J Cardiol* 1984;54:20–30.

Case 1361 A Starr-Edwards Model 6120 Mechanical Prosthesis in the Mitral Valve Position for 38 Years

Mark A. Peterman, MD, Michael S. Donsky, MD, Gregory J. Matter, MD, and William Clifford Roberts, MD*

The Starr-Edwards caged-ball prosthesis for cardiac valve replacement was first successfully used in the mitral position in September 1960. Because of swelling of the silicone rubber poppet due to lipid infiltration, the processing of the silicone rubber was altered in 1965 in hopes of preventing poppet degeneration. We describe findings in a woman who had mitral valve replacement in 1965 utilizing the revised silicone rubber poppet; the prosthesis remained in place for 38 years.

• • •

A 78-year-old woman was admitted to Baylor University Medical Center in August 2003 in functional class IV heart failure. At age 38 (1963), she had had aortic valve replacement with a Starr-Edwards mechanical prosthesis and mitral valve commissurotomy. At age 40 (1965), she had repeat aortic valve replacement and mitral valve replacement, both with Starr-Edwards mechanical prostheses. She did well until age 63 (1988), when a third aortic valve replacement, this time with a St. Jude Medical prosthesis, and a tricuspid valve annuloplasty were performed. She also had chronic anemia, for which she had received several transfusions.

On admission, blood pressure was 110/63 mm Hg, and heart rate was 82 beats/min. Her body mass index was 23 kg/m^2. A grade 3/6 systolic murmur was heard at the left sternal border and a grade 2/6 diastolic murmur at the cardiac apex. Rales were heard at the bases of both lungs. The liver was large, and the lower legs were severely edematous. The hemoglobin was 9.5 g/dl, and the hemotocrit was 29.5%.

An echocardiogram disclosed that her mean transmitral diastolic gradient was 18 mm Hg; the left ventricular ejection fraction was about 50%. The aortic pressure was 150/59 mm Hg, and the pulmonary artery pressure, 75/20 mm Hg. Coronary arteriography showed no significant coronary narrowings.

The Starr-Edwards model 6120/30 mm (3M) mechanical valve, which had been in the mitral position for 38 years, was excised and a porcine bioprosthesis was implanted via a right mini-thoracotomy approach. The patient recovered uneventfully and was discharged on the fifth postoperative day after reinitiation of warfarin therapy.

After photographing it, the excised Starr-Edwards prosthesis was sent to Edwards Lifesciences LLC (Irving, California), the laboratory that had originally produced the prosthesis. The prosthesis was disassembled to acquire the serial number of the valve, which confirmed it to be a model 6120. The poppet was deeply orange, swollen,

Departments of Internal Medicine (Cardiology Division), Cardiothoracic Surgery and Pathology, and the Baylor Heart & Vascular Institute, Baylor University Medical Center, Dallas, Texas. Manuscript received September 6, 2005; revised manuscript received and accepted October 11, 2005.
* Corresponding author: Tel: 214-820-7911; fax: 214-820-7533.
E-mail address: wc.roberts@BaylorHealth.edu (W.C. Roberts).

DOI: 10.1201/9781003409281-44

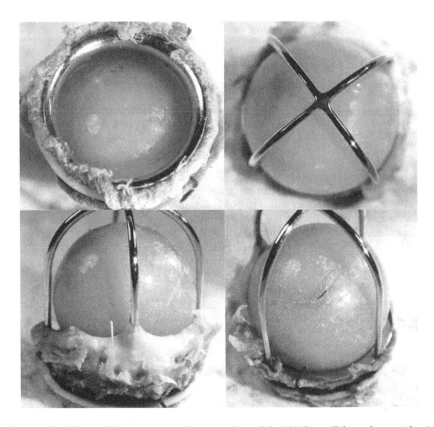

Figure 1 Views of the operatively excised model 6120 Starr-Edwards prosthesis that had been in place for 38 years.

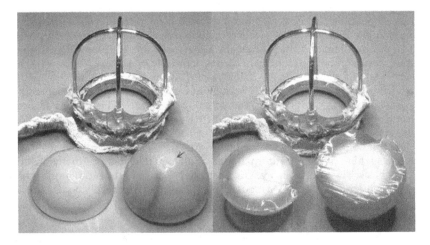

Figure 2 View of the poppet and age after incising the poppet in its mid-portion. The *arrow (left)* shows a region of elongated wear marks. The ball shows a demarcation of color probably corresponding to penetration of blood components, primarily lipids, by absorption *(right)*.

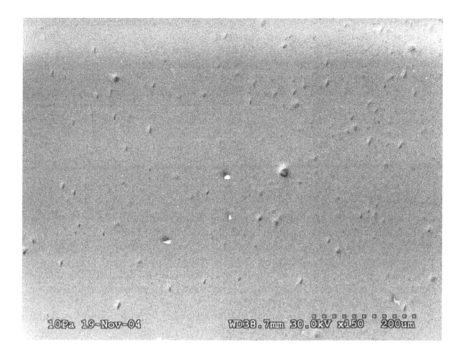

Figure 3 Scanning electron micrograph showing micropores on the poppet's surface (each ×500).

and moved only when significant pressure was applied (Figure 1). A senior scientist at the manufacturer's laboratory determined that the prosthetic poppet weighed 7.4 g, a gain of 0.9 g from its original weight (14% increase). After cutting the poppet in half, the maximal diameter was 21.8 mm, an increase of 1.7 mm (8% increase) from its original diameter (Figure 2). Several cuts were present on the poppet's surface, each about 1 mm long, and light wear groovings, due to restricted motion/rotation, also were present on the poppet's surface. Additionally, micropores were evident on the poppet's surface on scanning electron microscopy (Figure 3). The maximal excursion of the poppet was about 0.5 cm. There was also host tissue overgrowth covering about 50% of the aortic aspect of the prosthetic ring (Figure 1). (This tissue overgrowth combined with the poppet swelling restricted poppet motion leading to both prosthetic stenosis and erythrocyte hemolysis. The latter resulted from high shear jetting backflow from incomplete seating of the poppets.) Other than a local burnish region on 1 of the 4 metallic struts, corresponding to the sliding contact of the poppet as opposed to the normal rolling contact, the cage and the other 3 metallic struts showed no evidence of wear.

• • •

The first successful mechanical prosthesis in the mitral valve position in humans was the Starr-Edwards Model 6000.[1] This model had a significant incidence of systemic embolization as well as ball variance[1] (occasionally lethal[2]). The model 6120 Starr-Edwards mitral valve prosthesis was introduced in 1965 with a reduction in the surface area of metallic components, and an improved barium-impregnated poppet.[1] This model had a far lower incidence of systemic embolization (3% vs 38%)

217

compared with model 6000.[1] The next models (6300) were introduced in 1968 and added cloth covering to the stents. The modified cloth-covered series (model 6400 or track valve) was introduced in 1974 and discontinued in 1980, because results showed no advantage over the original 6120 model.

Although ball variance is usually discovered within 8 years of implantation, late ball variance has been described in early models in patients up to 20 years after implantation.[3] The longest interval previously reported from implantation to reoperation of a Starr-Edwards mitral prosthesis was 31 years in a cloth-covered model with a metal poppet.[4] To our knowledge, ball variance has not been reported in the model 6120 Starr-Edwards prosthesis. The present case is remarkable for the extremely late onset of prosthetic mitral valve stenosis and the occurrence of severe ball variance in a model 6120 Starr-Edwards mitral valve prosthesis.

REFERENCES

1. Freimanis I, Starr A. The unnatural history of valvular heart disease. Late results with silastic ball valve prostheses. *J Cardiovasc Surg* 1984;25:191–198.
2. Roberts WC, Levinson GE, Morrow AG. Lethal ball variance in the Starr-Edwards prosthetic mitral valve. *Arch Intern Med* 1970;126:517–521.
3. Grunkemeier GL and Starr A. Late ball variance with model 1000 Starr-Edwards aortic valve prosthesis. Risk analysis and strategy of operative management. *J Thorac Cardiovasc Surg* 1986;91:918–923.
4. Goshima M, Shiono M, Yamamoto T, Inoue T, Hata M, Sezai A, Niino T, Nakamura T, Ye Z, Negishi N, Sezai Y. Reoperation for a Starr-Edwards ball valve prosthesis implanted in mitral position 31 years ago. *Jpn J Thorac Surg* 2003;56:535–540.

Case 1374 Sudden Onset of "Cardiac" Symptoms, (?) Mild or Severe Aortic Valve Stenosis Involving a Congenitally Bicuspid Aortic Valve, and Nearly Normal Coronary Arteries in an Octogenarian

William C. Roberts, MD,[1-3] Paul A. Grayburn, MD[1-3]

An 86-year-old woman who lived alone was in good health until one evening, just after cleaning the kitchen, she suddenly noted palpitations, dizziness, weakness, and cool clammy skin while sitting. She called an ambulance service and was brought to a hospital. The symptoms resolved spontaneously after a few minutes. She was 61 inches tall and weighed 158 lb (body mass index, 29.8 kg/m²). A grade 2–3/6 systolic ejection murmur was heard over the precordium and best at the cardiac base and into both carotid arteries. An ECG showed sinus rhythm, atrial premature complexes, and no ST-segment or T-wave abnormalities. An echocardiogram (Figure 1) disclosed the following dimensions in centimeters: left ventricle end diastole was 4.3 and peak systole was 3.7, left ventricular and ventricular septal walls were each 1.3, and the left atrial cavity was 3.1. The calculated peak transvalvular aortic gradient was 47 mm Hg; blood hematocrit was 33% and hemoglobin was 10.9 g/dL. Serum total cholesterol was 260 mm Hg, low-density lipoprotein cholesterol 177 mm Hg, high-density lipoprotein cholesterol 88 mm Hg, and triglycerides 62 mg/dL. Troponins and creatine kinase levels were normal.

Cardiac catheterization disclosed the following pressures: pulmonary artery wedge A wave 29, V wave 36, mean 25; pulmonary artery, 54/26; right ventricle, 62/23; left ventricle, 206/33; and ascending aorta, 183/80 mm Hg. The peak transaortic valve gradient was 23 and the mean gradient was 29 mm Hg, the calculated aortic valve area was 0.61 cm² (index, 0.36 cm²/m²), and the left ventricular ejection fraction was 60%. The cardiac index was 2.2 L/min/m². Coronary angiogram disclosed no significant narrowings.

The aortic valve at operation was found to be congenitally bicuspid (Figure 2). It was excised virtually intact. It weighed 2.51 g: the raphe cusp weighed 1.74 g and the nonraphe cusp, 0.69 g[12]. Her postoperative course was uneventful.

COMMENTS

The above-described elderly woman who was known to have a precordial murmur for many years was asymptomatic until a single near-syncopal episode prompted hospitalization and cardiac evaluation. The transvalvular peak systolic pressure gradient across her aortic valve was only 23 mm Hg (mean gradient, 29 mm Hg) in

From the Departments of Internal Medicine, Division of Cardiology;[1] and Pathology;[2] and the Baylor Heart and Vascular Institute,[3] Baylor University Medical Center, Dallas, TX

Address for correspondence: William C. Roberts, MD, Baylor Heart and Vascular Institute, Baylor University Medical Center, 621 North Hall Street, Suite H-030, Dallas, TX 75226

E-mail: wc.roberts@baylorhealth.edu

DOI: 10.1201/9781003409281-45

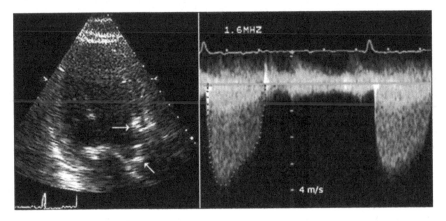

Figure 1 Left panel: Apical long-axis view showing extensive calcium along the ventricular septum (horizontal arrow) and the aortic valve leaflets (diagonal arrow). Right panel: Continuous wave Doppler spectral velocity signal across the aortic valve. The peak velocity was 3.8 m/sec and the mean transvalvular gradient was calculated as 36 mm Hg.

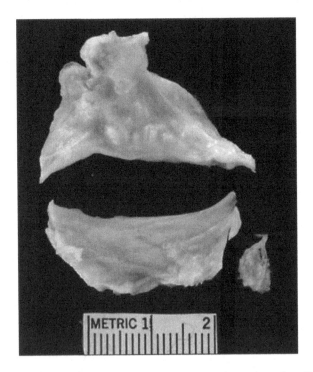

Figure 2 Photograph of the congenitally bicuspid aortic valve. Focal calcific deposits are present in each cusp.

the absence of associated aortic regurgitation and in the presence of a normal ejection fraction (60%), but the calculated aortic valve area was 0.61 cm². The valve area would, of course, indicate severe aortic valve stenosis, but the peak transvalvular gradient would indicate only mild aortic stenosis. Which is correct? Could the measured transvalvular gradient be incorrect or the calculated aortic valve area be incorrectly calculated? Although the patient's peak systolic left ventricular and aortic peak systolic pressures were high (206 and 183 mm Hg, respectively, indicating isolated systolic hypertension), her A peak-to-peak pressure gradient was only 23 mm Hg.[3]

There is some evidence that the calculated aortic valve area is not as accurate in patients with low transvalvular aortic pressure gradients as it is in patients with high transvalvular pressure gradients. Roberts and Ko[4] found that the peak transaortic pressure gradient correlated much better with the weight of the operatively excised stenotic aortic valve than did the calculated aortic valve area. Among women in whom the operatively excised stenotic aortic valve weighed <1 g, the peak transvalvular aortic pressure gradient averaged 28 mm Hg and the aortic valve area 0.83 cm²; of valves weighing >2–3 g (as in the present patient), the peak gradient averaged 63 mm Hg and the area, 0.58 cm²; of valves weighing >3–4 g, the peak gradient averaged 85 mm Hg and the valve area 0.51 cm². Thus, caution is needed in relying on the calculated aortic valve area in patients with small peak systolic pressure gradients.

In this patient, both echocardiography and catheterization yielded similar mean gradients and identical aortic valve areas in the setting of a low cardiac index (Table). This suggests that the low calculated valve area was an artifact of a low flow state rather than a technical error. Importantly, aortic valve area is notoriously misleading in the setting of a low transvalvular gradient.[5] Dobutamine challenge is recommended to recalculate both the mean gradient and aortic valve area at a higher level of flow (the numerator in both the Gorlin and continuity equations).[6] Given that the valve was only moderately abnormal by pathologic examination, it is likely that dobutamine would have resulted in a higher aortic valve area without an increased gradient, and surgery might have been avoided. The single episode of syncope, which prompted surgery, was probably not caused by aortic stenosis in this case. It must be remembered that syncope has many other causes, including vagal episodes, conduction system disease, and noncardiac etiologies. The echocardiogram showed large calcific deposits of the ventricular septum, which could indicate conduction system disease.

The above-described patient also raises the issue of the frequency of bicuspid aortic valves in octogenarians with aortic valve stenosis unassociated with significant mitral valve disease. Of 190 patients aged 80–89 years who had isolated aortic valve replacement for aortic valve stenosis in the past 12 years (1993–2005) at

Table 1: Echocardiographic and catheterization data

Variable	Echocardiography	Catheterization
Peak aortic velocity (m/sec)	3.8	—
Peak transvalvular gradient (mm Hg)*	58	23
Mean transvalvular gradient (mm Hg)	36	29
Aortic valve area (cm²)	0.6	0.6
Aortic regurgitation	Mild	—

*Peak gradient by Doppler represents the greatest difference in pressure between the left ventricle and aorta at any point in time. Peak gradient by catheterization represents the difference between the peak left ventricular pressure and the peak aortic pressure, which do not occur simultaneously due to a temporal delay in the peak aortic pressure (tardus). This explains why the peak gradient is less than the mean gradient at catheterization in this case.

Baylor University Medical Center (Dallas, TX), 54 (28%) had congenitally bicuspid aortic valves.[7] Of them, 20 (37%) were women (such as the present patient) and 34 (63%) were men.

REFERENCES

1. Roberts WC, Ko JM. Weights of operatively-excised stenotic unicuspid, bicuspid, and tricuspid aortic valves and their relation to age, sex, body mass index, and presence or absence of concomitant coronary artery bypass grafting. *Am J Cardiol* 2003;92:1057–1065.
2. Roberts WC, Ko JM. Weights of individual cusps in operatively-excised stenotic congenitally bicuspid aortic valves. *Am J Cardiol* 2004;94:678–681.
3. Roberts WC, Perloff JK, Costantino T. Severe valvular aortic stenosis in patients over 65 years of age. A clinico-pathologic study. *Am J Cardiol* 1971;27:497–506.
4. Roberts WC, Ko JM. Relation of weights of operatively excised stenotic aortic valves to preoperative transvalvular peak systolic pressure gradients and to calculated aortic valve areas. *J Am Coll Cardiol* 2004;44:1847–1855.
5. Carabello BA. Evaluation and management of patients with aortic stenosis. *Circulation* 2002;105:1746–1750.
6. Grayburn PA, Eichhorn EJ. Dobutamine challenge for low gradient aortic stenosis. *Circulation* 2002;106:763–765.
7. Roberts WC, Ko JM. Frequency by decade of unicuspid, bicuspid, and tricuspid aortic valves in adults having isolated aortic valve replacement for aortic stenosis, with or without associated aortic regurgitation. *Circulation* 2005;111:920–925.

Case 1390 Isolated Aortic Valve Replacement Without Coronary Bypass for Aortic Valve Stenosis Involving a Congenitally Bicuspid Aortic Valve in a Nonagenarian

William C. Roberts, MD,[1,2,4] Jong Mi Ko, BA,[4] Gregory John Matter, MD[3]

A 90-year-old man sought care because of rapidly progressing dyspnea and an episode of near syncope. Examination found him to be 71 inches tall and to weigh 180 lb (body mass index, 25 kg/m²). A grade 5/6 harsh systolic ejection precordial murmur was present, loudest over the right second intercostal space. A murmur of aortic regurgitation was not described. The blood hematocrit was 39%. Cardiac catheterization disclosed the following pressures (mm Hg): left ventricle, 207/15; aorta, 157/60; and peak transvalvular systolic pressure gradient, 50. The left ventricular ejection fraction was 50%, and the calculated aortic valve area was 0.64 cm². Angiogram disclosed wide open coronary arteries. The aortic valve was replaced with a 25-mm pericardial bioprosthesis (Baxter, Deerfield, IL). His postoperative course was uncomplicated. The operatively excised aortic valve was congenitally bicuspid, heavily calcified, and rigid, and it weighed 5.73 g. The patient was known to be alive 1507 days after valve replacement.

COMMENTS

The hitherto described patient had congenital heart disease, specifically a bicuspid aortic valve. Symptoms of aortic valve stenosis, namely those of heart failure and near syncope, did not develop until 90 years after birth. By this time, the bicuspid aortic valve was heavily calcified, quite stenotic, and replaced. The operatively excised valve was very heavy (5.73 g [normal, 0.5 g])[1] and immobile[2] (Figure 1).

Aortic stenosis, of course, is fairly common in older individuals, but it usually manifests itself symptomatically long before the age of 90, particularly when the stenosis involves a congenitally malformed valve. From 1993 to 2006, we studied operatively excised stenotic aortic valves in 9 nonagenarians: 3 had congenitally bicuspid aortic valves, including the present patient, and 6 had 3-cuspid aortic valves.[3] All but 1 patient survived the operative period; 1 died 874 days and 1 died 1011 days after valve replacement; 6 others have survived from 787 to 2324 days postoperatively as of June 29, 2006. The hitherto described patient is doing well 1507 days after valve replacement.

Why some patients with a congenitally bicuspid stenotic valve do not become symptomatic until their 90s and why others become symptomatic in early life is

From the Departments of Internal Medicine, Division of Cardiology,[1] Pathology,[2] and Cardiothoracic Surgery,[3] and the Baylor Heart and Vascular Institute,[4] Baylor University Medical Center, Dallas, TX

Address for correspondence: William C. Roberts, MD, Baylor Heart and Vascular Institute, Baylor University Medical Center, 621 North Hall Street, Suite H-030, Dallas, TX 75226

E-mail: wc.roberts@baylorhealth.edu

DOI: 10.1201/9781003409281-46

unclear. The stenosis is primarily the result of calcific deposits on the aortic aspects of the cusps. Those with higher serum cholesterol levels may develop calcific deposits on the valve cusps at an earlier age than the patients with lower serum cholesterol numbers. Unfortunately, we were unable to obtain the cholesterol values in the above-described patient. The fact that his coronary arteries were virtually free of plaque as determined by angiography suggests that his serum cholesterol levels were relatively low.

In patients with isolated aortic valve stenosis unassociated with mitral valve dysfunction, the absence of coronary narrowing by angiogram suggests that the underlying structure of the aortic valve is bicuspid rather than tricuspid, at least in patients aged 40–70 years.[4] Among 3 patients aged 90–91 years with isolated aortic stenosis and bicuspid aortic valves, 2 by angiogram had 1 or more epicardial coronary arteries narrowed >50% in diameter. In contrast, of 6 patients aged 90–91 years with isolated aortic valve stenosis superimposed on a 3-cuspid aortic valve, all had severe narrowing of 1 or more major epicardial coronary arteries by angiogram. Mautner and colleagues[4] examined the structure of stenotic aortic valves in adults and related the valve structure to several variables, including coronary arterial narrowing, useful in predicting that structure. One hundred eighty-eight patients having aortic valve replacement for isolated valvular aortic stenosis were studied. All patients were older than 40 years at the time of aortic valve replacement; all had coronary angiograms preoperatively; 182 (97%) had measurements of serum total cholesterol; and 184 (98%) had body mass index calculated. The structure of the operatively excised valve was classified as

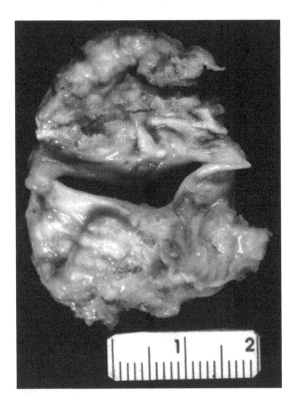

Figure 1 Congenitally bicuspid aortic valve in the 90-year-old patient described.

unicuspid or bicuspid (congenitally malformed) or as a tricuspid aortic valve. A logistic regression model was developed that found 4 factors (age, serum total cholesterol, angiographic coronary artery disease, and body mass index) to be predictive of aortic valve structure.[1] Patients with at least 3 or all 4 factors high or present (ie, age older than 65 years, serum total cholesterol >200 mg/dL, body mass index >29 kg/m^2, and coronary artery disease) had a low probability (10%–29%) of having a congenitally malformed valve[2] and patients with at least 3 or all 4 factors low or absent (ie, age 65 years or younger, serum total cholesterol <200 mg/dL, body mass index <29 kg/m^2, and no coronary artery disease) had a high probability (72%–90%) of having a congenitally malformed valve. Thus, the morphology of the operatively excised stenotic aortic valve can be predicted with knowledge of the age, serum total cholesterol, body mass index, and coronary artery status of the patient.

The presence of an elevated systolic systemic arterial pressure in an older person should not be interpreted to mean absent or only minimal or mild aortic valve stenosis. The peak systemic systolic pressure in the present patient at cardiac catheterization was 157 mm Hg and yet the peak left ventricular pressure was 207 mm Hg. We have observed the peak systemic systolic pressure to be as high as 200 mm Hg and yet the degree of aortic stenosis was severe, with a peak left ventricular systolic pressure of 300 mm Hg and a peak transvalvular gradient of 100 mm Hg.[5]

Aortic valve replacement even in nonagenarians is the procedure of choice for severe aortic stenosis. Bacchetta and associates[6] reported 18 patients aged 90 years or older who had aortic valve replacement for aortic stenosis, 13 of whom also had simultaneous coronary bypass grafting. All patients survived the 30-day operative period and, although the data are scant, at least up to 2.5 years postoperatively. Among 9 nonagenarians having aortic valve replacement for aortic stenosis at Baylor University Medical Center (Dallas, TX), all but 1 survived the 30-day postoperative period, 2 died nearly 2+ years later, and the others are alive up to 6+ years postoperatively.

REFERENCES

1. Silver MA, Roberts WC. Detailed anatomy of the normally functioning aortic valve in hearts of normal and increased weight. *Am J Cardiol* 1985;55:454–461.
2. Roberts WC, Ko JM, Hamilton C. Comparison of valve structure, valve weight, and severity of the valve obstruction in 1849 patients having isolated aortic valve replacement for aortic valve stenosis (with or without associated aortic regurgitation) studied at 3 different medical centers in 2 different time periods. *Circulation* 2005;112:3919–3929.
3. Roberts WC, Ko JM, Matter GJ. Aortic valve replacement for aortic stenosis in nonagenarians. *Am J Cardiol*. In press.
4. Mautner GC, Mautner SL, Cannon RO III, et al. Clinical factors useful in predicting aortic valve structure in patients > 40 years of age with isolated valvular aortic stenosis. *Am J Cardiol* 1993;72:194–198.
5. Roberts WC, Perloff JK, Costantino T. Severe valvular aortic stenosis in patients over 65 years of age. A clinicopathologic study. *Am J Cardiol* 1971;27:497–506.
6. Bacchetta MD, Ko W, Girardi LN, et al. Outcomes of cardiac surgery in nonagenarians: a 10-year experience. *Ann Thorac Surg* 2003;75:1215–1220.

Case 1423 Sudden Collapse in Aortic Stenosis

William Clifford Roberts, MD,[1,2,3] *Jong Mi Ko, BA,*[3] *Jeffrey M. Schussler, MD*[1]

A 78-year-old woman, who was born on May 3, 1928, and died on November 22, 2006, had been in her usual state of health until November 6, 2002, when, at age 74 years, she noted sudden left-sided weakness and was hospitalized. On examination, a right-gaze preference and left facial droop were noted as well as systemic hypertension (blood pressure 160/75 mm Hg), atrial fibrillation, and a grade 3/6 ejection-type murmur over the base of the precordium. A computed tomographic scan showed hyperdensity of the right middle cerebral artery. A thrombolytic agent was administered intra-arterially and the previously occluded artery opened to normal caliber. Echocardiography at the time disclosed a mass (thrombus) in the left atrial appendage, normal left ventricular function, and aortic valve stenosis (AS), with an estimated peak transvalvular gradient of 65 mm Hg and an aortic valve orifice area estimated at <0.4 cm² (Figure 1). At the time there were no symptoms of heart failure, syncope, or chest pain. She was started on warfarin sodium and lisinopril.

Thereafter, she was lost to follow-up until November 22, 2006 (age 78), when she was found on the floor of her home by her husband and was taken to the emergency room. On arrival, she was responsive but had left-sided weakness and slurred speech. Chest radiograph was consistent with heart failure. An electrocardiogram showed ventricular premature complexes. An echocardiogram showed severe AS and a low (20%) ejection fraction. None of the aortic valve cusps moved in either phase of the cardiac cycle. During the recording of the echocardiogram she became pulseless and resuscitative efforts were unsuccessful. The interval from the time she was found on the floor to the fatal cardiac arrest was 2.6 hours.

At necropsy, the heart weighed 440 g. The ventricular septum and left ventricular free wall were thickened (each 2.2 cm) but free of foci of fibrosis and necrosis. The 3 aortic valve cusps were severely thickened by both fibrous tissue and heavy calcific deposits and each was immobile; the posterior and left cusps were fused over a distance of 1.2 cm (Figure 2). All major epicardial coronary arteries were focally calcified, and the lumens of the right, left anterior descending, and left circumflex each were narrowed from 51% to 75% in cross-sectional area by plaque. Small calcific deposits were also present in the mitral annulus. The mitral leaflets and chordae were normal except for aging changes. The brain was grossly normal.

From the Department of Internal Medicine, the Division of Cardiology,[1] and the Department of Pathology,[2] and the Baylor Heart and Vascular Institute,[3] Baylor University Medical Center, Dallas, TX

Address for correspondence: William Clifford Roberts, MD, Baylor Heart and Vascular Institute, Baylor University Medical Center, 621 North Hall Street, Suite H-030, Dallas, TX 75226

E-mail: wc.roberts@baylorhealth.edu

    DOI: 10.1201/9781003409281-47

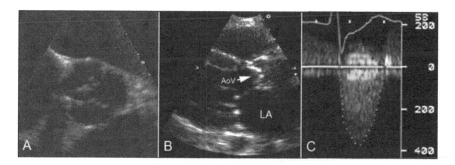

Figure 1 A, Transesophageal echocardiogram demonstrating thickened aortic valve leaflets and reduced aortic valve (AoV) orifice. B, During systole, the AoV leaflets have a significantly reduced opening. C, High velocity of the blood flowing through the AoV during systole is measured by Doppler interrogation during echocardiography. LA indicates left atrium.

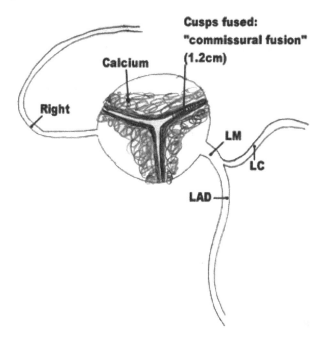

Figure 2 Tricuspid aortic valve, severely thickened by both fibrous tissue and heavy calcific deposits. Each cusp was immobile, and 2 cusps were fused at 1 commissural fusion (1.2 cm). LM indicates left main artery; LC, left circumflex artery; and LAD, left anterior descending artery.

COMMENTS

The patient described had severe AS. Her first symptom of the valvular problem appears to have been her last symptom, namely cardiac arrest. There had never been previous syncope, or chest pain, or dyspnea. Because the major epicardial coronary arteries were not severely narrowed, it is reasonable to attribute the sudden collapse to the AS.

In patients with severe AS, sudden death is a well-recognized consequence. Most patients with AS who die suddenly have had symptoms that could logically be attributed to the AS. Indeed, Braunwald[1] has emphasized ". . . that operative treatment is the most common cause of sudden death in asymptomatic patients with aortic stenosis . . . . Such patients should, in general, not be referred for surgical therapy but should be followed-up frequently and carefully. On the other hand, there has never been much argument that surgical treatment should be carried out promptly, as soon as the patient develops symptoms secondary to aortic stenosis."

Current guidelines for the management of patients with severe AS recommend valve replacement for patients who exhibit symptoms that can be related to the AS (chest pain, dyspnea, or syncope). In patients who have equivocal symptoms, stress testing can be performed to quantify their exercise response. Abnormal response to exercise in an otherwise asymptomatic individual with severe AS is an indication for valve replacement. In the truly asymptomatic individual, close clinical follow-up and at least a yearly echocardiogram is the current recommendation.[2]

One of us (WCR) has had an opportunity to study at necropsy 192 patients older than 15 years of age with AS unassociated with morphologic disease of the mitral valve (other than aging changes ± mitral annular calcium) and not treated operatively. Of the 192 patients, 47 (24%) died suddenly and unexpectedly. Of the 42 patients (of the 47) in whom good information was available on symptoms, 10 (24%) were considered asymptomatic before the sudden cardiac arrest. Of the 47 patients, the AS was considered to be severe in 36 (77%) and moderate (4 patients) or mild (7 patients) in the others. Of these 47 patients, 28 (60%) had a congenitally bicuspid aortic valve; 2 (4%) had a unicuspid acommissural valve, and 17 (36%) had a tricuspid valve. The patient described herein had a functionally bicuspid aortic valve because 2 of the 3 cusps were fused together at one commissure over a distance of 1.2 cm.

In summary, a patient with severe AS unassociated with significant mitral valve disease or severe coronary artery disease is presented whose symptom of AS was sudden death. Such cases are very uncommon.

REFERENCES

1. Braunwald E. On the natural history of severe aortic stenosis. *J Am Coll Cardiol* 1990;15:1018–1020.
2. Bonow RO, Carabello BA, Chatterjee K, et al. ACC/AHA 2006 guidelines for the management of patients with valvular heart disease: a report of the American College of Cardiology/American Heart Association Task Force on Practice Guidelines (Writing Committee to Revise the 1998 Guidelines for the Management of Patients with Valvular Heart Disease) developed in collaboration with the Society of Cardiovascular Anesthesiologists endorsed by the Society for Cardiovascular Angiography and Interventions and the Society of Thoracic Surgeons. *J Am Coll Cardiol* 2006;48:e1–e148.

Case 1445 Diagnosis of Congenital Unicuspid Aortic Valve by 64-Slice Cardiac Computed Tomography

Wende N. Gibbs, MD, Baron L. Hamman, MD, William C. Roberts, MD, and Jeffrey M. Schussler, MD

A 28-year-old man presented to our hospital with 3 days of intermittent, escalating dyspnea and chest tightness. He reported that he often experienced dyspnea when smoking, chewing tobacco, or exerting himself beyond the level of normal daily activity. His discomfort was partially relieved by his albuterol inhaler, which he used >10 times per day. As a child, he was told that he had a precordial murmur, but he had not sought medical attention. Five years prior to this evaluation, he was having similar symptoms and was treated with antibiotics. He was told at that time that he had mild asthma.

On examination, the patient was mildly dyspneic, with a harsh systolic murmur at the right upper sternal border. Transthoracic echocardiogram revealed left ventricular thickening with normal systolic and diastolic function and a left ventricular ejection fraction of 65%. A peak gradient of >4 meters per second was noted, with a calculated aortic valve area of <0.9 cm². The morphology of the valve was not clearly seen, but a unicuspid valve was suspected.

Transesophageal echocardiogram demonstrated a heavily calcified unicuspid aortic valve with reduced cuspid excursion and moderate to severe aortic regurgitation *(Figure 1A)*. Preoperative 64-slice computed tomographic coronary angiography (Lightspeed VCT, GE Healthcare) confirmed the valve morphology and demonstrated no significant coronary narrowing *(Figure 1B)*.

At operation, the valve was found to be unicuspid with one true unfused commissure. The free edge traversed the cusps without contact with the aortic wall

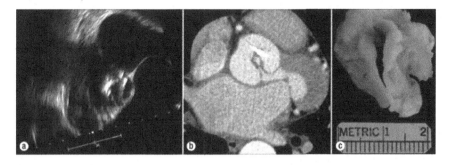

Figure 1 Unicuspid aortic valve evaluated with **(a)** transesophageal echocardiography, **(b)** computed tomography, and **(c)** gross pathology.

From the Department of Internal Medicine (Gibbs), Department of Thoracic Surgery (Hamman), Department of Pathology (Roberts), and Division of Cardiology (Schussler), Baylor University Medical Center, Dallas, Texas.

Corresponding author: Jeffrey M. Schussler, MD, 621 North Hall Street, Suite 500, Dallas, TX 75226 (e-mail: Jeffrey.Schussler@heartplace.com).

DOI: 10.1201/9781003409281-48

(Figure 1C). The patient received a St. Jude Medical mechanical prosthesis, and his postoperative course was uncomplicated.

The estimated incidence of unicuspid aortic valve is 0.02%.[1-3] During development, the aortic valve is formed from three tubercles, which each develop a cusp and sinus of Valsalva. Fusion of the cusps results in a unicuspid valve. Unicommissural unicuspid valves, as in our case, have one lateral attachment and an eccentric orifice. Acommissural unicuspid valves have no lateral attachment to the aorta.

REFERENCES

1. Novaro GM, Mishra M, Griffin BP. Incidence and echocardiographic features of congenital unicuspid aortic valve in an adult population. *J Heart Valve Dis* 2003;12(6):674–678.
2. Roberts WC, Ko JM. Frequency by decades of unicuspid, bicuspid, and tricuspid aortic valves in adults having isolated aortic valve replacement for aortic stenosis, with or without associated aortic regurgitation. *Circulation* 2005;111(7):920–925.
3. Roberts WC, Ko JM. Clinical and morphologic features of the congenitally unicuspid acommissural stenotic and regurgitant aortic valve. *Cardiology* 2007;108(2):79–81.

Case 1502 Comparison of the Quantity of Calcific Deposits in Bovine Pericardial Bioprostheses in the Mitral and Aortic Valve Positions in the Same Patient Late After Double-Valve Replacement

William Clifford Roberts, MD,[a,b,d] Carlos Ernesto Velasco, MD,[a] Jong Mi Ko, BA,[d] and Gregory John Matter, MD[c]
Dallas, Tex

Among patients undergoing cardiac valve replacement, the aortic valve is most commonly replaced, the mitral valve next, and, infrequently, both the mitral and aortic valves. When the latter situation occurs and when the substitute valves inserted are both bioprostheses, it is possible to compare the rates of degenerative change because one bioprosthesis serves as a control for the other. In 1983, Warnes and associates[1] reported on 5 patients with porcine bioprostheses in both the mitral and aortic valve positions from 18 to 107 months, and in each of the 4·patients in which the bioprosthesis was in place for greater than 18 months, the quantity of calcific deposits on the cusps of the bioprosthesis in the mitral valve position was much greater than that on the prosthesis in the aortic valve position. The present report was prompted by observing a patient who had a bovine parietal pericardial bioprosthesis in both the mitral and aortic positions explanted after they had been in place for 77 months; the quantity of calcium in the bioprosthesis in the aortic valve position was massive, and that in the bioprosthesis in the mitral position was minimal.

CLINICAL SUMMARY

A patient, who was born on March 25, 1949, had acute rheumatic fever in childhood and hypothyroidism since age 20 years. She was in her usual good health until April 2001 (age 52 years), when exertional dyspnea appeared, and it soon progressed to orthopnea, which prompted hospital admission. Echocardiographic and cardiac catheterization data are shown in Table 1. Electrocardiographic analysis disclosed sinus rhythm.

On May 22, 2001, both the mitral and aortic valves were replaced with Carpentier Edwards pericardial bovine bioprostheses treated with the XenoLogix

From the Departments of Internal Medicine (Division of Cardiology),[a] Pathology,[b] and Cardiothoracic Surgery,[c] and the Baylor Heart and Vascular Institute,[d] Baylor University Medical Center, Dallas, Tex.

Received for publication Jan 29, 2009; accepted for publication Feb 8, 2009; available ahead of print March 27, 2009.

Address for reprints: William C. Roberts, MD, Baylor Heart and Vascular Institute, Baylor University Medical Center, 3500 Gaston Ave, Dallas, TX 75246 (E-mail: wc.roberts@baylorhealth.edu).

J Thorac Cardiovasc Surg 2009;138:1448–50

doi:10.1016/j.jtcvs.2009.02.022

Table 1: Cardiac catheterization data in the patient presented

Variable	May 18, 2001 (before the first operation)	October 10, 2007 (before the second operation)
Pulmonary artery (mm Hg)	75/40	102/54
Right ventricle (mm Hg)	75/28	102/24
Right atrium (mm Hg)		
A wave	30	28
V wave	23	25
Mean	22	20
Pulmonary artery wedge (mm Hg)		
A wave	37	42
V wave	38	46
Mean	34	33
Left ventricle (mm Hg)	159/28	
Aorta (mm Hg)	165/95	130/82
Cardiac index (L · min^{-1} · m^2)	1.8	2.0
Ejection fraction (%)	40	
Body weight (lbs)	156	138
Height (inches)	62	62

−, No information available.

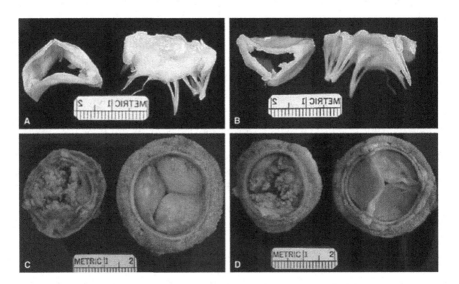

Figure 1 Native mitral and aortic valves (A and B) and bovine pericardial biopros-theses in the mitral and aortic valve positions (C and D) in the patient described. A, Anterior mitral leaflet from the atrial aspect and aortic valve from the ventricular aspect. B, Anterior mitral leaflet from the ventricular aspect and aortic valve from the aortic aspect. Both native valves are devoid of calcific deposits. C, Bioprosthesis in the mitral position from the atrial aspect and bioprosthesis in the aortic position from the aortic aspect. D, Bioprosthesis in the mitral position from the ventricular aspect and bioprosthesis in the aortic position from the ventricular aspect. Heavy calcific deposits are present on both surfaces of the bioprosthesis in the aortic valve position.

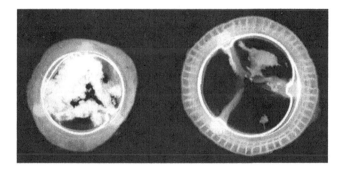

Figure 2   Radiograph of the bioprostheses excised from the aortic valve position *(left)* and the mitral valve position *(right)*. The calcific deposits are huge on the left and small on the right.

tissue treatment process (Edwards LifeSciences, Irvine, Calif), which removes approximately 98% of phospholipids, which are calcium-binding sites. The excised anterior mitral leaflet weighed 0.77 g, and the 3-cuspid aortic valve weighed 0.74 g (Figure 1, A and B). Both valves were free of calcium.

The patient was thereafter well until April 2002, when a febrile illness developed. *Streptococcus sanguis* was cultured from the blood. She was treated with antibiotics, and her usual health returned. Vegetations were never observed on either bioprosthesis by means of echocardiographic analysis. Another echocardiogram in March 2003 disclosed stenosis of the bioprosthesis in the aortic valve position.

She continued to be well until August 2007, when exertional dyspnea recurred, and within 3 weeks, she was essentially bedridden. She was rehospitalized on September 24, 2007, and repeat cardiac catheterization (Table 1) and echocardiographic analysis showed mild bioprosthetic mitral regurgitation and nearly nonmovable bioprosthetic cusps in the aortic valve position. The bioprosthesis in the aortic valve position could not be crossed at cardiac catheterization. The coronary arteries were normal on angiographic analysis.

On October 12, 2007, both bioprostheses were replaced with mechanical prostheses, and a tricuspid valve annuloplasty was performed. At the time of the operation, a small paravalvular leak was seen in the mitral position. The bioprosthesis in the mitral position (no. 25) weighed 4.04 g, and the bioprosthesis in the aortic position (no. 21) weighed 3.86 g (Figure 1, C and D). Radiographs of the operatively excised bioprostheses showed huge calcific deposits in the aortic prosthesis and small deposits in the mitral prosthesis (Figure 2). Her postoperative course was relatively uneventful. As of November 2008, she is active, and her activities are not limited. By means of echocardiographic analysis, her pulmonary arterial systolic pressure had decreased to 34 mm Hg, and left ventricular ejection fraction had increased to 55%. There was only trace tricuspid valve regurgitation.

DISCUSSION

The patient described had parietal pericardial bovine bioprostheses in both the mitral and aortic valve positions for 77 months and during that period developed huge quantities of calcium on the cusps of the bioprosthesis in the aortic valve position and only small quantities of calcium on the cusps of the bioprosthesis in the mitral valve position. Because the closing pressure on the mitral bioprosthesis is usually about a third higher than that on the aortic bioprosthesis (peak left ventricular systolic pressure vs end-diastolic aortic pressure; normally approximately 120 vs 80 mm Hg), it might be expected that the degeneration of a bioprosthesis in the mitral position would be greater (more calcium and more tears) and more rapid than that of a bioprosthesis in the aortic position, but the opposite was the case in the patient described herein. Why might that be the case? Some possibilities include the following:

1. Parietal pericardial bovine bioprostheses are not the same as porcine aortic valve bioprostheses. The former are thicker and less flexible and possibly withstand the left ventricular peak systolic pressure and the aortic end-diastolic pressure more easily than the more delicate porcine aortic cusps.
2. The bovine bioprosthesis in the aortic position was defective and not properly prepared, whereas the one in the mitral position was not.
3. The febrile illness the patient had beginning 11 months after the initial cardiac operation could have been active infective endocarditis that affected the bioprosthesis in the aortic position but not the bioprosthesis in the mitral position.
4. Smaller bovine parietal pericardial bioprostheses calcify more rapidly and more extensively than do larger bovine pericardial bioprostheses.
5. The paravalvular leak in the mitral position and the absence of a leak in the aortic position provided a "bypass shunt," diminishing the effect of the full force of the peak left ventricular systolic pressure on the bioprosthetic cusps in the mitral position.

None of these 5 possibilities can be proved or disproved, but this report might stimulate careful follow-up of similar patients to determine whether this distribution of calcium in the 2 left-sided bioprostheses is a pattern or an exception.

REFERENCE

1. Warnes CA, Scott ML, Silver GM, Smith CW, Ferrans VJ, Roberts WC. Comparison of late degenerative changes in porcine bioprostheses in the mitral and aortic valve position in the same patient. *Am J Cardiol* 1983;51:965–968.

Case 1506 Combined Mitral and Aortic Stenosis of Rheumatic Origin with Double-Valve Replacement in an Octogenarian

William Clifford Roberts[a,b,d,], Jong Mi Ko[d], John Ryan Schumacher[a],
Albert Carl Henry III[c]*

Replacement of both mitral and aortic valves in octogenarians is infrequent especially for combined mitral stenosis (MS) and aortic stenosis (AS) of rheumatic etiology. Such was the case, however, in the patient to be described herein.

An 81-year-old woman, who was born on 23 September 1925, had increasing dyspnea for several years because of what was believed to be "pulmonary fibrosis," worse in the lower lobes than the upper lobes. In December 2004, she was placed on home oxygen, and in January 2005, on continuous oxygen by nasal cannula. She had never smoked and had no history of acute rheumatic fever. Because of rather dramatic worsening of her dyspnea, she was hospitalized at Baylor University Medical Center on 1 May 2007. Her body mass index was 20 kg/m². Precordial examination disclosed an apical diastolic murmur and a basal ejection type systolic murmur. Electrocardiogram disclosed prolonged P-R interval and increased voltage compatible with left ventricular hypertrophy. Telemetric monitoring disclosed runs of atrial fibrillation.

Cardiac catheterization disclosed the following pressures in mm Hg: pulmonary artery wedge a-wave 21, v-wave 34, and mean 22; pulmonary artery, 68/26 (mean 39); left ventricle, 129/21 and aorta, 113/46; pulmonary arterial wedge—left ventricular mean diastolic gradient 8, and simultaneous left ventricular-aortic peak systolic gradient, 16. Cardiac index was 2.2 L/min/m². The calculated mitral valve area was 0.8 and the aortic valve area, 0.7 cm². Angiography disclosed insignificant coronary arterial narrowing.

On 4 May 2007, both left-sided cardiac valves (Figure 1) were replaced with St. Jude Medical prostheses: mitral #29, and aortic #19. The postoperative course was relatively smooth. The pulmonary arterial pressure fell dramatically, and she was discharged to the Baylor Specialty Hospital on 14 May 2007 where she remained for 17 days.

Thereafter, she did well until about 1 January 2008, when she noted pedal edema which progressed to anasarca and a weight gain from 112 to 148 lb. She was rehospitalized on 4 February 2008. The blood hemoglobin was 9.8 g/L and the

[a] *Department of Internal Medicine, Division of Cardiology, Baylor University Medical Center, Dallas, TX, United States*

[b] *Department of Pathology, Baylor University Medical Center, Dallas, TX, United States*

[c] *Department of Cardiothoracic Surgery, Baylor University Medical Center, Dallas, TX, United States*

[d] *Baylor Heart and Vascular Institute, Baylor University Medical Center, Dallas, TX, United States*
Received 29 October 2008; accepted 1 November 2008
Available online 30 November 2008
* Corresponding author. Department of Internal Medicine, Division of Cardiology, Baylor University Medical Center, Dallas, TX, United States.
E-mail address: wc.Roberts@baylorhealth.edu (W.C. Roberts).

DOI: 10.1201/9781003409281-50

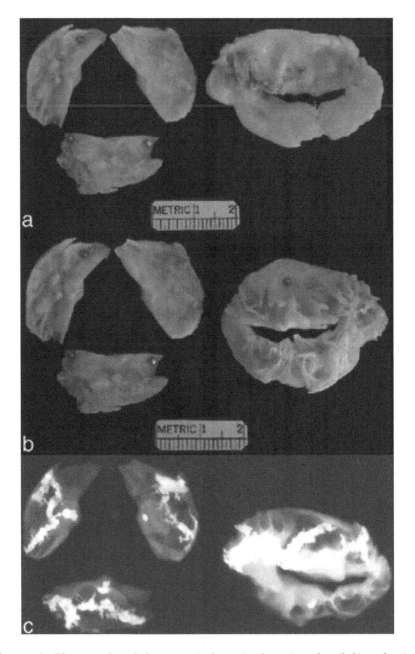

Figure 1 Photographs of the operatively excised aortic valve (left) and mitral valve (right). The mitral valve is shown from the atrial aspect in a and from the ventricular aspect in b. Radiographs of each valve are shown in c.

Table 1: Functional and anatomic classification of valvular heart disease in 1010 necropsy patients aged > =15 years[a]

Functional class	Patients	Anatomic class				
		AV	MV	MV-AV	TV-MV	TV-MV-AV
1. Aortic stenosis (AS)	292 (29%)	256 (88%)	0	35 (12%)	0	1 (0.3%)
2. Mitral stenosis (MS)	189 (19%)	0	117 (62%)	40 (21%)	13 (7%)	19 (10%)
3. MS+AS	152 (15%)	0	0	120 (79%)	0	32 (21%)
4. Aortic regurgitation (AR)[b]	119 (12%)	107 (90%)	0	10 (8%)	0	2 (2%)
5. Mitral regurgitation (MR)	97 (10%)	0	85 (88%)	8 (8%)	1 (1%)	3 (3%)
6. MS+AR	65 (6%)	0	52 (80%)	0	0	13 (20%)
7. MR+AR	45 (4%)	0	0	39 (87%)	0	6 (13%)
8. AS + MR	23 (2%)	0	0	21 (91%)	0	2 (9%)
9. Tricuspid stenosis+MS±AS	28 (3%)	0	0	0	4 (14%)	24 (86%)
Totals	1010 (100%)[c]	363 (36%)	254 (25%)	273 (27%)	18 (2%)	102 (10%)

AV = aortic valve; MV = mitral valve; TV = tricuspid valve.
Reproduced with permission from Elsevier and the author (Roberts WC. Am J Cardiol 1983;51:1005–1028).

[a] Excludes patients with mitral regurgitation secondary to coronary heart disease (papillary muscle dysfunction), carcinoid heart disease, hypertrophic cardiomyopathy, and those with infective endocarditis limited to 1 or both right-sided cardiac valves. Tricuspid valve regurgitation was present in many patients in most of the 9 functional groups. All patients were in functional class III or IV (New York Heart Association), and more than half had 1 or more cardiac operations.

[b] In many patients, the aortic valve cusps were normal or nearly normal and the regurgitation was the result of disease of the aorta (Marfan and Marfan-like syndrome, syphilis, systemic hypertension, healed aortic dissection).

[c] The hearts in all 1010 patients were examined and classified by WCR.

hematocrit, 30.3%. With diuretic therapy she lost 30 lb and returned home feeling much better. She was now in persistent atrial fibrillation. As of October 2008, she was doing well.

Although now infrequent in the Western world, combined MS and AS of rheumatic origin was relatively common when acute rheumatic fever was far more prevalent. Roberts[1] collected 1010 cases at autopsy of valvular heart disease studied from approximately 1955 to 1980: isolated AS (with or without regurgitation) was the most frequent valve lesion (29%); isolated MS (with or without mitral regurgitation) was next (19%), and combined MS and AS was in third place (15%) (Table 1). None of the patients with combined MS and AS, however, was > 80 years of age. In the last 3 decades, combined MS and AS of rheumatic etiology was infrequent in the Western world.

Combined MS and AS is particularly rare in octogenarians. Uricchio et al.[2] in 1959 reported 141 patients with combined MS and AS, all of whom had undergone both mitral and aortic commissurotomy: their ages ranged from 23 to 67 years.

Katznelson et al.[3] studied 22 patients ranging in age from 23 to 61 years (mean 45); the average age of onset of symptoms of cardiac dysfunction was 40. Honey[4] studied 35 patients and their ages ranged from 24 to 54 years (mean 40). Reid et al.[5] studied 15 patients aged 26 to 48. Morrow et al.[6] studied 8 patients aged 20 to 48, all of whom had combined mitral and aortic valvulotomy. Zitnik et al.[7] studied 10 such patients who ranged in age from 34 to 55 (mean 42). Roberts and Sullivan[8] studied at necropsy 30 such patients who died within 60 days of double valve replacement for combined MS and AS: one was an octogenarian, aged 83, but the others were younger (mean age 57). Berman et al.[9] performed combined percutaneous mitral and aortic valvulotomy in 6 patients, aged 60 to 83. Thus, only 2 of the 267 patients in those studies with combined MS and AS were octogenarians.

Combined MS and AS is more common in women than in men. Of the 267 patients reported in the previously mentioned 8 studies,[2-9] 171 (64%) were women.

Several studies have examined cardiac hemodynamics in patients with combined MS and AS.[2-9] Although there are exceptions, the degree of AS when combined with MS is not as great (transvalvular peak systolic gradient) as in patients with isolated AS. Furthermore the MS, as emphasized by Zitnik et al.,[7] can mask the presence of AS. If the AS is missed in this circumstance and mitral valve commissurotomy or replacement is performed and the downstream AS is neglected dire consequences can ensue. Obviously, it is best to diagnose both MS and AS preoperatively, but if one lesion is to be missed, it is far better to miss the upstream problem (MS) than the downstream problem (AS).

And finally, combined MS and AS can produce an operative challenge. First, the patients are most commonly women, some of whom, as in the present patient, are of small stature and, consequently, have relatively small hearts.[8] In combined MS and AS, neither the left ventricular cavity nor the ascending aorta is dilated, a circumstance which provides less space for either the mitral or the aortic mechanical prosthesis or bioprosthesis compared to the space provided in patients with isolated AS who often have congenitally bicuspid aortic valves and dilated ascending aortas.

ACKNOWLEDGMENT

The authors of this manuscript have certified that they comply with the Principles of Ethical Publishing in the International Journal of Cardiology.[10]

REFERENCES

1. Roberts WC. Morphologic features of the normal and abnormal mitral valve. *Am J Cardiol* 1983;51:1005–1028.
2. Uricchio JF, Goldberg H, Sinha KP, Likoff W. Combined mitral and aortic stenosis: clinical and physiologic features and results of surgery. *Am J Cardiol* 1959;4:479–491.
3. Katznelson G, Jreissaty RM, Levinson GE, Stein SW, Abelmann WH. Combined aortic and mitral stenosis. *Am J Med* 1960;29:242–256.
4. Honey M. Clinical and haemodynamic observations on combined mitral and aortic stenosis. *Brit Heart J* 1961;23:545–555.
5. Reid JM, Stevenson JG, Barclay RS, Welsh TM. Combined aortic and mitral stenosis. *Brit Heart J* 1962;24:509–515.
6. Morrow AG, Awe WC, Braunwald E. Combined mitral and aortic stenosis. *Brit Heart J* 1962;24:606–612.
7. Zitnik RS, Piemme TE, Messer RJ, Reed DP, Haynes FW, Dexter L. The masking of aortic stenosis by mitral stenosis. *Am Heart J* 1965;69:22–30.

8. Roberts WC, Sullivan MF. Clinical and necropsy observations early after simultaneous replacement of the mitral and aortic valves. *Am J Cardiol* 1986;58:1067–1084.
9. Berman AD, Weinstein JS, Safian RD, Diver DJ, Grossman W, McKay RG. Combined aortic and mitral balloon valvuloplasty in patients with critical aortic and mitral valve stenosis: results in six cases. *J Am Coll Cardiol* 1988;11:1213–1218.
10. Coats AJ. Ethical authorship and publishing. *Int J Cardiol* 2009;131:149–150.

Case 1531 Carcinoid Heart Disease Without the Carcinoid Syndrome but with Quadrivalvular Regurgitation and Unsuccessful Operative Intervention

William Clifford Roberts, MD[a,b,d,]*, Cyril Abie Varughese, DO[e], Jong Mi Ko, BA[d], Paul A. Grayburn, MD[b,d], Robert Frederick Hebeler, Jr., MD[c], and Elizabeth C. Burton, MD[a]

A 53-year-old woman is described who underwent mitral and aortic valve replacement and tricuspid valve annuloplasty for pure regurgitation at all 3 valve sites for unrecognized carcinoid heart disease without the carcinoid syndrome 22 days before death. Metastatic carcinoid was not recognized until necropsy, which disclosed a probable ovarian primary but with large hepatic metastases and left-sided cardiac involvement either greater than or equal to the right-sided involvement. Pulmonary hypertension, very unusual in carcinoid heart disease, persisted postoperatively and probably played a role in the patient's early death. Hepatic metastasis with ovarian primary is most unusual in this circumstance. © 2011 Elsevier Inc. All rights reserved.

(Am J Cardiol 2011;107:788–792)

It was in 1930, 80 years ago, when the first patient with a metastasizing carcinoid neoplasm associated with fibrous lesions on the right side of the heart was described.[1] In 1931, the first patient with metastasizing carcinoid syndrome (head and upper chest flushes and diarrhea) associated with fibrous lesions not only on the tricuspid and pulmonic valves but also on the anterior mitral leaflet and left ventricular mural endocardium was described.[2] Subsequently, of course, numerous reports have appeared describing clinical and morphologic features of the carcinoid syndrome and carcinoid heart disease.[2,3] Most patients have the primary carcinoid in the small intestine, widespread metastases, and specific carcinoid plaques limited to the right side of the heart.[2,3] The present report was prompted by study of a patient with severe mitral and aortic regurgitation leading to double valve replacement but without symptoms of the carcinoid syndrome but with metastasizing carcinoid.

CASE DESCRIPTION

A 53-year-old mother of 6, who was born May 5, 1955, and died February 18, 2009, had been well until November 2008, when she noted exertional dyspnea, subcutaneous peripheral edema, and recurring palpitations, which proved to be runs of atrial fibrillation. The symptoms gradually worsened, with episodes of rapid heart rate, each lasting several minutes. On January 26, 2009, cardiac catheterization disclosed the following pressures in mm Hg: pulmonary arterial wedge mean 22, a wave 30, v wave 28; pulmonary trunk 56/10; right ventricle 56/18; right atrial mean 9, a wave 15, v wave 10; left ventricle 130/26; and aorta 127/58. Left ventriculography

[a]Departments of Pathology, [b]Internal Medicine (Cardiology), and [c]Cardiothoracic Surgery; [d]Baylor Heart and Vascular Institute, Baylor University Medical Center; and [e]Department of Internal Medicine, Methodist Dallas Medical Center, Dallas, Texas, USA. Manuscript received September 1, 2010; revised manuscript received and accepted October 11, 2010.
[*] Corresponding author: Tel: 214-820-7911; fax: 214-820-7533.
E-mail address: wc.roberts@baylorhealth.edu (W.C. Roberts).

DOI: 10.1201/9781003409281-51

disclosed a normal-sized left ventricular cavity, with an ejection fraction of 60% and 4+/4+ mitral regurgitation. Aortography disclosed 4+/4+ aortic regurgitation. The coronary arteries were angiographically normal. Echocardiography showed thickened mitral and aortic valve cusps and a normal-sized left ventricle (Figure 1).

On January 27, 2009, the mitral and aortic valves were replaced with mechanical prostheses (#20 ATS Medical [Minneapolis, Minnesota] in the aortic position and #29 St. Jude Medical [St. Paul, Minnesota] in the mitral position). A Maze procedure was also performed as well as tricuspid valve annuloplasty. The operatively excised valves are shown in Figures 2 and 3. The 6-day postoperative hospital course was characterized by a weight gain of 6.6 kg (from 76.7 to 83.3 kg), sinus rhythm, and gradual ambulation.

On February 13, 2009, the patient was rehospitalized because of increasing weakness and dyspnea, evidence of gastrointestinal bleeding (on warfarin with an international normalized ratio of 4.7), and large pleural and pericardial effusions. The blood hemoglobin level was 11.1 g/dl, and the hematocrit was 35%. The serum bilirubin level was 1.4 mg/dl; alkaline phosphatase, 295 U/L; aspartate aminotransferase, 210 U/L; and alanine aminotransferase, 147 U/L. The blood urea nitrogen level was 17 mg/dl and glucose 96 mg/dl. The brain natriuretic peptide level was 430 pg/ml (normal range <100). Echocardiography now showed a normal-sized, normally functioning left ventricle, a very dilated and dysfunctional right ventricle, and large pericardial and right pleural effusions (Figure 4). Approximately 1,800 ml of serous fluid was drained from the right pleural space. Shortly thereafter, the patient had a cardiac arrest and died.

At necropsy, classic carcinoid neoplasms were present in the right ovary (2.3 × 2.1 × 1.9 cm), the liver (2 hemorrhagic and necrotic carcinoid masses, 10 × 9 × 9 and 3 × 3 × 3 cm; liver weight 2,100 g); the serosa of the bowel (1 nodule) and uterus (1 nodule); the adrenal glands (multiple small nodules); the pancreas (1 nodule, 0.3 cm); and the heart (multiple microscopic-sized nodules). Sections of the tumors in the liver, ovary, and adrenal glands were positive for neuron-specific enolase.

The heart (Figures 5 to 8) weighed 370 g. The coronary arteries were free of atherosclerotic plaque. The left ventricular cavity was small, and the right ventricular cavity was very dilated. No myocardial foci of fibrosis or necrosis were present,

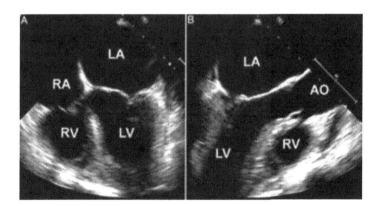

Figure 1 Preoperative (1 day) echocardiograms in the patient are described. *(A)* Four-chamber view showing the thickened mitral and tricuspid leaflets and the normal-sized right ventricular and left ventricular cavities. *(B)* Long-axis view again showing the thickened mitral leaflets and also a thickened aortic valve cusp. AO = aorta; LA = left atrium; LV = left ventricle; RA = right atrium; RV = right ventricle.

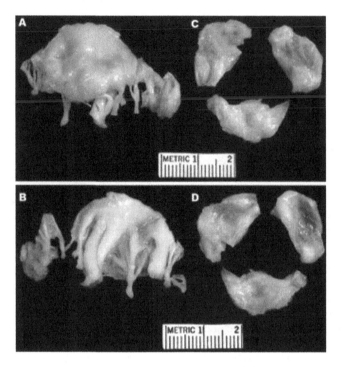

Figure 2 Photographs of the operatively excised mitral *(A,B)* and aortic *(C,D)* valves. *(A)* View of the atrial aspect of the anterior mitral leaflet. *(B)* View of the ventricular aspect of the anterior mitral leaflet with marked fibrous thickening of the chordae tendineae. A fragment of posterior leaflet with attached papillary muscle is also visible. *(C)* Focally thickened ventricular aspect of the tricuspid aortic valve. *(D)* Aortic aspect.

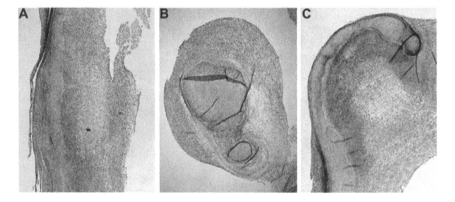

Figure 3 Photomicrograph of anterior mitral leaflet *(A)*, chordae tendineae *(B)*, and aortic valve cusp *(C)*. The underlying leaflet and chordae are normal, but both are quite thickened by superimposed cellular fibrous tissue devoid of elastic fibrils. The sinus portion of the aortic valve is filled with cellular fibrous tissue devoid of elastic fibers (C). Elastic van Gieson's stains (100×).

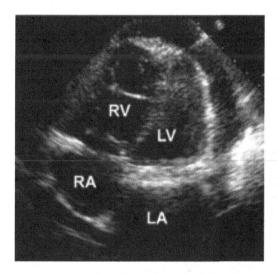

Figure 4 Four-chamber echocardiogram shortly before death in the patient described. The right ventricular cavity is severely dilated, whereas the left ventricle (LV) is not dilated. LA = left atrium; RA = right atrium; RV = right ventricle.

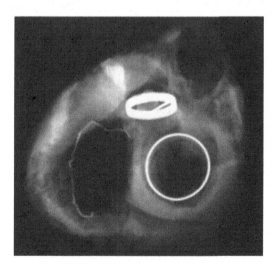

Figure 5 X-ray of the heart at necropsy. Prostheses are present in the mitral and aortic valve positions, and a ring is in the tricuspid valve annular position. The left ventricular cavity is not dilated, whereas the right ventricular cavity is considerably dilated.

except in the posteromedial left ventricular papillary muscle, which was fibrotic. Both atria were dilated, the right more than the left. The pulmonic valve cusps were thickened, and the anterior cusp was rigid and immobile. The foramen ovale was closed.

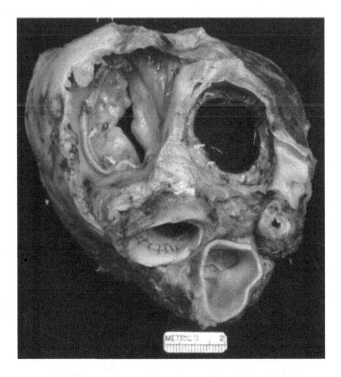

Figure 6 View of heart after removing the atrial walls and most of the ascending aorta and pulmonary trunk. The prosthesis in the mitral position fills the entire "floor" of the left atrium. The cloth-covered ring is visible in the tricuspid valve annulus.

COMMENTS

Our patient underwent mitral and aortic valve replacement and tricuspid valve annuloplasty for pure mitral, aortic, and tricuspid valve regurgitation. Examination of the operatively excised valves suggested an appearance similar to that described in patients having taken fenfluramine-phentermine for weight reduction. The patient, however, denied having ever taken that medication. Postoperatively, the patient's condition worsened, and she died 22 days after the operation. Necropsy disclosed carcinoid tumors in 1 ovary, both adrenal glands, the liver, the pancreas, the serosal surfaces of the uterus and bowel, and the heart (intramyocardial). There was never evidence of the carcinoid syndrome (flushing, diarrhea), and the presence of the carcinoid neoplasm was not diagnosed until necropsy, which also disclosed evidence of carcinoid heart disease involving both right-sided cardiac valves as well as both left-sided valves.

The primary in the patient described was not certain, but the ovary appeared to be the most logical site. Only 1 of the 2 ovaries was involved, and the cancerous nodule was >2 cm in diameter. Hepatic metastasis of carcinoid with ovarian primary, however, is quite unusual.[4,5] Chatterjee and Heather[6] found hepatic carcinoid metastases in only 1 of 35 reported cases with primary carcinoid in the ovary. Although our patient had only 2 carcinoid metastases in the liver, both were large.

In our patient, carcinoid heart disease involved all 4 cardiac valves: the pulmonic valve to a worse extent than the aortic valve, but the mitral valve to a worse extent

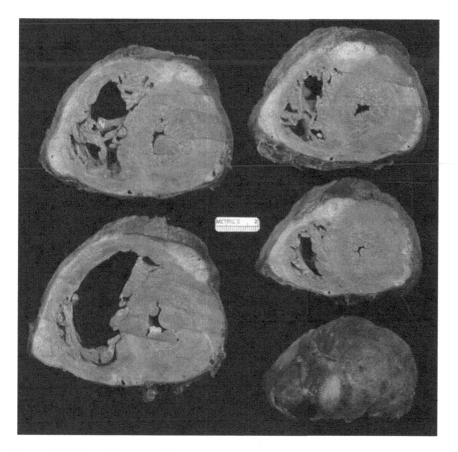

Figure 7 View of various "slices" of the cardiac ventricles showing the very small left ventricular cavity and the very dilated right ventricular cavity.

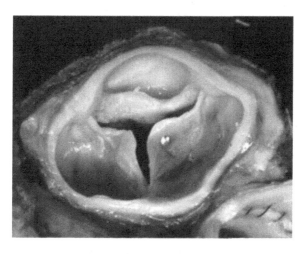

Figure 8 View of the pulmonic valve from above. The anterior cusp is very thick and immobile. The other 2 cusps are only mildly thickened by fibrous tissue.

245

than the tricuspid valve. Although the pulmonic valve was heavily involved by the carcinoid process, there was no pressure gradient across the valve, although the end-diastolic pressures in both the pulmonary trunk and the right ventricle were similar, indicating pure pulmonic regurgitation.

Is the electrocardiogram helpful in patients with malignant carcinoid in diagnosing carcinoid heart disease? No. Ross and Roberts[3] examined electrocardiograms in 34 patients with the carcinoid syndrome: the total 12-lead QRS voltages[7] in the 19 patients with carcinoid heart disease ranged from 58 to 227 mm (mean 105; standardization 10 mm) and in the 15 patients without carcinoid heart disease from 89 to 192 mm (mean 132). Twelve-lead QRS voltages in 16 men aged 44 to 74 years (mean 55) without cardiovascular disease ranged from 84 to 159 mm (mean 124) and heart weight from 288 to 392 g (mean 351).[8] Thus, in groups of patients with the carcinoid syndrome, those with carcinoid heart disease have lower total 12-lead QRS voltages, but much overlap occurred between the 2 groups. Our patient had a total 12-lead QRS voltage of 127 mm. The duration of the P-R, QRS, and Q-T intervals and heart rates at rest were similar in the 2 groups with and without carcinoid heart disease.

The presence of pulmonary hypertension in our patient is most unusual in carcinoid heart disease and reasonably can be attributed to the left-sided mitral disease.[9] The reason for its persistence postoperatively is unclear. The patient's symptoms worsened considerably postoperatively. The discs of the prostheses in both mitral and aortic positions moved without interference.

Cardiac valve replacement and/or "repair" for carcinoid heart disease is becoming more accepted, but nevertheless, outcomes are not always favorable.[9] In an early report from the Mayo Clinic, 9 of 26 patients died in the early perioperative period and 9 others a mean of 19 months postoperatively. Only 4 of their 26 patients had mitral or aortic valve replacement, and none had both valves replaced, as did our patient. Although the mortality was higher, late operative survival (8 of 26 patients) resulted in considerable decrease (2 patients) or elimination (6 patients) of symptoms.[9] A later report from the same institution summarized results in 11 patients with carcinoid heart disease who underwent operation for left- and right-sided valve disease:[10] the tricuspid valve was replaced in all 11, the pulmonic in 3 (valvectomy in 7), the mitral valve in 6 (repair in 1), and the aortic valve in 4 (repair in 2). There were 2 perioperative deaths and 4 additional deaths in a mean follow-up period of 41 months. All but 1 operative survivor improved by >1 functional class. In retrospect, had the presence of carcinoid been recognized preoperatively or at operation in our patient, both tricuspid and pulmonic valves probably also would have been replaced (quadruple valve replacement).[11]

ACKNOWLEDGMENT

We thank Brad J. Roberts, BS, RCS, RDCS, for his help in preparing the echocardiogram.

REFERENCES

1. Cassidy MA. Abdominal carcinomatosis with probable adrenal involvement. *Proc Roy Soc Med* 1930;24:139–141.
2. Roberts WC, Sjoerdsma A. The cardiac disease associated with the carcinoid syndrome (carcinoid heart disease). *Am J Med* 1964;36:5–34.
3. Ross EM, Roberts WC. The carcinoid syndrome: comparison of 21 necropsy subjects with carcinoid heart disease to 15 necropsy subjects without carcinoid heart disease. *Am J Med* 1985;79:339–353.
4. Chaoqalit N, Connolly HM, Schaff HV, Webb MJ, Pellikka PA. Carcinoid heart disease associated with primary ovarian carcinoid tumor. *Am J Cardiol* 2004;93:1314–1315.

5. Rabban JT, Lerwill MF, McCluggage WG, Grenert JP, Zaloudek CJ. Primary ovarian carcinoid tumors may express CDX-2: a potential pitfall in distinction from metastatic intestinal carcinoid tumors involving the ovary. *Int J Gynecol Pathol* 2009;28:41–48.

6. Chatterjee K, Heather JC. Carcinoid heart disease from primary ovarian carcinoid tumors. *Am J Med* 1968;45:643–648.

7. Siegel RJ, Roberts WC. Electrocardiographic observations in severe aortic valve stenosis: correlative necropsy study to clinical, hemodynamic, and ECG variables demonstrating relation of 12-lead QRS amplitude to peak systolic transaortic pressure gradient. *Am Heart J* 1982;103:210–221.

8. Odom H II, Davis L, Dinh HA, Baker BJ, Roberts WC, Murphy ML. QRS voltage measurements in autopsied men free of cardiopulmonary disease: a basis for evaluating total QRS voltage as an index of left ventricular hypertrophy. *Am J Cardiol* 1986;58:801–804.

9. Connolly HM, Nishimura RA, Smith HC, Pellikka PA, Mullany CJ, Kvols LK. Outcome of cardiac surgery for carcinoid heart disease. *J Am Coll Cardiol* 1995;25:410–416.

10. Connolly HM, Schaff HV, Mullany CJ, Rubin J, Abel MD, Pellikka PA. Surgical management of left-sided carcinoid heart disease. *Circulation* 2001;104:I36–I40.

11. Arghami A, Connolly HM, Abel MD, Schaff HV. Quadruple valve replacement in patients with carcinoid heart disease. *J Thorac Cardiovasc Surg* 2010;140:1432–1434.

Case 1559 43.3-Year Durability of a Smeloff-Cutter Ball-Caged Mitral Valve

Stuart J. Head, BS, Jamie Ko, Rajeev Singh, MD, William C. Roberts, MD, and Michael J. Mack, MD

Extended durability of mechanical heart valves has been documented for many years. We describe a case of a ball-caged mechanical valve implanted 43.3 years previous to developing valve dysfunction. The patient presented with both prosthetic valve stenosis and insufficiency. This Smeloff-Cutter valve (Cutter Laboratories, Berkeley, CA) in the mitral position was dysfunctional due to lipid absorption, which resulted in ball variance and concomitant pannus growth prevented optimal seating of the ball in its cage. This is the longest length of time in which a Smeloff-Cutter mechanical valve has been originally implanted.

(Ann Thorac Surg 2011;91:606–8) © 2011 by The Society of Thoracic Surgeons

In the early 1960s, heart valves were introduced for heart valve replacement, which resulted in the first mechanical valve prosthesis implantation of a Starr-Edwards valve (Edwards Lifesciences, Irvine, CA) in the mitral position in 1961.[1] After this, newly developed ball-caged valves followed in quick succession, manufactured by a number of companies producing aortic and mitral valve prostheses. The Smeloff-Cutter valve (Cutter Laboratories, Berkeley, CA) was introduced in 1964, being the first "full-flow" valve, which was achieved by including an additional smaller cage on which the ball could rest during valve closure.[2]

"Ball variance" is a previously documented cause of valve dysfunction,[3] in which lipid absorption in the ball causes it to grow and form surface irregularities, increasing the risk of thromboembolic events and valve dysfunction. We report a case in which ball variance and pannus overgrowth caused a 43.3-year implanted Smeloff-Cutter ball-caged valve to fail. This case is the longest implantation time of this type of valve.

At age 13, mitral valve stenosis developed in the patient, due to rheumatic fever. Therefore, the patient underwent a valve replacement. Recently, the 56-year-old woman presented with New York Heart Association functional class IV symptoms of heart failure and palpitations as a result of long-standing persistent atrial fibrillation. Transthoracic and transesophageal echocardiography (Figure 1) revealed moderate to severe mitral valve regurgitation and severe mitral stenosis with a valve area of 0.7 cm^2 and a mean gradient of 15 mm Hg. There was decreased left ventricular function with an ejection fraction of 40%, systemic pulmonary hypertension, and severe tricuspid regurgitation.

Cardiopulmonary Research Science and Technology Institute, Dallas, Texas, Department of Cardio-Thoracic Surgery, Erasmus University Medical Center, Rotterdam, the Netherlands, Department of Pathology, The Baylor Heart and Vascular Institute, Dallas, Department of Cardiology, The Diagnostic Clinic of Longview, Longview, and Heart Hospital Baylor Plano, Plano, Texas

Accepted for publication June 29, 2010.

Address correspondence to Dr Mack, Heart Hospital Baylor Plano, 1100 Allied Dr, Plano, TX 75093; e-mail: mmack@csant.com.

DOI: 10.1201/9781003409281-52

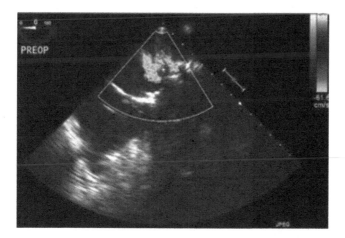

Figure 1 Preoperative echocardiogram showing both mitral stenosis and insufficiency.

The patient had been noncomplaint with warfarin therapy until suffering a stroke in 1988 after discontinuing therapy, which left her with a significant residual right hemipharesis. However, this event subsequently made her extremely diligent in taking the anticoagulant with good control and no further clinical events. For this reason, she opted for another mechanical valve.

At the time of the redo mitral valve replacement, a pre-cardiopulmonary bypass transesophageal echocardiographic finding consisted of the mitral valve prosthesis in a good position with severe mitral valve regurgitation. A 2.4 m/s maximum velocity was measured across the valve, calculating to a peak gradient of 23 mm Hg and a mean gradient of 9 mm Hg. The valve area was 2.3 cm² by pressure halftime and 0.7 cm² measured by continuity equation. Furthermore, a left ventricular ejection fraction of 40% was obtained. All measurements are consistent with preoperative findings.

The limited access procedure was performed exposing only the aorta and right atrium. A superior septal approach to the mitral valve was performed. Inspection of the valve revealed some erosion of the ball (Figure 2). Pannus formation built up around the valve prevented the ball to seat completely in its cage. There was an extensive amount of calcium built up both in the annulus and the ventricular muscle below the annulus. The 43.3-year-old valve was replaced with a 25-mm On-X bi-leaflet mechanical valve (On-X Life Technologies Inc, Austin, TX). After the valve was implanted, transesophageal echocardiography measured a maximum velocity across the valve of 1.3 m/s, with a peak-to-peak gradient of 7 mm Hg and a mean gradient of 3 mm Hg. By pressure half-time the valve area had improved to 3.5 cm². Concomitant tricuspid valve annuloplasty with a 26-mm tricuspid annulus ring and a full left-sided and right-sided Cryo maze procedure were performed. Her postoperative course was uneventful. She was discharged home on postoperative day 6. The patient is in New York Heart Association functional class I at her most recent follow-up at 6 weeks postoperatively.

COMMENT

Valve dysfunction after extended durability can be the result of a wide variety of causes, including lipid absorption into the ball and pannus formation, causing tissue impingement as the two most common. Absorption increases the

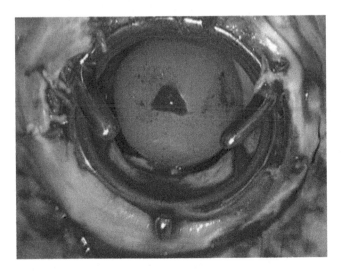

Figure 2 The 43.3-year-old Smeloff-Cutter valve in the mitral position. The valve was dysfunctional due to ball variance and pannus formation, both visible here. The ball shows signs of wear, having lost its perfect round shape and showing erosion.

size of the ball and causes it to lose its round shape.[3] This can cause denting, increasing the risk of complications, such as thrombus formation and hemolysis. Dysfunction occurs because ball variance can make it impossible for the ball to move freely with regurgitation as a result, or can cause it to stick in the cage in the closed position. However, many causes of late valve dysfunction are not related to the design of the valve. Ozkokeli and colleagues[4] reported a case in which a 37-year implanted Starr-Edwards valve (Edwards Lifesciences) (model 1000–9A) developed acute prosthetic valve endocarditis, a complication unrelated to the implantation time. Also, indiscriminate to years of implantation is the formation of tissue overgrowth. An article by Butany and colleagues[5] describes pannus growth in a DeBakey Surgitool (Travenol Laboratories Inc, Morton Grove, IL) mechanical aortic valve prosthesis implanted for 32 years. The valve itself did not show any signs of wear, but it became dysfunctional due to the excessive tissue. Schmitto and colleagues[6] reported a suboptimal but satisfactory working Starr-Edwards ball-caged valve at 39 years after initial implantation. However, a post-valvular ascending aortic aneurysm of 6.0 × 6.5 cm made it necessary to perform a Bentall procedure.[6]

A few cases have been reported of patients with a mechanical aortic or mitral valve in place for more than 30 years in which the nonprosthetic valve in the systemic circulation was regurgitating, not the prosthesis.[8] In these cases, the prostheses were working satisfactory, but in many cases the decision was made to prophylactically replace the valve.

Reports of prolonged ball-caged valve durability are mostly Starr-Edwards valves, with survival of greater than 43 years in a number of cases (Table 1). In the literature, it is reported that Smeloff-Cutter valves have been explanted after as long as 37 years.[8] Until further results have been published, we believe that this case reports the longest implanted Smeloff-Cutter mechanical valve of 43.3 years.

Table 1: Valve implantation times ≥43 years

Valve Type	Position	Age at Surgery	Years in Position
Starr-Edwards	Aortic	19	46.3
Starr-Edwards[7]	Mitral	24	44
Starr-Edwards	Aortic	28	43.8
Starr-Edwards	Aortic and mitral	31	43.7
Smeloff-Cutter	Mitral	13	43.3
Starr-Edwards	Aortic	19	43.1
Starr-Edwards	Aortic	16	43.1
Starr-Edwards	Aortic	19	43

REFERENCES

1. Starr A, Edwards M. Mitral replacement: clinical experience with a ball-valve prosthesis. *Ann Surg* 1961;154:726–740.
2. Gott VL, Alejo DE, Cameron DE. Mechanical heart valves: 50 years of evolution. *Ann Thorac Surg* 2003;76:S2230–S2239.
3. Peterman MA, Donsky MS, Matter GJ, Roberts WC. A Starr-Edwards model 6120 mechanical prosthesis in the mitral valve position for 38 years. *Am J Cardiol* 2006;97:756–758.
4. Ozkokeli M, Ates M, Ekinci A, Akcar M. Thirty-seven-year durability of a Starr-Edwards aortic prosthesis. *Tex Heart Inst J* 2005;32:99–101.
5. Butany J, Naseemuddin A, Nair V, Feindel CM. DeBakey Surgitool mechanical heart valve prosthesis, explanted at 32 years. *Cardiovasc Pathol* 2004;13:345–346.
6. Schmitto JD, Ortmann P, Popov AF, et al. Bentall procedure 39 years after implantation of a Starr-Edwards aortic cagedball-valve prosthesis. *J Cardiothorac Surg* 2010;5:12.
7. Fernandez J, Farivar RS. Explantation of a 44-year-old Starr-Edwards mitral valve for delayed hemolysis. *J Thorac Cardiovasc Surg* 2010;140:e35–e36.
8. Si MS, Zapolanski A. A 37-year-old Smeloff-Cutter aortic valve. *Ann Thorac Surg* 2009;87:628–629.

Case 1589 Combined Congenitally Bicuspid Aortic Valve and Mitral Valve Prolapse Causing Pure Regurgitation

William C. Roberts, MD, Saleha Zafar, MD, Jong Mi Ko, Melissa M. Carry, MD, and Robert F. Hebeler, MD

Described herein is a patient with a purely regurgitant congenitally bicuspid aortic valve and a purely regurgitant prolapsing mitral valve. Although it is well established that the bicuspid aortic valve is a congenital anomaly, it is less well appreciated that mitral valve prolapse is almost certainly also a congenital anomaly. The two occurring in the same patient provides support that mitral valve prolapse is also a congenital anomaly.

It is well appreciated that the bicuspid aortic valve (BAV) is usually of congenital origin. It is less well appreciated that mitral valve prolapse (MVP) is usually of congenital origin. Most patients with a congenitally BAV (unless complicated by superimposed infective endocarditis) have a structurally normal mitral valve. It is most unusual for a patient with a congenitally BAV, particularly one that is purely regurgitant, to have associated MVP. Such was the case, however, in the patient described herein.

CASE DESCRIPTION

A 64-year-old white man with a doctorate, who was born in June 1947, had been well until November 2011, when he had the first of several episodes of syncope. During hospitalization for acute appendicitis, an electrocardiogram disclosed the presence of atrial fibrillation. Another syncopal episode and the appearance of exertional and nocturnal dyspnea in 2012 prompted a visit to a cardiologist. His body mass index was 30 kg/m². A grade 2/6 basal precordial systolic murmur and a grade 4/6 blowing apical systolic murmur with radiation into the left axilla were heard. The initial electrocardiogram showed supraventricular tachycardia with a ventricular rate of 140 beats a minute. An echocardiogram showed MVP with a flail P_2 portion of the posterior leaflet and severe mitral regurgitation. The aortic valve was bicuspid, and moderate aortic regurgitation was present. The left ventricular cavity was of normal size, and its ejection fraction was 60%. Cardiac catheterization disclosed the following pressures in mm Hg: left ventricle, 136/33; aorta, 139/70; pulmonary artery wedge, a wave 23, v 38, mean 11; pulmonary artery, 34/13; right ventricle, 39/14; and right atrium, a wave 14, v wave 13, mean 11. The cardiac index was 2.9 L/min/m². Coronary angiogram disclosed no luminal narrowing; the right coronary was the dominant artery. Left ventricular cavity size and contractility were normal. The aortic regurgitation was graded 2+/4+.

Five days later the purely regurgitant aortic valve was replaced with a #29 Mosaic porcine xenograft. The mitral valve was repaired by resecting P_2, replacing two chordae, and inserting a #37 ATS annuloplasty ring *(Figures 1–3)*. Additionally,

From the Divison of Cardiology, Department of Internal Medicine (Roberts, Zafar, Ko, Carry), and Department of Cardiothoracic Surgery (Hebeler), Baylor Heart and Vascular Hospital and Baylor University Medical Center at Dallas.

Corresponding author: William C. Roberts, MD, Baylor Heart and Vascular Institute, 621 North Hall Street, Dallas, TX 75226 (e-mail: wc.roberts@baylor-health.edu).

DOI: 10.1201/9781003409281-53

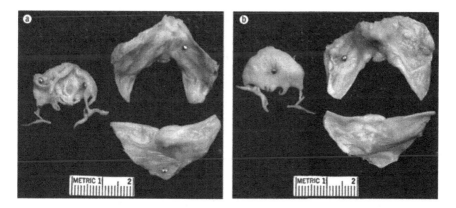

Figure 1 Mitral and aortic valves of the patient described. **(a)** Ventricular aspect of the resected portion of the posterior mitral leaflet and of the congenitally bicuspid aortic valve. Several chordae are missing, indicating that they had ruptured in the past and later became incorporated in the superimposed fibrous tissue on the ventricular aspect of the leaflet (see Figure 2). **(b)** Atrial aspect of the mitral leaflet and aortic aspect of a congenitally bicuspid aortic valve.

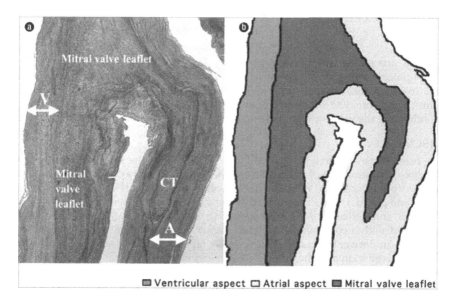

Figure 2 (a) Photomicrograph of a portion of the posterior mitral valve leaflet and attached chordae tendineae (CT). The leaflet and chordal thickening is the result of superimposed fibrous tissue on both atrial (A) and ventricular (V) aspects of the leaflet and surrounding the chordae. The leaflet itself consists primarily of the fibrosa element; the spongiosa element is minimal. These histological features are characteristic of mitral valve prolapse. Elastic von Gieson stain, ×40. **(b)** A color-coded replica with green representing the ventricular aspect, yellow representing the atrial aspect, and red representing the mitral valve leaflet.

253

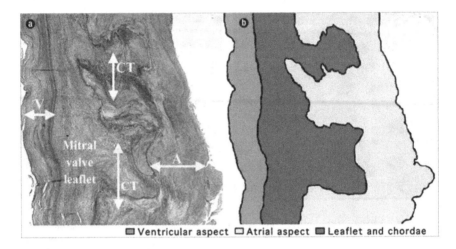

☐ Ventricular aspect ☐ Atrial aspect ☐ Leaflet and chordae

Figure 3 (a) Photomicrograph of a portion of the mitral leaflet and chordae tendineae (CT) with superimposed fibrous tissue on the atrial (A) aspect and on the ventricular (V) aspect. The underlying normal leaflet and chordae tendineae are outlined by a black-staining elastic membrane. It is likely that the chordae had ruptured in the distant past and later the portion closest to the leaflet was covered by fibrous tissue. Elastic von Gieson stain, ×40. **(b)** A color-coded replica with green representing the ventricular aspect, yellow representing the atrial aspect, and red representing the leaflet and chordae.

a Maze procedure was performed. Seven days postoperatively, because of the development of complete atrioventricular disassociation, a dual-chamber pacemaker was inserted. Electrocardiogram in July 2012 disclosed sinus rhythm (75 beats a minute) and complete left bundle branch block. When seen on September 11, 2012, 3 months after the valve operation, the patient was asymptomatic and "feeling great."

DISCUSSION

The occurrence of both a congenitally BAV and MVP in the same patient suggests that both conditions are of congenital origin. That the BAV is a congenital anomaly is well accepted, but that MVP is also likely a congenital anomaly—at least some of the leaflet and chordal tissue is congenitally deficient—is less well appreciated.

Iqbal and colleagues[1] in 1980 appear to have been the first to report MVP associated with a congenital BAV. They described two patients, one a 39-year-old man who underwent mitral and aortic valve replacement for combined mitral and aortic regurgitation and the other, a 23-year-old man with mitral regurgitation and a normally functioning congenitally BAV.

Chisholm[2] in 1981 found a congenitally BAV in 8 of 257 black patients with MVP. None of his 8 patients had either mitral or aortic dysfunction severe enough to warrant operative intervention. All 8 patients had evidence of trace aortic regurgitation, and none had evidence of aortic stenosis. None apparently had significant mitral regurgitation. The cardiac size in all 8 patients was normal.

In 1994 Fernicola and Roberts[3] described 11 patients who underwent aortic valve replacement for a dysfunctioning congenitally BAV and mitral replacement for a purely regurgitant mitral valve. In 2012 Roberts and colleagues[4] described another 16 patients at another institution who had aortic valve replacement for a

Table 1: Previously reported patients having simultaneous aortic and mitral valve operations for a dysfunctioning congenitally bicuspid aortic valve and a dysfunctioning mitral valve*

Valve dysfunction	Patients (n)	Ages, years: Range (mean)	IE	IC	RHD	MVP	Unknown
			Etiology of MR				
AS + MS	6	46–74 (59)	0	0	4	0	2
AS + MR	13	52–84 (66)	2	2	0	4	5
AR + MS	0	0	0	0	0	0	0
AR + MR	9	24–66 (46)	7	0	0	1	1
Totals	28	24–84 (56)	9	2	4	5	8

*From Fernicola and Roberts, 1994 (3) and Roberts et al, 2012 (4).
AR indicates aortic regurgitation; AS, aortic stenosis; IC, ischemic cardiomyopathy; IE, infective endocarditis; MR, mitral regurgitation; MS, mitral stenosis; MVP, mitral valve prolapse; RHD, rheumatic heart disease.

dysfunctioning congenitally BAV and simultaneous mitral valve operation for a dysfunctioning mitral valve. The *Table* summarizes the findings in the combined studies by Fernicola and Roberts[3] and by Roberts et al.[4] Of their 28 patients, the BAV was stenotic in 19 (68%) and purely regurgitant in 9 (32%); the mitral valve was stenotic in 6 (21%) and purely regurgitant in 22 (79%). Of the 19 patients with stenotic BAVs, at least 4 (21%) had MVP; of the 9 patients with a purely regurgitant BAV, only 1 (11%) had MVP, as did the patient described herein.

REFERENCES

1. Iqbal MZ, Eybel CE, Messer JV. Mitral valve prolapse associated with bicuspid aortic valve. *Cardiovasc Rev Rep* 1980;1:465–468.
2. Chisholm JC. Mitral valve prolapse syndrome associated with congenital bicuspid aortic valve. *J Natl Med Assoc* 1981;73(10):921–923.
3. Fernicola DJ, Roberts WC. Pure mitral regurgitation associated with a malfunctioning congenitally bicuspid aortic valve necessitating combined mitral and aortic valve replacement. *Am J Cardiol* 1994;74(6):619–624.
4. Roberts WC, Janning KG, Vowels TJ, Ko JM, Hamman BL, Hebeler RF Jr. Presence of a congenitally bicuspid aortic valve among patients having combined mitral and aortic valve replacement. *Am J Cardiol* 2012;109(2):263–271.

Case 1611 Infective Endocarditis Superimposed On a Massively Calcified Severely Stenotic Congenitally Bicuspid Aortic Valve

Syed Sarmast, MD, Jeffrey M. Schussler, MD, Jong M. Ko, BA, and William C. Roberts, MD

We describe a 55-year-old man who presented with a stroke resulting from active infective endocarditis (IE) involving a heavily calcified bicuspid aortic valve. The case highlights the infrequency of IE involving a heavily calcified valve, the inability of the infection to penetrate the calcific deposits, and the ability of the infection to spread to the adjacent soft tissues, leading to ring abscess and its multiple complications.

The aortic valve is the most common site for one or more vegetations to form in infective endocarditis (IE).[1] Since the introduction of corticosteroids and the increased frequency of immunotherapy and intravenous drug addiction, infection involving the aortic valve has most commonly involved a previously structurally normal valve. The next most common aortic valve to be involved by IE was a congenitally malformed bicuspid aortic valve that had functioned normally or had only mild dysfunction.[2] IE involving a previously calcified valve is unusual and particularly so when the aortic valve is massively calcified. The present report was prompted by study of a patient who developed IE on a previously heavily calcified, severely stenotic aortic valve.

CASE DESCRIPTION

A 55-year-old white man, on chronic hemodialysis for end-stage renal disease believed to be secondary to diabetes mellitus, was hospitalized because of the sudden onset of confusion. Diabetes mellitus was diagnosed when he was 43 years old (2001), requiring insulin therapy by age 49. Systemic hypertension was diagnosed at age 50. He had a sedentary lifestyle and was obese (body mass index 35 kg/m²). Twelve months earlier, hemodialysis had been initiated; 7 months earlier, a malfunctioning right arm arteriovenous fistula had been repaired; and 1 month earlier, he presented with fever, nausea, vomiting, and abdominal pain. Methicillin-resistant *Staphylococcus aureus* bacteremia related to a right internal jugular PermaCath infection was diagnosed. During that admission, a grade 2/6 precordial systolic ejection murmur was heard. Echocardiography revealed a calcified stenotic bicuspid aortic valve with trace aortic regurgitation, and a small mobile mass attached to the aortic valve was seen. An aortic root abscess also was seen. He was discharged home to receive intravenous vancomycin for 6 weeks and then returned because of confusion. Repeat blood cultures again grew *Staphylococcus aureus*. He was treated with daptomycin.

From the Division of Cardiology, Department of Internal Medicine, Baylor University Medical Center at Dallas and the Jack and Jane Hamilton Heart and Vascular Hospital, Dallas, Texas.

Corresponding author: Syed Sarmast, MD, Baylor Heart and Vascular Hospital, 621 N. Hall Street, Dallas, TX 75226 (e-mail: Syed.Sarmast@BaylorHealth.edu).

DOI: 10.1201/9781003409281-54

On July 31, 2010, the aortic valve (bioprosthesis) and proximal portion of the ascending aorta were replaced (the latter was a homograft), the paravalvular abscess was debrided, and the coronary ostial sites were implanted into the homograft. The excised stenotic and infected aortic valve weighed 8.36 g and was congenitally bicuspid *(Figure 1)*. Culture of the excised valve grew methicillin-resistant *Staphylococcus aureus*. The patient's early postoperative course was complicated by episodes of paroxysmal atrial fibrillation and nonsustained ventricular tachycardia.

One month following the operation, the patient was back at home and continuing his hemodialysis treatments 3 times a week. A successful renal transplant was performed on September 13, 2012, and hemodialysis was discontinued. As of October 2013, he remains active and exercises 30 minutes a day at least 3 times a week. He is currently unemployed and on disability.

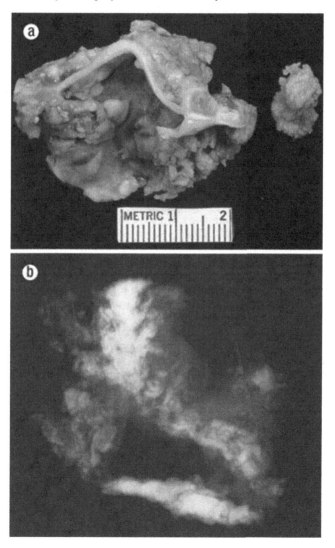

Figure 1 (a) Photograph of the operatively excised stenotic aortic valve and **(b)** radiograph of the valve in the patient described.

DISCUSSION

The patient described herein with end-stage renal disease requiring chronic hemodialysis had a heavily calcified stenotic congenitally bicuspid aortic valve and developed superimposed IE initiated as a result of infection at the percutaneous dialysis entry site. The infection, unable to grow well in the calcified valve, rapidly spread to the adjoining soft tissue, producing a ring abscess.

The unusual feature of the present patient is the development of IE on a massively calcified aortic valve. The normal aortic valve weighs about 0.4 g. Thus, the valve in the present patient (8.36 g) was 20 times heavier than normal, and most of that excessive weight was the result of the calcific deposits, not the superimposed vegetative material. Roberts and Ko[3] initially reported weights of operatively excised stenotic aortic valves in 2003 and from January 1998 to August 2013 had weighed 1726 stenotic aortic valves: only 12 (0.7%) weighed >8 g, and none of the other 11 patients had IE. Indeed, the lighter the aortic valve, the greater the likelihood of its being complicated by IE.[2]

IE involving a stenotic aortic valve is far less common than IE involving a nonstenotic aortic valve. Fernicola and Roberts[4] studied at necropsy 96 patients with active IE involving the aortic valve: 25 (26%) had underlying stenosis and 71 (74%) had an underlying nonstenotic valve. Of the 25 with underlying stenosis, 21 (84%) had a ring abscess and 10 (40%) had an underlying congenitally bicuspid valve; of the 71 with a nonstenotic aortic valve, 37 (52%) had a ring abscess ($P = 0.005$) and 21 (30%), a congenitally bicuspid valve (ns).

The patient described had two reasons for having a heavily calcified aortic valve: 1) the underlying bicuspid condition,[2] and 2) the presence of end-stage renal disease with chronic hemodialysis.[5]

REFERENCES

1. Arnett EN, Roberts WC. Pathology of active infective endocarditis: a necropsy analysis of 192 patients. *Thorac Cardiovasc Surg* 1982;30(6):327–335.
2. Roberts WC, Vowels TJ, Ko JM. Natural history of adults with congenitally malformed aortic valves (unicuspid or bicuspid). *Medicine (Baltimore)* 2012;91(6):287–308.
3. Roberts WC, Ko JM. Weights of operatively-excised stenotic unicuspid, bicuspid, and tricuspid aortic valves and their relation to age, sex, body mass index, and presence or absence of concomitant coronary artery bypass grafting. *Am J Cardiol* 2003;92(9):1057–1065.
4. Roberts WC, Oluwole BO, Fernicola DJ. Comparison of active infective endocarditis involving a previously stenotic versus a previously nonstenotic aortic valve. *Am J Cardiol* 1993;71(12):1082–1088.
5. Roberts WC, Taylor MA, Shirani J. Cardiac findings at necropsy in patients with chronic kidney disease maintained on chronic hemodialysis. *Medicine (Baltimore)* 2012;91(3):165–178.

Case 1636 Clues to Diagnosing Carcinoid Heart Disease as the Cause of Isolated Right-Sided Heart Failure

Carey Camille Roberts, BS[a,b], Rohit J. Parmar, MD[b,c], Paul A. Grayburn, MD[b,c], Gautam R. Patankar, MD[b,c], Jong Mi Ko, BA[b], Baron L. Hamman, MD[d], and William Clifford Roberts, MD[b,c,e],*

Described herein is a 67-year-old woman who underwent replacement of both tricuspid and pulmonic valves because of severe isolated right-sided systolic heart failure. The cause of the heart failure preoperatively was believed to be the result of left breast radiation a year earlier. At operation, however, the pulmonic valve was excised and a biopsy of the stiff-walled right atrium was performed, and histologic examination of each was classic of carcinoid heart disease. She never awoke postoperatively. Postoperatively, computed tomography disclosed numerous masses in the liver. Retrospectively, clues to the presence of carcinoid heart disease include thickening of both the tricuspid and pulmonic valve leaflets by echocardiogram, a pressure gradient, albeit small, across the pulmonic valve, the plastering of the septal tricuspid-valve leaflet to the ventricular septum, the total absence of left-sided heart disease, and the presence of extremely low 12-lead QRS electrocardiographic voltage. © 2014 Elsevier Inc. All rights reserved.

(Am J Cardiol 2014;114:1623–1626)

The most common cause of right-sided heart failure is left-sided heart failure. Isolated right-sided heart failure is far less common than that associated with left-sided heart failure, and usually results from pulmonary disease (parenchymal, vascular and/or bellows-system abnormalities), all of which produce pulmonary hypertension. Constrictive pericardial diseases and isolated congenital pulmonic-valve stenosis are far less common causes. Carcinoid heart disease as a cause of right-sided heart failure is rare, but distinctive clues to its presence are usually discernible[1-6] (Figure 1). This report describes a patient with undiagnosed carcinoid heart disease and discusses certain clinical clues which may have established the proper diagnosis and prevented the unsuccessful right-sided double-valve replacement.

CASE DESCRIPTION

This 67-year-old white woman apparently had been in her usual state of health until age 57 when she had a knee replacement (December 2001) because of osteoarthritis. An electrocardiogram at the time showed total 12-lead QRS voltage to be 158 mm (measured with normal [10 mm] standardization [10 mm = 1 mV])

[a]Second Year, Georgetown University School of Medicine, Washington, DC and [b]The Baylor Heart and Vascular Institute, Departments of [c]Internal Medicine (Division of Cardiology), [d]Cardiothoracic Surgery, and [e]Pathology, Baylor University Medical Center, Dallas, Texas. Manuscript received July 23, 2014; revised manuscript received and accepted August 15, 2014.

Support for this investigation was provided by the Baylor Health Care System Foundation through the Cardiovascular Research Review Committee in cooperation with the Baylor Heart and Vascular Institute.

* Corresponding author: Tel: (214) 820–7911; fax: (214) 820–7533.

E-mail address: wc.roberts@baylorhealth.edu (W.C. Roberts).

DOI: 10.1201/9781003409281-55

259

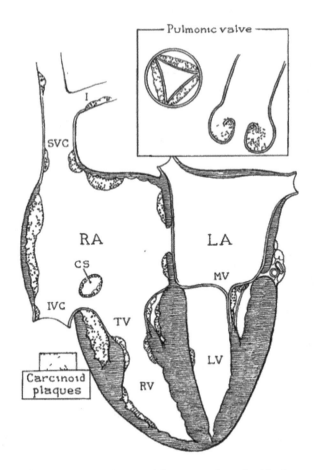

Figure 1 Diagram showing the usual location of carcinoid plaques in patients with carcinoid heart disease. CS = coronary sinus ostium; I = innominate vein; IVC = inferior vena cava; LA = left atrium; LV = left ventricle; MV = mitral valve; RA = right atrium; RV = right ventricle; SVC = superior vena cava; TV = tricuspid valve. Reproduced with permission from the authors (Ross EM and Roberts WC) and the publisher (Elsevier).[4]

(Figure 2). At age 66 (2012), she underwent left breast lumpectomy for confirmed cancer and received radiation to that breast and to the left axillary region. At age 67, peripheral edema, abdominal swelling, and weight gain appeared and each progressively worsened over a 6-month period during which time she gained 40 pounds. Examination in August 2013 confirmed the presence of anasarca. Facial flushing, diarrhea or labile blood pressure, if present, was not recorded. A precordial murmur was described as absent. An electrocardiogram now showed total 12-lead QRS of 51 mm; incomplete right bundle branch block and atrial premature complexes (Figure 2). Echocardiogram disclosed both pulmonic and tricuspid valve regurgitation, thickening of both valvular leaflets, immobility of the tricuspid valve leaflets, severe dilatation of both right sided chambers, and no dilatation of the left-sided chambers (Figure 3). Cardiac catheterization disclosed the following pressures in mm Hg: pulmonary artery, 30/10; right ventricle,

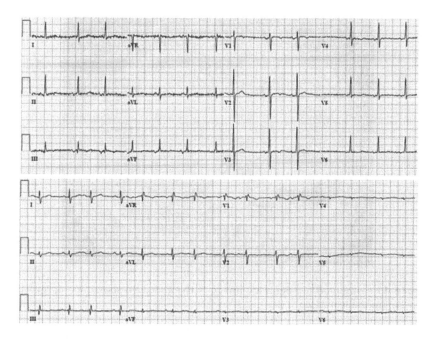

Figure 2 Electrocardiograms of the described patient at age 57 (December 2001) *(upper)* showing total 12-lead QRS voltage to be 158 mm (measured with normal [10 mm] standardization [10 mm = 1 mV]). Electrocardiogram from same patient 11 years later at age 66 (2012) *(lower)* with right-sided heart failure showing total 12-lead QRS voltage to be 51 mm, the presence of incomplete right bundle branch block, and atrial premature complexes.

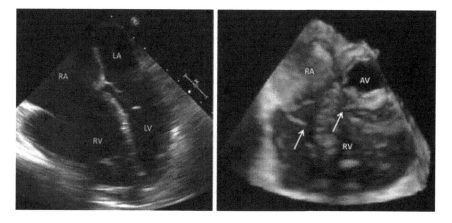

Figure 3 Transesophageal echocardiographic 4-chamber view showing right ventricular volume overload pattern with dilated right ventricle (RV) and right atrium (RA) and paradoxical ventricular septal motion. Left ventricle (LV) and left atrium (LA) are of normal size and there was no atrial septal defect *(left)*. Three-dimensional short-axis view of the right atrium (RA), right ventricle (RV) and aortic valve (AV). The tricuspid leaflets *(arrows)* are shortened, thickened and immobile, consistent with carcinoid heart disease *(right)*.

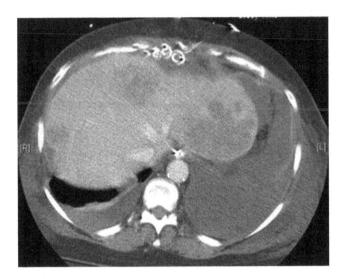

Figure 4 Computed tomographic image of the abdomen showing enlarged liver with innumerable masses.

43/18; right atrial mean 18 with V wave 25 and pulmonary arterial wedge mean 8. The cardiac index was 1.4 L/min/m². The left ventricular ejection fraction was approximately 60%. Coronary angiography disclosed insignificant narrowing (<30% diameter reduction).

In September 2013, the pulmonic valve was replaced with a homograft and the tricuspid valve, with a bioprosthesis (Edwards, Magna Ease). The tricuspid valve leaflets and chordae were sclerotic. Early postoperatively, excessive bleeding necessitated reexploration. Computed tomographic examination of the heart during the postoperative period disclosed an enlarged liver (23 cm in greatest dimension) containing innumerable masses (Figure 4) and "focal thickening of the cecum and terminal ileum." During the entire 10-day post-operative period, the patient never awoke and had fatal multi-organ "failure".

Examination of the operatively-excised thickened pulmonic valve and of a portion of the thickened right atrial wall disclosed classic changes of carcinoid heart disease (Figure 5). Necropsy was not performed.

DISCUSSION

The patient described had some clinical features suggesting the presence of carcinoid heart disease. These features included severe isolated right-sided heart failure (anasarca), thickened pulmonic and tricuspid valve leaflets with severe regurgitation of both valves and some stenosis of the pulmonic valve, the absence of left-sided heart disease, the absence of pulmonary disease including the absence of pulmonary hypertension, the presence of extremely low total 12-lead QRS voltage on electrocardiogram, and, the clincher, the presence of classic superimposed fibromuscular tissue on the operatively excised pulmonic valve cusps and on the mural endocardium of the right atrium (which was biopsied).[1–6]

A major clue to diagnosis was the echocardiogram which showed severe right-sided dilatation unassociated with any left-sided dilatation or atrial septal defect. Additionally, both tricuspid and pulmonic valve leaflets were thickened and the tricuspid leaflets immobile, something not seen in patients with cor pulmonale. The echocardiogram also suggested the absence of pulmonary hypertension, a

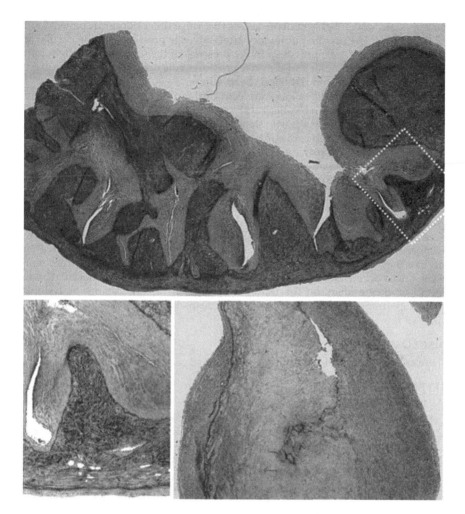

Figure 5 Histologic section of wall of right atrium *(top, lower left)* and pulmonic valve cusp *(lower right)*. Carcinoid plaque *(stained green)* is superimposed on the mural endocardium of the right atrium and on the cusp and endocardium of the pulmonic valve. Movat stains: x20 *(upper)*; x100 *(lower left)*; x40 *(lower right)*.

requirement for the presence of cor pulmonale. And, most important, there was no evidence of any pulmonary disease.

Because the patient had received radiation a year earlier for cancer of the left breast, the thickening of the right-sided valves was attributed clinically to the radiation-induced heart valve disease. An earlier study, however, had suggested that significant cardiac valve thickening secondary to radiation takes years as a rule to occur after completion of the radiation therapy.[7] The interval between the 2 events in our patient was no more than 1 year. Moreover, the radiation was limited to the left breast and axilla, yet only the right-sided heart valves were involved, a pattern more consistent with carcinoid heart disease than radiation injury.

Hemodynamic clues that carcinoid heart disease was the cause of the isolated right-sided heart failure was the pressure gradient—albeit small (13 mm Hg)—across the pulmonic valve. Such gradients across this valve do not occur in patients with cor pulmonale. The normal pulmonary arterial wedge pressure and the normal left ventricular end-diastolic pressures in the presence of the very elevated right atrial mean and right ventricular end-diastolic pressures rule out constrictive pericarditis as the cause of the isolated rightsided heart failure.

The extremely low QRS voltage on electrocardiogram fits the picture of carcinoid heart disease. Roberts and colleagues[8] studied total 12-lead QRS voltage in 11 different cardiac conditions (aortic stenosis, pure aortic regurgitation, pure mitral regurgitation, hypertrophic cardiomyopathy, idiopathic dilated cardiomyopathy, amyloid heart disease, cardiac adiposity and the carcinoid syndrome among others) and found that the 19 patients with carcinoid heart disease had the lowest 12-lead QRS voltage (mean 105) except for the 30 patients with cardiac amyloidosis who had a total 12-lead mean QRS voltage of 104 mm (measured with normal [10 mm] standardization [10 mm = 1 mV]). Our patient near the end of life preoperatively had a total 12-lead QRS voltage of 51 mm!

And finally, the finding by computed tomography of multiple masses in the liver occurs in nearly 100% of patients with the carcinoid syndrome with or without carcinoid heart disease.[4] In contrast, metastasis to the liver of a patient with carcinoma of the breast occurs in only about 20%.[9-13] The superimposed fibromuscular tissue devoid of elastic fibers on the mural endocardium of right atrium and similar tissue superimposed on the pulmonic valve cusps is diagnostic of carcinoid heart disease.[1-6]

DISCLOSURES

There are no conflicts of interest for any author.

REFERENCES

1. Roberts WC, Sjoerdsma A. The cardiac disease associated with the carcinoid syndrome (carcinoid heart disease). *Am J Med* 1964;36:5–34.
2. Roberts WC, Mason DT, Wright LD Jr. The non-distensible right atrium of carcinoid disease of the heart. *Am J Clin Pathol* 1965;44:627–631.
3. Ferrans VJ, Roberts WC. The carcinoid endocardial plaque. An ultrastructural study. *Hum Pathol* 1976;7:387–409.
4. Ross EM, Roberts WC. The carcinoid syndrome: comparison of 21 necropsy subjects with carcinoid heart disease to 15 necropsy subjects without carcinoid heart disease. *Am J Med* 1985;79:339–354.
5. Roberts WC. A unique heart disease associated with a unique cancer: carcinoid heart disease. *Am J Cardiol* 1997;80:251–256.
6. Roberts WC, Varughese CA, Ko JM, Grayburn PA, Hebeler RF Jr, Burton EC. Carcinoid heart disease without the carcinoid syndrome but with quadrivalvular regurgitation and unsuccessful operative intervention. *Am J Cardiol* 2011;107:788–792.
7. Brosius FC 3rd, Waller BF, Roberts WC. Radiation heart disease. Analysis of 16 young (aged 15 to 33 years) necropsy patients who received over 3,500 rads to the heart. *Am J Med* 1981;70:519–530.
8. Roberts WC, Filardo G, Ko JM, Siegel RJ, Dollar AL, Ross EM, Shirani J. Comparison of total 12-lead QRS voltage in a variety of cardiac conditions and its usefulness in predicting increased cardiac mass. *Am J Cardiol* 2013;112:904–909.
9. Van Walsum GAM, de Ridder JAM, Verhoef C, Bosscha K, van Gulik TM, Hesselink EJ, Ruers TJM, van den Tol MP, Nagtegaal ID, Brouwers M, van Hillegersberg R, Porte RJ, Rijken AM, Strobbe LJA, de Wilt JHW. Resection of liver metastases in patients with breast cancer: survival and prognostic factors. *EJSO* 2012;38:910–917.

10. Mariani P, Servois V, Rycke YD, Bennett SP, Feron JG, Alumbarak MM, Reyal F, Baranger B, Pierga JY, Salmon RJ. Liver metastases from breast cancer: surgical resection or not? A case-matched control study in highly selected patients. *EJSO* 2013;39:1377–1383.
11. Kim JY, Park JS, Lee SA, Kim JK, Jeong J, Yoon DS, Lee HD. Does liver resection provide long-term survival benefits for breast cancer patients with liver metastasis? A single hospital experience. *Yonsei Med J* 2014;55:558–562.
12. Cummings MC, Simpson PT, Reid LE, Jayanthan J, Skerman J, Song S, McCart Reed AE, Kutasovic JR, Morey AL, Marquart L, O'Rourke P, Lakhani SR. Metastatic progression of breast cancer: insights from 50 years of autopsies. *J Pathol* 2014;232:23–31.
13. Elsberger B, Roxburgh CS, Horgan PG. Is there a role for surgical resections of hepatic breast cancer metastases? *Hepatogastroenterology* 2014;61:181–186.

Case 1723 The Mitral Valve 16 Months After Operative Insertion of the Alfieri Stitch

*Samreen Fathima, MD, Shelley A. Hall, MD, Paul A. Grayburn, MD, and William C. Roberts, MD**

We describe considerable fibrous thickening of the mitral leaflets 16 months after insertion of an Alfieri stitch in a previously anatomically normal but functionally regurgitant mitral valve. Whether this type of mitral thickening will occur after percutaneous insertion of the mitral clip for pure mitral regurgitation remains to be determined. © 2018 Elsevier Inc. All rights reserved.
(Am J Cardiol 2019;123:695–696)

In the early 1990s, Alfieri et al[1] introduced what became known as "The Alfieri Stitch," a bowtie procedure or edge-to-edge mitral valve repair for patients with pure mitral regurgitation. The operation usually decreased the severity of the mitral regurgitation and it usually reduced the pulmonary arterial pressure. The procedure, however, was not without complications, a major one being the conversion of the previous mitral regurgitation to mitral stenosis. Subsequently, of course, percutaneous transcatheter mitral valve repair has proved to be effective and has replaced the operative approach.[2–5] Only 1 published photo late after insertion of "the stitch" has been found.[6] The present report describes another patient who had "the stitch" operatively inserted months earlier.

CASE DESCRIPTION

A 19-year-old man, who was born in January 1998, had heart failure (HF) shortly after birth. The degree of HF waxed and waned during the next 15 or so years. By June 2016 (age 17), the HF had reached the point that a left ventricular assist device was inserted and at the same procedure an Alfieri stitch was placed on the mitral leaflets to decrease the degree of functional mitral regurgitation. Neither the left ventricular assist device nor the Alfieri stitch proved to be beneficial. The patient gained 40 pounds during the next several months because of worsening HF. An echocardiogram 6 months before the heart transplant showed mild mitral regurgitation, thickening of the distal third of the mitral leaflets, severe dilatation of both ventricular cavities, and severe tricuspid valve regurgitation (Figure 1). Echocardiographic findings before and after placement of the Alfieri stitch are summarized in Table 1. In October 2017 (age 18), heart transplantation was performed. Examination of the native heart showed it to be typical of idiopathic dilated cardiomyopathy. It weighed 330 g. The mitral leaflets, which had been anatomically normal at the time of insertion of the Alfieri stitch, were now quite thickened by fibrous tissue, particularly in their distal halves (Figure 2). When contacted in November 2018, 13 months after the heart transplant, the patient was asymptomatic and working.

Baylor Scott & White Heart and Vascular Institute, the Departments of Pathology and Internal Medicine (Division of Cardiology), Baylor University Medical Center, Dallas, Texas. Manuscript received August 7, 2018; revised manuscript received and accepted November 12, 2018.

* Corresponding author: Tel: (214) 820–7911; fax: (214) 820–7533.
E-mail address: William.Roberts1@bswhealth.org (W.C. Roberts).

 DOI: 10.1201/9781003409281-56

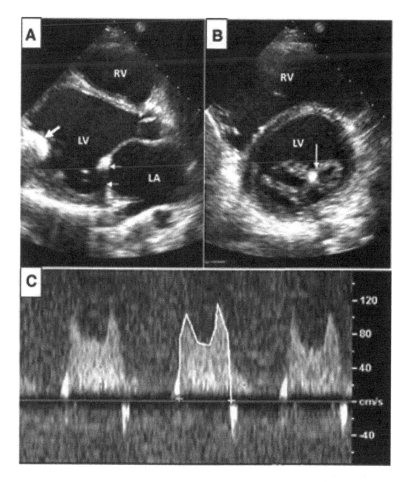

Figure 1 Echocardiographic images after insertion of a left ventricular assist device (LVAD) and Alfieri stitch. (*A*) Parasternal long-axis view showing thickened mitral leaflets with restricted diastolic excursion (*small arrows*). Both ventricular cavities and the left atrium are dilated (left ventricle at end-diastole = 6.2 cm, and at peak systole = 5.9 cm). The LVAD cannula is seen at lower left (*large arrow*). (*B*) Parasternal short-axis view showing Alfieri stitch (*arrow*) with double orifice mitral valve. (*C*) Mean transmitral gradient is 3 mm Hg by continuous wave Doppler.

DISCUSSION

Described in this report is considerable fibrous thickening of the mitral leaflets after insertion of an Alfieri stitch 16 months earlier. Today, the Alfieri stitch operation is infrequently performed but the insertion of the mitral clip by the percutaneous route is now frequently performed.[2–4] Whether the percutaneous approach will also cause the leaflets to thicken and potentially convert an occasional patient from pure mitral regurgitation to mitral stenosis remains to be seen.

DISCLOSURES

The investigators have no conflicts of interest to disclose.

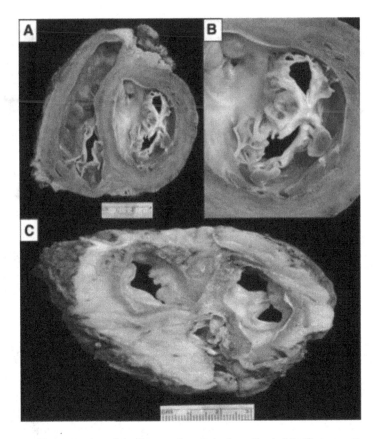

Figure 2 Photographs of the heart of patient described. (*A*). Cross section of the ventricles at the level of tricuspid and mitral valves showing the ventricular aspect of the Alfieri stitch. (*B*) A close-up of the mitral valves from the ventricular aspect. (*C*) View of the tricuspid and mitral valves after "deroofing" the atrial walls. The quantity of adipose tissue in the atrioventricular sulci is excessive.

Table 1: Echocardiographic data before and after placement of the Alfieri stitch

	Pre-OP (days)	Post-OP (days)	
Variable	−10	+1	+330
Peak velocity in early diastolic transmitral flow (m/s)	1.8	1.1	1.0
Decel time (m/s)	230	89	282
Mean gradient (mm Hg)	0	6	3
Mitral regurgitation (0–3+)	3+	1+	3+
Left ventricular internal diameter end diastole (mm)	83	74	62
Left ventricular posterior wall, peak systole (mm)	69	–	59
Left ventricular posterior wall, end diastole (mm)	7	8	6
Left ventricular ejection fraction (%)	37	34	10

REFERENCES

1. Alfieri O, Maisano F, De Bonis M, Stefano PL, Torracca L, Oppizzi M, La Canna G. The double-orifice technique in mitral valve repair: a simple solution for complex problems. *J Thorac Cardiovasc Surg* 2001;122:674–681.
2. Feldman T, Kar S, Rinaldi M, Fail P, Hermiller J, Smalling R. Percutaneous mitral repair with the MitraClip system: safety and midterm durability in the initial EVEREST (endovascular valve edge-to-edge repair study) cohort. *J Am Coll Cardiol* 2009;54:686–694.
3. Maisano F, La Canna G, Colombo A, Alfieri O. The evolution from surgery to percutaneous mitral valve interventions: the role of the edge-to-edge technique. *J Am Coll Cardiol* 2011;58:2174–2182.
4. Feldman T, Foster E, Glower DD, Glower DG, Kar S, Rinaldi MJ, Fail PS, Smalling RW, Siegel R, Rose GA, Engeron E, Loghin C, Trento A, Skipper ER, Fudge T, Letsou GV, Massaro JM, Mauri L. EVEREST II Investigators. Percutaneous repair or surgery for mitral regurgitation. *N Engl J Med* 2011;364:1395–1406.
5. Stone GW, Lindenfeld JA, Abraham WT, Kar S, Lim DS, Mishell JM, Whisenant B, Grayburn PA, Rinaldi M, Kapadia SR, Rajagopal V, Sarembock IJ, Brieke A, Marx SO, Cohen DJ, Weissman NJ, Mack MJ, for the COAPT Investigators. Transcatheter mitral-valve repair in patients with heart failure. *N Engl J Med* 2018;379:2307–2318.
6. Privitera S, Butany J, Cusimano RJ, Silversides C, Ross H, Leask R. Alfieri mitral valve repair clinical outcome and pathology. *Circulation* 2002;106:173–174.

Case 1727 Orthotopic Heart Transplantation for Ankylosing Spondylitis Masquerading as Nonischemic Cardiomyopathy

Samarthkumar J. Thakkar, MD[a], Paul A. Grayburn, MD[a,b], Shelley Anne Hall, MD[a,b], and William C. Roberts, MD[a,b,c]

Described herein is a 48-year-old man who underwent orthotopic heart transplantation because of severe heart failure considered clinically due to idiopathic dilated cardiomyopathy, but examination of the operatively excised native heart disclosed classic features of ankylosing spondylitis. Orthotopic heart transplantation for this condition has not been reported previously. © 2019 Elsevier Inc. All rights reserved.

(Am J Cardiol 2019;123:1732–1735)

We recently studied the heart of a patient who had undergone orthotopic heart transplantation (OHT) for presumed idiopathic dilated cardiomyopathy and examination of the operatively excised heart disclosed it to have classic morphologic features of ankylosing spondylitis.[1,2] The patient clinically had aortic regurgitation, complete heart block, and periodic low back pain. Search of PubMed failed to disclose any report of OHT for ankylosing spondylitis. A description of this patient is the purpose of this report.

CASE DESCRIPTION

A 48-year-old male roofer, who was born in March 1970, had been well until May 2011 (age 41) when he developed the sudden onset of dyspnea and was hospitalized. His systolic blood pressure was about 200 mm Hg, his coronary arteries were free of obstructive lesions, and his left ventricular ejection fraction was about 15%. He was started on valsartan, carvedilol, isosorbide dinitrate, and amlodipine, but despite these medicines, he had frequent episodes of acute heart failure. During one episode in March 2015, he was found to have abnormal kidney function and an atrophic left kidney (cause unknown) that was excised. The main artery to the right kidney was found to be stenotic and a stent was inserted. At that time, he developed complete heart block and a dual chamber pacemaker was inserted. In July 2016, he was started on peritoneal dialysis and 2 months later, hemodialysis. In July 2017, cardiac resynchronization therapy defibrillator was inserted.

In April 2018, he developed cardiogenic shock and pulmonary edema and was transferred to Baylor University Medical Center at Dallas. On arrival, his blood pressure was 160/80 mm Hg. A precordial murmur was not heard but his respirations were extremely rapid. The electrocardiogram (Figure 1) showed

[a]Baylor Scott and White Heart and Vascular Institute, Baylor University Medical Center, Dallas, Texas; [b]Department of Internal Medicine (Division of Cardiology), Baylor University Medical Center, Dallas, Texas; and [c]Department of Pathology, Baylor University Medical Center, Dallas, Texas. Manuscript received November 1, 2018; revised manuscript received and accepted February 11, 2019.

[*] Corresponding author: Tel: (214) 820–7911; fax: (214) 820–7533.

E-mail address: william.roberts1@BSWHealth.org (W.C. Roberts).

DOI: 10.1201/9781003409281-57

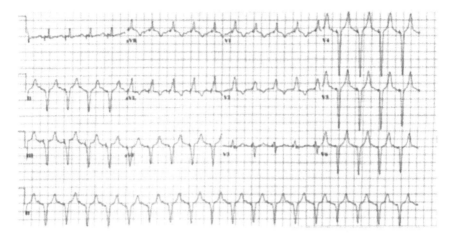

Figure 1 Electrocardiogram, recorded at the time of presentation, showing atrial-sensed ventricular-paced rhythm, biventricular pacemaker, and the total 12-lead QRS voltage of 152 mm.

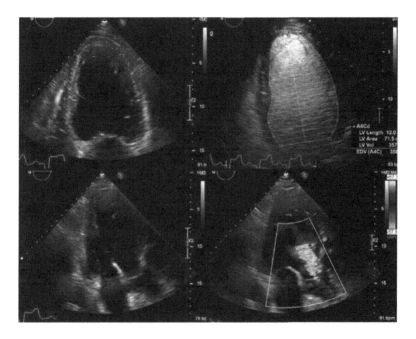

Figure 2 *Top left:* Apical 4-chamber view showing severely dilated, elongated left ventricle (LV) with normal right ventricular (RV) size and systolic function. An ICD lead is seen in the RV (arrow). *Top right:* Apical 4-chamber end-diastolic frame with ultrasound contrast. LV end-diastolic volume was 358 ml with LVEF 19% by biplane Simpson's method. *Bottom left:* Apical long-axis view showing severely thickened, restricted anterior mitral leaflet (yellow arrow). The posterior leaflet (white arrow) was of normal thickness and motion. *Bottom right:* Apical long-axis view with color Doppler imaging showing severe aortic regurgitation (AR).

Table 1: Pertinent admission laboratory findings in the patient described

B-type natriuretic peptide (pg/ml)	1895
Creatinine (mg/dl)	18
Blood urea nitrogen (mg/dl)	77
Estimated GFR (ml/min/1.73 m2)	3
Sodium (meq/L)	136
Potassium (meq/L)	5.2
Calcium (mg/dl)	8.7
Magnesium (mg/dl)	2.2
Phosphorous (mg/dl)	2.0
Total cholesterol (mg/dl)	219
Low density lipoprotein cholesterol (mg/dl)	151
High density lipoprotein cholesterol (mg/dl)	35
Triglyceride (mg/dl)	241
Hemoglobin A1c (%)	5.8
Rheumatic factor ([IU]/ml)*	8
ANA*	Negative
HLA-B 27*	Negative
C-reactive protein (mg/dl)*	0.5

GFR = glomerular filtration rate.
*Test performed 6 months after the orthotopic heart transplant.

atrial-sensed ventricular-paced rhythm and total 12-lead QRS voltage of 152 mm (10-mm standard).[3] The echocardiogram (Figure 2) showed the left ventricular chamber to be severely dilated, the ejection fraction to be about 20%, and severe aortic regurgitation to be present. At cardiac catheterization, the cardiac index was 1.5 L/min/m². Certain laboratory findings are listed in Table 1.

He underwent combined heart and kidney transplant in May 2018. The native heart weighed 675 g (Figures 3 and 4). The left ventricular cavity was considerably dilated longitudinally: the distance from the base of the right aortic valve cusp to the apex was 9.5 cm. The anterior mitral leaflet was severely thickened by dense fibrous tissue, and the posterior mitral leaflet was normal. The bases of each aortic cusp were thickened by similar fibrous tissue which extended cephalad onto the aorta in the areas of the commissures. The epicardial coronary arteries were free of atherosclerotic plaques.

DISCUSSION

Described herein is a 48-year-old man who underwent OHT because of severe heart failure attributed clinically to idiopathic dilated cardiomyopathy. Study of his explanted native heart, however, disclosed classic (specific) morphologic findings of ankylosing spondylitis,[1,2] distinctive and different from other cardiac conditions (Figure 5). Before OHT, echocardiogram disclosed severe aortic regurgitation. Although the degree of aortic regurgitation in our patient was severe by echocardiogram, a precordial murmur was not detected while in severe heart failure, probably the result of his rapid respiratory rate and his obesity (body mass index 33 kg/m²). A precordial murmur had been present earlier when he was not in heart failure. His pulse pressure when hospitalized at our institution was 80 mm Hg.

Aortic regurgitation appears to occur in about 20% of patients with ankylosing spondylitis[4] and it usually appears after the appearance of the orthopedic consequences, although the reverse occurs, as in the present patient, on occasion.

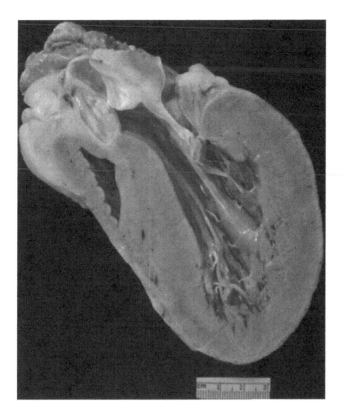

Figure 3   Shown here is the heart of a 48-year-old man showing a dilated left ventricular cavity with thickened left ventricular walls, enlarged papillary muscles, and thickened anterior mitral leaflet. The posterior mitral leaflet is normal (not thickened).

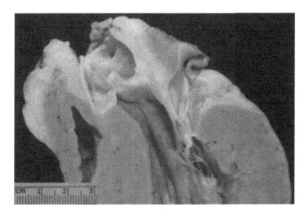

Figure 4   Shown here is a closer view of the mitral and aortic valve showing the remarkably thickened anterior mitral leaflet which is extending into the base of the posterior aortic valve cusp. The posterior mitral leaflet is normal.

273

The severe thickening of the anterior mitral leaflet in ankylosing spondylitis in the absence of thickening of the posterior mitral leaflet as shown in the present patient is diagnostic (Figure 5). Although all 8 patients (all men) with ankylosing spondylitis studied by Buckley and Roberts[1] at necropsy had extremely severe aortic regurgitation, only one of the 187 patients with ankylosing spondylitis studied clinically by Klingberg et al[4] had "severe" aortic regurgitation; 24 others had "mild", and 9 had "moderate" aortic regurgitation.

Interview of the patient and his wife 3 months after the OHT revealed that the patient indeed had had low back pain periodically for years, but he attributed it to

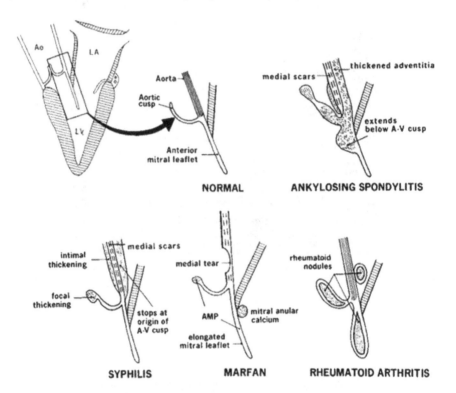

Figure 5 Diagram showing the distinctive morphologic features of 4 different cardiac conditions including *ankylosing spondylitis*. In *cardiovascular syphilis*, the aortic wall behind the sinuses of Valsalva is spared and the adventitial scar tissue does not extend below the aortic valve or involve mitral valve or ventricular septum. Only the distal margins of the aortic valve cusps are thickened in syphilis, not the proximal portions which are always involved in ankylosing spondylitis. In *rheumatoid arthritis*, the distinctive nodules similar to subcutaneous nodules, may infiltrate pericardium, myocardium and mural and valvular endocardium. If the valvular tissue is involved, regurgitation usually of only mild degree results. In the *Marfan syndrome*, aortic regurgitation is a consequence of disease of aortic wall, not of aortic valve; the aorta is thinner, and usually contains intimal-medial tears. The ascending aorta is diffusely involved, and dilatation of the aortic root causes the aortic regurgitation, which is usually severe. The mitral and rarely the aortic valve cusps may be redundant in patients with the Marfan syndrome.

Abbreviations: Ao = aorta; A-V = atrioventricular; LA = left atrium; LV = left ventricle.
Reproduced with permission from the authors and the publisher.[1]

his kidney disease rather than to the arthritic problem. Thus, the cardiac features of ankylosing spondylitis in this patient probably appeared after the clinical onset of his orthopedic back problem. Lateral chest radiograph, however, did not show changes of ankylosing spondylitis.

The dense fibrous tissue—characteristic of ankylosing spondylitis—was present in the membranous ventricular septum just above the location of the atrioventricular node and its presence in that location appears to be the cause of the patient's complete heart block diagnosed initially about 2 years before the OHT.

We were unable to find a previous publication of a patient with ankylosing spondylitis having an OHT.

DISCLOSURES

The authors have no conflicts of interest to disclose.

REFERENCES

1. Bulkley BH, Roberts WC. Ankylosing spondylitis and aortic regurgitation. Description of the characteristic cardiovascular lesion from study of eight necropsy patients. *Circulation* 1973;48:1014–1027.
2. Roberts WC, Hollingsworth JF, Bulkley BH, Jaffe RB, Epstein SE, Stinson EB. Combined mitral and aortic regurgitation in ankylosing spondylitis. Angiographic and anatomic features. *Am J Med* 1974;56:237–243.
3. Roberts WC, Filardo G, Ko JM. Comparison of total 12-lead QRS voltage in a variety of cardiac conditions and its usefulness in predicting increased cardiac mass. *Am J Cardiol* 2013;112:904–909.
4. Klingberg E, Sveälv BG, Täng MS, Bech-Hanssen O, Forsblad-D'Elia H, Bergfeldt L. Aortic regurgitation is common in ankylosing spondylitis: Time for routine echocardiography evaluation? *Am J Med* 2015;128:1244–1250.

Case 1729 Effect of Progressive Left Ventricular Dilatation on Degree of Mitral Regurgitation Secondary to Mitral Valve Prolapse

William C. Roberts, MD[a,b,c]*, Paul A. Grayburn, MD[a,c], Stuart R. Lander, MD[d], Dan M. Meyer, MD[e,c], and Shelley A. Hall, MD[c]

Described herein is a 71-year-old man who at age 61 was found by echocardiogram to have severe mitral regurgitation (MR) from mitral valve prolapse. During the subsequent 9 years the MR progressively lessened as his left ventricular cavity dilated and his ejection fraction progressively fell such that just before orthotopic heart transplantation the degree of MR was no longer severe, and the prolapse of the mitral leaflets had disappeared. This report describes this unique patient. © 2019 Published by Elsevier Inc.

(Am J Cardiol 2019;123:1887–1888)

To our knowledge, the resolution of severe mitral regurgitation (MR) from mitral valve prolapse (MVP) as the cardiac output progressively fell and the left ventricular cavity progressively dilated has not been described. Such is the purpose of this report.

CASE DESCRIPTION

A 71-year-old white man, who was born in December 1946, was told when in his 40s that he had a "heart murmur" from MVP. Because of the precordial murmur an echocardiogram was done when he was 61 years old (April 2008), and it confirmed MVP with marked leaflet thickening, severe leaflet prolapse, and severe MR; additionally, the left ventricular size and function were normal. The tricuspid valve also had evidence of prolapse. Thereafter, he was asymptomatic and working out regularly with a trainer until age 70 (October 2016), when experiencing an upper respiratory infection, he also noted exertional dyspnea, orthopnea, and lower leg edema. Examination in January 2017 disclosed no precordial murmur; echocardiogram showed the left ventricular ejection fraction to be 20% (Figure 1). The thickened mitral leaflets were tented toward the left ventricular wall without prolapse and there was moderate MR. The electrocardiogram showed atrial fibrillation, ventricular premature complexes, left ventricular hypertrophy with strain, and prolonged Q-T interval. Cardiac catheterization disclosed angiographically normal coronary arteries and the following pressures (in mm Hg): mean pulmonary artery wedge 26; right ventricle 35/3, mean right atrium 6; left ventricle 95/17, and aorta 105/75. The cardiac index (Fick) was 1.3 L/min/m². The left ventricular end-diastolic dimension

---

ᵃBaylor Scott & White Heart and Vascular Institute, Baylor Scott & White Health, Dallas, Texas; ᵇDepartments of Pathology, Baylor Scott & White Health, Dallas, Texas; ᶜInternal Medicine (Division of Cardiology), Baylor University Medical Center, Baylor Scott & White Health, Dallas, Texas; ᵈBaylor Scott & White Heart and Vascular Hospital, Baylor Scott & White Health, Dallas, Texas; and ᵉDepartment of Cardiac Surgery, Baylor Scott & White Health, Dallas, Texas. Manuscript received February 26, 2019; and accepted February 27, 2019.
* Corresponding author: Tel: (214) 820–7911; fax (214) 820–7533.

E-mail address: William.Roberts1@bswhealth.org (W.C. Roberts).

                                    DOI: 10.1201/9781003409281-58

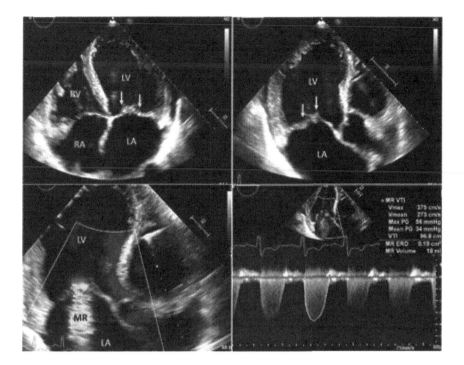

Figure 1 *Top left:* Apical 4-chamber view at end-systole showing 4-chamber dilation with thickened mitral leaflets (arrows) that never prolapsed into the left atrium (LA). The LA is bowed toward the right atrium (RA) consistent with high LA pressure. RV = right ventricle. *Top right:* Apical long-axis view showing thickened mitral leaflets (arrows) without prolapse. *Bottom left:* Apical long-axis view of centrally directed mitral regurgitation (MR) jet. *Bottom right:* Continuous wave doppler of the MR jet showing a low peak velocity—3.75 m/s, suggesting very elevated LA pressure. The calculated EROA was 0.19 cm², a value suggesting only mild MR.

was 7.1 cm, and its systolic diameter, 6.4 cm. His B-type natriuretic peptide was 1440 pg/ml. He was placed for the first time on full heart failure medications.

Repeat echocardiogram in November 2017 showed the left ventricular ejection fraction to be 10% and the MR was only of mild degree and no mitral prolapse was seen. An intracardiac defibrillator was inserted and the atrioventricular node ablated. Heart failure medications and apixaban were continued. Because of lack of improvement from either the medications or devices, orthotopic heart transplant was performed in June 2018. The explanted heart weighed 620 g. The epicardial coronary arteries were devoid of any narrowing. The myocardium was devoid of grossly visible lesions. The mitral valve leaflets were classic for MVP (Barlow syndrome type), and the tricuspid valve also had evidence of prolapse (Figure 2).

When contacted in December 2018, he was asymptomatic and back to work!

COMMENTS

Described herein is a patient with classic MVP known to be present for at least 3 decades. Several years before heart transplantation when the left ventricular function was normal the echocardiogram showed severe MR. With time, the left ventricular ejection fraction and cardiac output progressively fell, and the left ventricular cavity progressively dilated such that just before heart transplantation

277

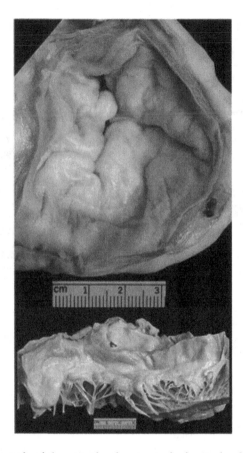

Figure 2 Photograph of the mitral valve, typical of mitral valve prolapse, in the explanted native heart. *Top*: View from the left atrium. *Bottom*: View of the opened mitral valve.

there was no precordial murmur, no mitral valve prolapse, and only mild MR by echocardiogram. As the left ventricular cavity dilated, the mitral chordae were pulled laterally preventing the mitral leaflets from prolapsing into the left atrial cavity. Current guidelines support mitral valve repair before the left ventricular ejection fraction falls below 60% to avoid the inevitable consequence of LV failure.[1] We are not aware of a similar published report describing the resolution of MVP and severe reduction in MR from classic MVP with progressive worsening of left ventricular function.

REFERENCE

1. Nishimura RA, Otto CM, Bonow RO, Carabello BA, Erwin JP 3rd, Fleisher LA, Jneid H, Mack MJ, McLeod CJ, O'Gara PT, Rigolin VH, Sundt TM 3rd, Thompson A. 2017 AHA/ACC focused update of the 2014 AHA/ACC guideline for the management of patients with valvular heart disease: a report of the American College of Cardiology/American Heart Association Task Force on Clinical Practice Guidelines. *J Am Coll Cardiol* 2017;70:252–289.

Case 1733 Libman-Sacks Endocarditis Involving a Bioprosthesis in the Aortic Valve Position in Systemic Lupus Erythematosus

William C. Roberts, MD[a,b],*, Andy Y. Lee, MD[b], Stuart R. Lander, MD[b], Charles S. Roberts, MD[c], and Baron L. Hamman, MD[c]

Described herein is a 39-year-old man with systemic lupus erythematosus not receiving corticosteroid therapy who developed Libman-Sacks endocarditis causing stenosis of a bioprosthesis in the aortic valve position. © 2019 Elsevier Inc. All rights reserved.

(Am J Cardiol 2019;124:316–318)

Libman and Sacks described what later became known as Libman-Sacks (L-S) endocarditis in 1924,[1] and its relation to systemic lupus erythematosus (SLE) was described by Gross in 1940.[2] Lipman and Sacks initially described 4 patients at necropsy and noted that the endocarditis could involve any of the 4 cardiac valves. The "endocarditis" was described as deposits of fibrin not containing microorganisms or leukocytes on either side of a valvular leaflet but more commonly on the atrial side (atrioventricular valve), or aortic side (semilunar valve). Once patients with SLE were treated with corticosteroids the L-S fibrin lesions were uncommonly seen, the medication presumably converting the fibrin deposits into fibrous thickenings.[3,4] We recently encountered a man with known SLE not treated with corticosteroids who developed aortic valve regurgitation, underwent replacement of that valve with a bioprosthesis, which became stenotic because of development of L-S endocarditis on both sides of the bioprosthetic cusps within 8 months of its implantation. A description of this unusual patient is the purpose of this report.

CASE DESCRIPTION

A 39-year-old Hispanic man, who was born in April 1979, had been well until age 26 when he noted tender nodules and a rash on his legs, and pain in some joints. A diagnosis of SLE was made. He was advised to take prednisone but during the next 13 years he failed to do so. At age 39, he developed signs of heart failure, was found to have aortic regurgitation, and in May 2018 underwent replacement of his aortic valve with a bioprosthesis and insertion of a bypass conduit in his narrowed left anterior descending coronary artery. About 6 months later, symptoms of heart failure reoccurred and it rapidly progressed. On admission to Baylor University Medical Center in December 2018, echocardiogram showed the velocity across his bioprosthesis to be 3.9 m/s; mean transbioprosthetic gradient 35 mm Hg; left

[a]Baylor Scott and White Heart and Vascular Institute, Departments of Internal Medicine and Heart Surgery, Baylor University Medical Center, Baylor Scott and White Health, Dallas, Texas; [b]Departments of Internal Medicine (Division of Cardiology) and Cardiac Surgery, Baylor University Medical Center, Baylor Scott and White Health, Dallas, Texas; and [c]Cardiothoracic Surgery, Department of Cardiology, Baylor University Medical Center, Baylor Scott and White Health, Dallas, Texas. Manuscript received and accepted April 4, 2019.
* Corresponding author: Tel: (214) 820–7911.
E-mail address: William.roberts1@bswhealth.org (W.C. Roberts).

DOI: 10.1201/9781003409281-59

ventricular ejection fraction 30%; left ventricular end-diastolic diameter 6.7 cm, and systolic diameter, 6.3 cm. Mild mitral regurgitation was also found. The left internal mammary arterial conduit to the left anterior descending coronary artery was wide open. The left circumflex ostium was narrowed about 50%. The right coronary artery was wide open. His blood pressure was 115/70 mm Hg. His body mass index was 37 kg/m^2. The bioprosthesis was replaced with a mechanical prosthesis (#25 On-X). Multiple laboratory values just before replacement of the bioprosthesis are listed in Table 1.

The operatively-excised bioprosthesis is shown in Figure 1. Thrombi are present on both the aortic and ventricular aspects of the cusps. Histologic study of the thrombi revealed that they consisted of fibrin within which were scattered monocytes, mainly plasma cells (Figure 2). The surgeon incised the bioprosthesis to facilitate its removal.

Table 1: Laboratory valves in the 39-year-old patient just before replacement of the bioprosthesis in the aortic valve position

Variable	Case
Hemoglobin (g/dl)	9
Hematocrit (%)	28
Platelets per mcL (ml)	109,000
Erythrocyte sedimentation rate (mm/hour)	79
C-reative protein (mg/dl)	2.1
Creatinine (mg/dl)	2.1
Total cholesterol (mg/dl)	154
Low-density lipoprotein cholesterol (mg/dl)	116
Urine protein/creatinine ratio	1:6
Antinuclear antibodies (ANA)	Negative
Antineutrophil cytoplasmic antibodies (ANCA)	Negative
Anti-DNA antibody titer	01:40
Anti-SSA	Negative
Anti-SSB	Negative
Anti-RNP	Negative
Anti-SM	Negative
Anti-Jol	Negative
Anti-Scl70	Negative
HIV	Negative
Anti-cardiolipin IgA (APL 'U/ml)	14
Anti-cardiolipin IgG (GPL 'U/ml)	72
Anti-cardiolipin IgM (MPL 'U/ml)	<10
B2-glycoprotein Ab IgA (SAU)	>150
B2-glycoprotein Ab IgG (SGU)	143
B2-glycoprotein Ab IgM (SMU)	<10
Phosphatidylserine Ab IgA (APS 'U/ml)	7
Phosphatidylserine Ab IgG (GPL 'U/ml)	>100
Phosphatidylserine Ab IgM (MPL 'U/ml)	6
Complement C3 (mg/dl)	108
Complement C4 (mg/dl)	18
Lupus anticoagulant	Positive
Prothrombin time (s)	11
Activated partial thromboplastin time (s)	39
Thrombin time (s)	16
Dilute Russell viper venom time	139

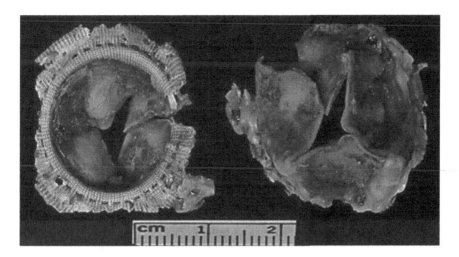

Figure 1 Bioprosthesis viewed from both the ventricular (left) and aortic (right) aspects in the patient described. Typical Libman-Sacks lesions are present on both sides of the bioprosthetic cusps.

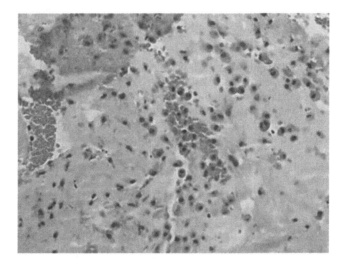

Figure 2 Photomicrograph of the Libman-Sacks lesion from the patient described. The lesion consists of fibrin within which are some mononuclear cells, mainly plasmacytes. Hematoxylin/eosin stain; × 400.

DISCUSSION

Described herein is a patient who at age 26 years was diagnosed with SLE. Although advised to do so, he never took a corticosteroid drug. At age 39, he underwent replacement of his native aortic valve because it was purely regurgitant. It is unclear if the operatively-excised native aortic valve contained superimposed fibrin deposits. Several months after replacement of the native aortic valve he developed heart failure and the bioprosthesis was found to be stenotic. Accordingly, just 8 months after implanting the bioprosthesis in the aortic valve position it was excised and replaced with a bileaflet mechanical prosthesis. The cusps of the operatively-excised bioprosthesis contained fibrin thrombi typical of L-S endocarditis.

Although it has been reported on native aortic and mitral valves on many occasions and leading to valve replacement,[5-15] L-S endocarditis involving a bioprosthesis in the aortic or mitral valve position is rare.[16-20] Niaz and Butany[17] described a 32-year-old woman who developed L-S endocarditis causing stenosis on a bioprosthesis in the aortic valve position in place for 8 years. The patient had not been on corticosteroid therapy. Both Moriski et al[19] and Sladak and Ausla[20] described young (ages 45 and 36 years) patients with L-S endocarditis involving a bioprosthesis in the mitral valve position and in each patient the bioprosthesis was made stenotic. L-S endocarditis occurs not only in patients with well-documented SLE but also in patients with the antiphospholipid syndrome without SLE.[21-23]

It is important to emphasize the apparent effect on corticosteroid drug therapy in patients with either SLE or the antiphospholipid syndrome. These medications appear to convert the fibrin thrombi of L-S endocarditis to fibrous lesions leading to thickening of the underlying valvular leaflet. The present patient never received corticosteroid therapy and presumably as a consequence developed full-blown L-S lesions without much underlying fibrous thickening of the cusps.

As a final note, coronary artery disease, as occurred in the present patient, is far more common in SLE patients than in subjects of similar age and sex without SLE.[24]

DISCLOSURES

All authors have participated in the work and have reviewed and agree with the content of the article and have no conflict of interests to disclose.

REFERENCES

1. Libman E, Sack B. A hitherto undescribed form of valvular and mural endocarditis. *Arch Intern Med* 1924;33:701–737.
2. Gross L. The cardiac lesions in Libman-Sacks disease: with a consideration of its relationship to acute diffuse lupus erythematosus. *Am J Pathol* 1940;16:375–408.
3. Bulkley BH, Roberts WC. The heart in systemic lupus erythematosus and the changes induced in it by corticosteroid therapy: a study of 36 necropsy patients. *Am J Med* 1975;58:243–264.
4. Roberts WC, High ST. The heart in systemic lupus erythematosus. *Curr Probl Cardiol* 1999;24:1–56.
5. Moynihan T, Hanse R, Troup P, Olinger G. Simultaneous aortic and mitral valve replacement for lupus endocarditis: report of a case and review of the literature. *J Thorac Cardiovasc Surg* 1988;1:142–145.
6. Alameddine AK, Schoen FJ, Yanagi H, Couper GS, Collins JJ Jr., Cohn LH. Aortic or mitral valve replacement in systemic lupus erythematosus. *Am J Cardiol* 1992;70:955–956.
7. Kumar S, Sinha B, Ravikumar E. Emergency aortic valve replacement in systemic lupus erythematosus. *Heart Lung Circ* 2006;15:397–399.
8. Sasahashi N, Harada H, Saji Y, Marui A, Nishina T, Komeda M. Aortic valve replacement for aortic regurgitation in a patient with antiphospholipid antibody syndrome. *Gen Thorac Cardiovasc Surg* 2007;55:293–296.
9. Dandekar UP, Watkin R, Chandra N, Kirkpatrick CS, Bhudia S, Pitt M, Rooney SJ. Aortic valve replacement for Libman-Sacks endocarditis. *Ann Thorac Surg* 2009;88:669–671.
10. Bouma W, Klinkenberg TJ, van der Horst IC, Wijdh-den Hamer IJ, Erasmus ME, Bijl M, Suurmeijer AJ, Zijlstra F, Mariani MA. Mitral valve surgery for mitral regurgitation caused by Libman-Sacks endocarditis: a report of four cases and a systematic review of the literature. *J Cardiothorac Surg* 2010;5:13.

11. Barreiro Delgado Y, García Méndez I, Martín Alemany N, Calabia Martinez J, Morales Fornos M, Fuertes M, Valles Prats M. Libman-Sacks endocarditis and severe aortic regurgitation in a patient with systemic lupus erythematosus on peritoneal dialysis. *Nefrologia* 2011;31:619–621.
12. Yashiki N, Yamaguchi S, Moriyama H, Kato H, Takago S, Tanaka N, Yoshizumi K, Ohtake H, Watanabe G. Severe aortic insufficiency due to a huge leaflet perforation in Libman-Sacks syndrome: report of a case. *Surg Today* 2011;41:399–401.
13. D'Alessandro LCA, Paridon SM, Gaynor JW. Successful repair of aortic valve perforation in pediatric Libman–Sacks endocarditis. *J Thorac Cardiovasc Surg* 2012;144:e151–e153.
14. Gouya H, Cabanes L, Mouthon L, Pavie A, Legmann P, Vignaux O. Severe mitral stenosis as the first manifestation of systemic lupus erythematosus in a 20-year-old woman: the value of magnetic resonance imaging in the diagnosis of Libman-Sacks endocarditis. *Int J Cardiovasc Imaging* 2014;3:959–960.
15. Keenan JB, Rajab TK, Janardhanan R, Larsen BT, Khalpey Z. Aortic valve replacement for Libman-Sacks endocarditis. *BMJ Case Rep* 2016(October 4):1–3.
16. Gordon RJ, Weilbaecher D, Davy SM, Safi HJ, Quinones MA, DeFelice CA, Zoghbi WA. Valvulitis involving a bioprosthetic valve in a patient with systemic lupus erythematosus. *J Am Soc Echocardiogr* 1996;9:104–107.
17. Niaz A, Butany J. Antiphospholipid antibody syndrome with involvement of a bioprosthetic heart valve. *Can J Cardiol* 1998;14:951–954.
18. Saito S, Ikeguchi H, Yamamoto H, Koike A, Yamaguchi K, Takeuchi E. Does antiphospholipid antibody syndrome affect bioprosthetic heart valve? Midterm echocardiographic report. *Jpn J Thorac Cardiovasc Surg* 2005;53:36–38.
19. Morisaki A, Hirai H, Sasaki Y, Hosono M, Sakaguchi M, Nakahira A, Seo H, Suehiro S. Mitral bioprosthetic valve stenosis in a patient with antiphospholipid antibody syndrome and systemic lupus erythematosus. *Gen Thorac Cardiovasc Surg* 2012;60:822–826.
20. Sladek EH, Accola KD. Antiphospholipid syndrome and Libman-Sacks endocarditis in a bioprosthetic mitral valve. *Ann Thorac Surg* 2016; 101:e29–e31.
21. Ziporen L, Goldberg I, Arad M, Hojnik M, Ordi-Ros J, Afek A, Blank M, Sandbank Y, Vilardell-Tarres M, de Torres I, Weinberger A, Asherson RA, Kopolovic Y, Shoenfeld Y. Libman-Sacks endocarditis in the antiphospholipid syndrome: immunopathologic findings in deformed heart valves. *Lupus* 1996;5:196–205.
22. Koniari I, Siminelakis SN, Baikoussis NG, Papadopoulos G, Goudevenos J, Apostolakis E. Antiphospholipid syndrome; its implication in cardiovascular diseases: a review. *J Cardiothorac Surg* 2010;5:101.
23. Denas G, Jose SP, Bracco A, Zoppellaro G, Pengo V. Antiphospholipid syndrome and the heart: a case series and literature review. *Autoimmun Rev* 2015;14:214–222.
24. Haider YS, Roberts WC. Coronary arterial disease in systemic lupus erythematosus: quantification of degrees of narrowing in 22 necropsy patients (21 women) aged 18 to 37 years. *Am J Cardiol* 1981;70:775–781.

Case 1735 Smeloff-Cutter Mechanical Prosthesis in the Aortic Position for 49 Years

Robin A. Chalkley, MD[a,b,c], Chong W. Kim, MD[a,b,c], James W. Choi, MD[a,b,c], William C. Roberts, MD[a,b,c], and Jeffrey M. Schussler, MD[a,b,c],*

We describe a 76-year-old male physician who at age 27 underwent replacement of his stenotic aortic valve with a Smeloff-Cutter mechanical prosthesis which functioned normally for 49 years. He died of a noncardiac condition. A normally functioning substitute cardiac valve for this length of time has not been previously reported. © 2019 Published by Elsevier Inc.

(Am J Cardiol 2019;124:457–459)

Smeloff-Cutter valve first design began production in 1964; a second design was implemented in 1966 and was produced until the end of 1989 at which time the Smeloff-Cutter valve was no longer manufactured.[1] It was one of the first commercially available prosthetic heart valves and the first with double cage design.[1] The double cage design was intended to reduce the risk of thromboembolism secondary to the "self-washing" effect.[2] The Smeloff-Cutter was a popular ball-in-cage valve and had 72,000 valves implanted.[3] It was mostly used in aortic position.[3] Smeloff-Cutter valve durability was comparable to the more popular Starr-Edwards valve and had 25 year survival of 31%.[4] Longest reported implanted Smeloff-Cutter valve was 43 years reported in publications.[5] We recently encountered a physician who had the Smeloff-Cutter valve implanted for 49 years in the aortic position without any complications secondary to the Smeloff-Cutter valve and who died of noncardiac causes. A description of Smeloff-Cutter valve implanted for this length of time has not been previously described.

CASE DESCRIPTION

This 76-year-old man underwent replacement of his stenotic aortic valve for congenital bicuspid aortic stenosis at age 27 years by Dr. Denton A. Cooley. During the 49 years that followed, he took warfarin intermittently; he did not take warfarin for approximately a decade because of recurrent gastrointestinal bleeding. No episodes occurred that suggested prosthetic thrombosis or systemic embolism. Later in life, he developed coronary artery disease for which he received 3 drug-eluting stents for unstable angina, and heart failure due to ischemic cardiomyopathy for which he received an implantable cardioverter defibrillator. Weeks before his death, echocardiogram revealed a peak left ventricular outflow velocity of 2.18 m/sec, an aortic valve velocity time integral of 44.2 cm, an aortic valve peak transvalvular gradient of 19 mm Hg and an aortic valve area of 2.9 cm². His mechanical valve type was identified while he was living using a radiographic guide developed by Mehlman and Resnekov[6] and confirmed at necropsy to be a Smeloff-Cutter type cage in ball. The patient died from chronic renal failure.

[a]Baylor Scott & White Heart and Vascular Hospital, Dallas, Texas; [b]Baylor University Medical Center, Dallas, Texas; and [c]Texas A&M College of Medicine, Dallas, Texas. Manuscript received February 15, 2019; revised manuscript received and accepted May 6, 2019.
* Corresponding author: Tel: 469-800-7400; fax: 469-800-7401.

E-mail address: Jeffrey.Schussler@BSWHealth.org (J.M. Schussler).

DOI: 10.1201/9781003409281-60

The patient was originally from South Korea where he graduated from Seoul National Medical School. He eventually came to the United States where he practiced internal medicine for 40 years. He was strongly desirous that his mechanical prosthesis be examined after his death. The excised poppet of the prosthesis was discolored but its surface was smooth and devoid of indentions and cracks. The poppet moved normally in its cage.

COMMENTS

The Smeloff-Cutter valve was first produced in 1964.[1] It was the first substitute valve to have a double cage in which the silicone rubber ball moved.[1] It also had a "self-washing" effect thought to reduce the risk of thrombosis.[2] This first design (produced from 1964 to 1966) was plagued with poppet malfunction. The poppet absorbed lipids which caused it to swell, a situation that could lead to immobility of the poppet in the cage.[1,5] The second iteration (produced from 1966 to 1989) included changes to the silicon rubber processing (as it did for many other ball and cage valves including the more popular Starr-Edwards valve) and the cage was changed slightly.[1] In the newer version, the housing was titanium and the ball was silicone rubber.[1] The incidence of thromboembolism in patients with this valve in the aortic position without anticoagulation was 1% per patient year.[2] Of the 72,000 valves implanted (the Starr-Edwards poppet-in-cage 250,000 has been implanted).[3] The 10, 20, and 25 year survival postvalve implantation was 69%, 47%, and 31%, respectively.[1] The 10, 20, and 25 actuarial freedom rate of valve complication, reoperations or

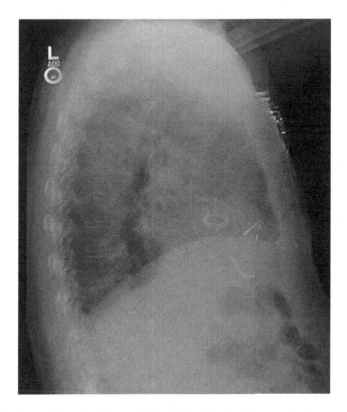

Figure 1 Lateral chest radiograph the distinctive double cage design.

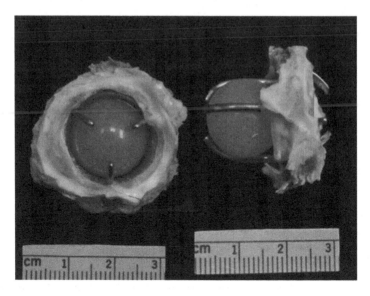

Figure 2 Smeloff-Cutter valve post mortem; note the ball discoloration from lipid absorption.

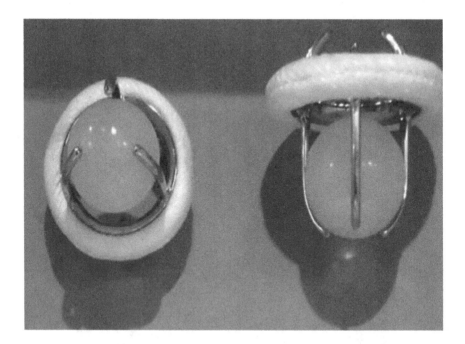

Figure 3 New Smeloff-Cutter valve.

death was 73%, 47%, and 20% respectively.[1] These rates are similar to Starr-Edwards valve.[1] That our patient suffered no complications with his mechanical prosthesis is testament to the durability of the design of the Smeloff-Cutter valve, particularly in the aortic position (Figures 1–4).

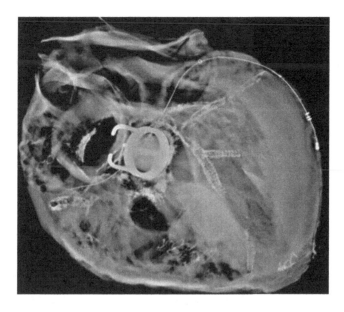

Figure 4   Post mortem radiograph of the heart.

DISCLOSURES

·The authors have no conflicts of interest to disclose.

REFERENCES

1. Gott VL, Alejo DE, Cameron DE. Mechanical heart valves: 50 years of evolution. *Annal Thora Surg* 2003;76:S2230–S2239.
2. Gometza B, Duran CM. Ball valve (Smeloff-Cutter) aortic valve replacement without anticoagulation. *Annal Thor Surg* 1995;60:1312–1316.
3. Belenkie I, Carr M, Schlant R, Nutter D, Symbas P. Malfunction of a Cutter-Smeloff mitral ball valve prosthesis: diagnosis by phonocardiography and echocardiography. *Am. Heart J* 1973;86:399–403.
4. Godje O, Fischlein T, Adelhard K, Mair H, Reichart B. 25 years follow-up of patients after replacement of the aortic valve with a Smeloff-Cutter prosthesis. *Thora Card Surg* 1996;44:234–238.
5. Head SJ, Ko J, Singh R, Roberts WC, Mack MJ. 43.3-year durability of a Smeloff-Cutter ball-caged mitral valve. *Annal Thora Surg* 2011;91:606–608.
6. Mehlman DJ, Resnekov L. A guide to the radiographic identification of prosthetic heart valves. *Circulation* 1978;57:613–623.

Case 1740 Management of Adults with Normally Functioning Congenitally Bicuspid Aortic Valves and Dilated Ascending Aortas

William C. Roberts, MD[a,b,c]*, Shaffin Siddiquiz[d], Aldo E. Rafael-Yarihuaman, MD[e], and Charles S. Roberts, MD[e]

We describe herein a 65-year-old woman who underwent resection of a dilated (5.1 cm) ascending aorta associated with a normally functioning congenitally bicuspid aortic valve. The patient provided the framework to discuss proper management—operative versus nonoperative—of the dilated ascending aorta associated with a normally functioning bicuspid aortic valve. Unfortunately, there is inadequate data to provide an unequivocal answer to this dilemma. Operative intervention requires that the short-term risk of the prophylactic procedure be considerably lower than the long-term risk of aortic dissection/ rupture without operative intervention. Because there is no proof that operative intervention provides less morbidity and lower mortality, nonoperative management at this time seems to be the better approach. © 2019 Elsevier Inc. All rights reserved.

(Am J Cardiol 2020;125:157–160)

During the last 3 decades, numerous articles have appeared detailing proper management of the dilated ascending aorta in patients with a dysfunctioning bicuspid aortic valve (BAV).[1-5] In contrast, few studies have focused on the proper management of the dilated ascending aorta in adults with normally functioning BAVs.[6-8] Such is the purpose of this report based on a description of clinical and morphologic findings in a single patient with a dilated ascending aorta and a normally functioning BAV.

CASE DESCRIPTION

A 65-year-old nonsmoking, asthmatic, white woman with known Raynaud's disease was otherwise well until about 2 years earlier when occasional exertional dyspnea and "sharp stabbing" chest pains unassociated with exertion appeared. Because the chest pains worsened markedly in a 2-week period, she sought medical care. Examination disclosed no precordial murmur or subcutaneous edema. Her body mass index was 25 kg/m². Electrocardiogram showed normal sinus rhythm and total 12-lead QRS voltage of 75 mm (with 10 mm standard).[9] Computed tomographic study disclosed a 5.1 cm aneurysm of the tubular portion of the ascending aorta and

[a]Baylor Scott & White Heart and Vascular Institute, Baylor University Medical Center, Baylor Scott & White Health, Dallas, Texas; [b]Department of Internal Medicine (Cardiology), Baylor University Medical Center, Baylor Scott & White Health, Dallas, Texas; [c]Department of Pathology, Baylor University Medical Center, Baylor Scott & White Health, Dallas, Texas; [d]Princeton University, Princeton, New Jersey; and [e]Department of Cardiac Surgery, Baylor University Medical Center, Baylor Scott & White Health, Dallas, Texas. Manuscript received August 19, 2019; revised manuscript received and accepted September 23, 2019.
* Corresponding author: Tel: (214) 820–7911; fax: (214) 820–7533.
E-mail address: william.roberts1@bswhealth.org (W.C. Roberts).

DOI: 10.1201/9781003409281-61

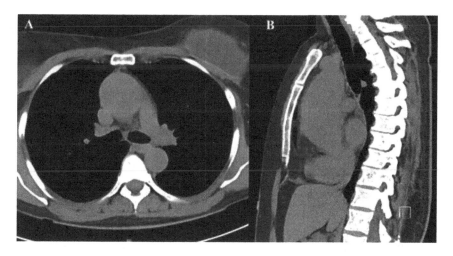

Figure 1 Shown here are (A) axial and (B) sagittal computed tomographic images of the patient, depicting the ascending aortic aneurysm 3 days before resection. The aneurysm measured 5.1 cm in maximal diameter.

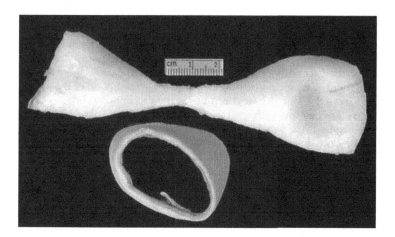

Figure 2 Photograph of fragments of the resected ascending aorta from the patient described. The aorta is grossly normal and histologic examination of its wall proved to show its wall to be normal.

a normal sized heart (Figure 1). Cardiac catheterization with angiography showed normal epicardial coronary arteries and trace aortic regurgitation. Simultaneous left ventricular and aortic pressures were 122/13 and 119/59 mm Hg, respectively. The left ventricular ejection fraction was about 60%. The aortic aneurysm was resected (Figure 2) and the aortic valve, which was congenitally bicuspid, left in place. Histologic study of the aneurysm wall disclosed normal intima, media, and adventitia (Figure 3). A total of 25 cm of Movat-stained sections were examined. When contacted 2 months after the aneurysmal resection, she was asymptomatic without physical limitations. The postoperative course was uneventful.

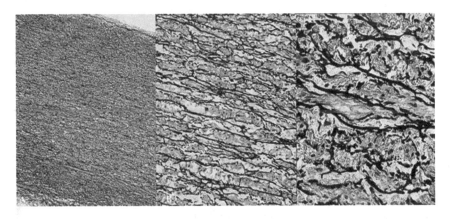

Figure 3 Photomicrographs of the wall of the resected ascending aorta, showing it to be normal histologically. Movat stains ×100 *(A)*, ×400 *(B)*, and ×1000 *(C)*.

DISCUSSION

Before about 1995, few patients with a malfunctioning (stenotic or purely regurgitant) congenitally BAV had simultaneous resection of the ascending aorta irrespective of whether it was dilated or not.[2] Beginning in the 1990s, some cardiac surgeons began advocating resection of the dilated ascending aorta at the time of replacement of a dysfunctioning congenitally BAV to prevent the later occurrence of aortic dissection or rupture. Thereafter, in both the cardiologic and cardiac surgical communities, resection of the ascending aorta (if dilated) was advocated. There ensued much debate whether the magic aortic diameter to warrant resection of the aorta was 4.5, 5.0, 5.5, or 6.0 cm.[10–19] That debate continues to the present-day time.

What we are dealing with in this report is whether a dilated ascending aorta should be excised in patients with normally functioning BAVs. The present patient is the only one encountered at our institution in the last 25 years in whom a dilated ascending aorta was resected in the presence of a normally functioning BAV. Previous reports on this topic, in our view, do not provide an unequivocal answer, mainly because the normally functioning BAV cases are intermixed with the malfunctioning ones, either stenosis or pure regurgitation. Additionally, little data is available on results of histologic study of the wall of the aortic aneurysm in association with a normally functioning BAV. The only report that isolated histologic analysis of normally functioning BAVs from malfunctioning BAVs was that of Leone et al[20] who described results of histologic study of the walls of dilated ascending aortas in 16 patients stated to have "absent valvulopathy"; the aortic media was histologically normal in 11 (69%) and mildly abnormal in 5 (31%). In contrast, considerable published information is available on histologic structure of the walls of resected ascending aortas in patients with malfunctioning congenitally BAVs.[20, 21]

The dilemma (Figure 4) here is balancing the frequency of aortic dissection or rupture of a dilated ascending aorta in association with a BAV in adults not undergoing aortic resection versus the frequency of prevention of aortic dissection or rupture if the dilated aorta is resected, along with the added operative risk of resection of the dilated aorta. The presently available data, in our view, favor nonresection over resection of the dilated aorta in patients with BAVs. La Canna et al[22] reported 27 patients with normally functioning BAVs and dilated ascending aortas (mean diameter 4.7 ± 0.5 cm), 11 of whom began the study with ascending aortic diameters >5 cm: 25 of the 27 patients did not undergo resection of the

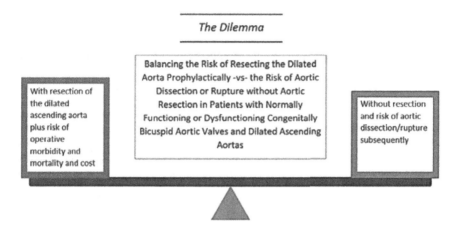

Figure 4 The dilemma presented by the present case.

ascending aorta, and none developed aortic dissection/rupture during a follow-up of 1 to 11 years (mean 3). Etz et al[23] studied 158 patients with BAVs and dilated ascending aortas (3.7 to 6.6 cm in diameter [mean 4.6]), and all apparently had normally functioning BAVs; of the 71 in whom the dilated ascending aorta was not resected, aortic dissection/rupture was not known to have occurred in any patient during follow-up (mean 4.2 years). In a meta-analysis including 1,342 adults with BAVs and dilated ascending aortas (3.5 to 5.6 cm [mean 4.2]), Guo et al[24] reported that the aorta was not replaced in 1,120 patients (83%); during follow-up (2.5 to 14.7 years [mean 4.1]), 9 patients (0.8%) developed aortic dissection or rupture. The number of patients in this meta-analysis with normally functioning BAVs, however, is unclear. The most robust data demonstrating the infrequency of dissection/rupture in patients with malfunctioning BAVs come from McKellar et al[2] who followed (0 to 38 years [median 12]) 1,286 patients, all of whom underwent aortic valve replacement for dysfunctioning BAVs without concomitant resection of the ascending aorta, irrespective of its size: 507 patients (39%) had aortic diameters >4.0 cm and 779 (61%) patients had aortic diameters <4.0 cm at aortic valve replacement; only 11 patients (0.08%) underwent resection of the ascending aorta during follow-up but reoperation in 9 of them was precipitated by malfunction of the mechanical prosthesis or bioprosthesis in the aortic valve position; 13 of the 1,286 patients (1%) were documented to have aortic dissection during follow-up.

Now to the frequency of prevention of aortic dissection/rupture by excising the dilated ascending aorta prophylactically in adults with BAVs. Etz et al[23] followed 87 adults with "well-functioning" BAVs and dilated ascending aortas (3.7 to 7.4 cm [mean 5.2]), all of which were resected along with 63 (72%) aortic valves; during follow-up (mean 3.4 years), 3 (3.4%) died within 60 days of operation and 2 later (stroke and myocardial infarction). Yazdchi et al[25] reported, in abstract form, 205 patients with "well-functioning" BAVs and dilated ascending aortas (mean diameter 5.1 cm), all of which were resected, and, of them, 118 patients (58%) had "minimally repaired" aortic valves; by 5 years, 12 patients (6%) had died, and by 10 years postoperatively, 25 patients (12%) had died. Russo et al,[26,27] in 2 different studies, described 82 adults with "normally functioning" BAVs, all of whom had the dilated ascending aorta (mean diameter 5.4 cm) resected and 26 (32%) of whom had concomitant aortic valve repair; by 5 years postoperatively, 6 patients (7.3%) had died, and by 10 years, 18 patients (21%) had died.

The present patient was 65 years of age, and a woman of that age in the USA would be expected to live to age 86, an additional 21 years.[28] The chances of ascending aortic rupture/dissection in her in the next 20 years without resection of the aneurysm are unknown but it must be extremely small. If the patient, however, had been 40 years of age (expected survival to age 83 years),[28] one potentially could more reasonably justify resection of the ascending aorta if its maximal diameter, as in our patient, was >5 cm. Additionally, if there had been evidence of rapid enlargement of the aneurysm in a relatively short period of time, operative intervention might be more reasonable. In our patient, no information is available on the rate of enlargement of her aneurysm. In addition, the size of the aneurysm could be followed for a period of time to see if rapid progression occurred, and then aortic resection reconsidered.

It is appreciated that the frequency of aortic dissection may be 5 to 10 times higher in patients with congenitally unicuspid or bicuspid aortic valves than in patients with tricuspid aortic valves, irrespective of valve function.[29] Nevertheless, aortic dissection is extremely uncommon whether the aortic valve is congenitally malformed or 3-cuspid. Although the operative risk associated with resection of ascending aortic aneurysm is quite low, especially in high-volume centers, the surgical risk, of course, must be considerably lower than the chance of aortic dissection or rupture to justify operation. Because there is no proof that operative intervention provides less morbidity and lower mortality, nonoperative management at this time seems to be the better approach for a dilated ascending aorta with a normally functioning BAV.

DISCLOSURES

The authors have no conflict of interest to declare.

REFERENCES

1. Davies RR, Kaple RK, Mandapati D, Gallo A, Botta DM Jr, Elefteriades JA, Coady MA. Natural history of ascending aortic aneurysms in the setting of an unreplaced bicuspid aortic valve. *Ann Thorac Surg* 2007;83:1338–1344.
2. McKellar SH, Michelena HI, Li Z, Schaff HV, Sundt TM 3rd. Long-term risk of aortic events following aortic valve replacement in patients with bicuspid aortic valves. *Am J Cardiol* 2010;106:1626–1633.
3. Roberts WC. Prophylactic replacement of a dilated ascending aorta at the time of aortic valve replacement of a dysfunctioning congenitally unicuspid or bicuspid aortic valve. *Am J Cardiol* 2011;108:1371–1372.
4. Sievers HH, Stierle U, Mohamed SA, Hanke T, Richardt D, Schmidtke C, Charitos EI. Toward individualized management of the ascending aorta in bicuspid aortic valve surgery: the role of valve phenotype in 1362 patients. *J Thorac Cardiovasc Surg* 2014;148:2072–2080.
5. Rinewalt D, McCarthy PM, Malaisrie SC, Fedak PW, Andrei AC, Puthumana JJ, Bonow RO. Effect of aortic aneurysm replacement on outcomes after bicuspid aortic valve surgery: validation of contemporary guidelines. *J Thorac Cardiovasc Surg* 2014;148:2060–2069.
6. Nistri S, Sorbo MD, Marin M, Palisi M, Scognamiglio R, Thiene G. Aortic root dilatation in young men with normally functioning bicuspid aortic valves. *Heart* 1999;82:19–22.
7. Nkomo VT, Enriquez-Sarano M, Ammash NM, Melton LJ 3rd, Bailey KR, Desjardins V, Horn RA, Tajik AJ. Bicuspid aortic valve associated with aortic dilatation: a community-based study. *Arterioscler Thromb Vasc Biol* 2003;23:351–356.
8. Michelena HI, Khanna AD, Mahoney D, Margaryan E, Topilsky Y, Suri RM, Eidem B, Edwards WD, Sundt TM 3rd, Enriquez-Sarano M. Incidence of aortic complications in patients with bicuspid aortic valves. *JAMA* 2011;306:1104–1112.

9. Roberts WC, Filardo G, Ko JM, Siegel RJ, Dollar AL, Ross EM, Shirani J. Comparison of total 12-lead QRS voltage in a variety of cardiac conditions and its usefulness in predicting increased cardiac mass. *Am J Cardiol* 2013;112: 904–909.

10. Midulla PS, Ergin A, Galla J, Lansman SL, Sadeghi AM, Levy M, Griepp RB. Three faces of the Bentall procedure. *J Card Surg* 1994;9:466–481.

11. Borger MA, Preston M, Ivanov J, Fedak PW, Davierwala P, Armstrong S, David TE. Should the ascending aorta be replaced more frequently in patients with bicuspid aortic valve disease? *J Thorac Cardiovasc Surg* 2004;128:677–683.

12. Pape LA, Tsai TT, Isselbacher EM, Oh JK, O'Gara PT, Evangelista A, Fattori R, Meinhardt G, Trimarchi S, Bossone E, Suzuki T, Cooper JV, Froehlich JB, Nienaber CA, Eagle KA, International Registry of Acute Aortic Dissection (IRAD) Investigators. Aortic diameter > 5.5 cm is not a good predictor of type A aortic dissection: observations from the International Registry of Acute Aortic Dissection (IRAD). *Circulation* 2007;116:1120–1127.

13. Sundt TM 3rd. Replacement of the ascending aorta in bicuspid aortic valve disease: where do we draw the line? *J Thorac Cardiovasc Surg* 2010;140(6 Suppl): S41–S44.

14. Pisano C, Maresi E, Balistreri CR, Candore G, Merlo D, Fattouch K, Bianco G, Ruvolo G. Histological and genetic studies in patients with bicuspid aortic valve and ascending aorta complications. *Interact Cardiovasc Thorac Surg* 2012;14:300–306.

15. Sundt TM. Sound arguments, true premises, and valid conclusions. *J Thorac Cardiovasc Surg* 2014;148:2070–2071.

16. Sundt TM. Aortic replacement in the setting of bicuspid aortic valve: how big? How much? *J Thorac Cardiovasc Surg* 2015;149(2 Suppl): S6–S9.

17. Kim JB, Spotnitz M, Lindsay ME, MacGillivray TE, Isselbacher EM, Sundt TM 3rd. Risk of aortic dissection in the moderately dilated ascending aorta. *J Am Coll Cardiol* 2016;68:1209–1219.

18. Sundt TM. Drawing the line on prophylactic aortic replacement: Primum non nocere. *JAMA Netw Open* 2018;1:e181289.

19. Heng E, Stone JR, Kim JB, Lee H, MacGillivray TE, Sundt TM. Comparative histology of aortic dilatation associated with bileaflet versus trileaflet aortic valves. *Ann Thorac Surg* 2015;100:2095–2101, discussion 2101.

20. Leone O, Biagini E, Pacini D, Zagnoni S, Ferlito M, Graziosi M, Di Bartolomeo R, Rapezzi C. The elusive link between aortic wall histology and echocardiographic anatomy in bicuspid aortic valve: implications for prophylactic surgery. *Eur J Cardiothorac Surg* 2012;41:322–327.

21. Roberts WC, Vowels TJ, Ko JM, Filardo G, Hebeler RF Jr, Henry AC, Matter GJ, Hamman BL. Comparison of the structure of the aortic valve and ascending aorta in adults having aortic valve replacement for aortic stenosis versus for pure aortic regurgitation and resection of the ascending aorta for aneurysm. *Circulation* 2011;123:896–903.

22. La Canna G, Ficarra E, Tsagalau E, Nardi M, Morandini A, Chieffo A, Maisano F, Alfieri O. Progression rate of ascending aortic dilation in patients with normally functioning bicuspid and tricuspid aortic valves. *Am J Cardiol* 2006;98:249–253.

23. Etz CD, Zoli S, Brenner R, Roder F, Bischoff M, Bodian CA, DiLuozzo G, Griepp RB. When to operate on the bicuspid valve patient with a modestly dilated ascending aorta. *Ann Thorac Surg* 2010;90:1884–1890.

24. Guo MH, Appoo JJ, Saczkowski R, Smith HN, Ouzounian M, Gregory AJ, Herget EJ, Boodhwani M. Association of mortality and acute aortic events with ascending aortic aneurysm: a systematic review and meta-analysis. *JAMA Netw Open* 2018;1:e181281.

25. Yazdchi F, Roselli EE, Lowry A, Rajeswaran J, Rodriguez L, Pettersson GB, Svensson LG, Blackstone EH. Abstract 13308: preserving well-functioning bicuspid aortic valves in ascending aortic aneurysm repair. *Circulation* 2013;128(22 Suppl):A13308.
26. Russo M, Bertoldo F, Nardi P, D'Annolfo A, Saitto G, Pellegrino A, Chiariello L. Fate of normally functioning bicuspid aortic valve in patients undergoing ascending aorta surgery. *J Heart Valve Dis* 2015;24:570–576.
27. Russo M, Saitto G, Nardi P, Bertoldo F, Bassano C, Scafuri A, Pellegrino A, Ruvolo G. Bicuspid aortic root spared during ascending aorta surgery: an update of long-term results. *J Thorac Dis* 2017;9:1634–1638.
28. Arias E, Xu J. *United States Life Tables, 2017.* National Vital Statistics Reports, 68. Hyattsville, MD: National Center for Health Statistics; 2019.
29. Roberts CS, Roberts WC. Dissection of the aorta associated with congenital malformation of the aortic valve. *J Am Coll Cardiol* 1991;17:712–716.

Case 1753 Cardiovascular Ochronosis

Nuvaira Ather[a], William C. Roberts[a, b, c], *

1. INTRODUCTION

Ochronosis, a manifestation of alkaptonuria, a rare autosomal recessive metabolic disorder caused by a deficiency of homogentisate oxidase, was first described by Virchow in 1866 and the entity subsequently has predictably created instant interest among physicians because of its characteristic staining of various body tissues.[1] Consequently, at least 66 case reports on this topic have been published (Table 1).[1-62] This article summarizes contributions of a number of prominent historical figures to this topic and adds an additional 2 cases of black pigment in one or more cardiovascular structures to those already published.

1.1. Case Description

Pertinent clinical and cardiovascular findings in the 2 patients are summarized in Table 2 and illustrated in Figure 1. Both patients had systemic hypertension and hypothyroidism; both were overweight, and both had focally black operatively excised aortic valves. The aortic valve in case #2 weighed 4.6 times that of case #1 and yet the transvalvular aortic valve gradients were similar. The valve in case #1 weighed only 0.79 g (normal about 0.4 g[63]) such that the valve in this patient was only about twice normal size, an occurrence that produces only minimal or mild aortic stenosis with few exceptions.[64] Both patients had resection of portions of the ascending aorta and black pigment was present focally on their intimal surfaces where minimal atherosclerotic plaque was present. When contacted 6 and 2 months postoperatively, both patients were asymptomatic, and their activities were not limited.

2. DISCUSSION

Ochronosis has an interesting history, mainly because of the extremely prominent figures who have written about it. Virchow (1821–1902) was the first to describe this entity (1866), and he named it ochronosis based on its "translucent brown or yellowish [deposits] [histologically] . . . [that] largely adhered to the intercellular substance." He beautifully described at autopsy the deposits as "black as ink" in

---

[a] *Baylor Scott & White Heart and Vascular Institute, Baylor University Medical Center, Baylor Scott & White Health, Dallas, Texas, USA*

[b] *Department of Pathology, Baylor University Medical Center, Baylor Scott & White Health, Dallas, Texas, USA*

[c] *Department of Internal Medicine (Division of Cardiology), Baylor University Medical Center, Baylor Scott & White Health, Dallas, Texas, USA*

* Corresponding author. Baylor Scott & White Heart and Vascular Institute, 621 N. Hall Street, Suite H-030, Dallas, TX 75226, USA
E-mail address: William.Roberts1@BSWHealth.org (W.C. Roberts).

ARTICLE INFO
Article history:
Received 10 October 2019
Revised 10 February 2020
Accepted 28 February 2020

Table 1: Previously reported cases in English of ochronosis with black pigment in a cardiovascular structure confirmed by anatomic examination

#	First author	Year published	Age (y)	Sex	Ochronosis diagnosed clinically	Black deposits				A/S	Dysfunction		CAD disease
						AV	MV	Aorta	Other arteries (location)		AV (type)	MV (type)	
1	Virchow[1,a]	1866	67	Man	0	0	0	+	0	A	0	0	0
2	Galdston[2]	1952	65	Man	+	+	+	+	0	A	–	–	–
3	"	1952	60	Man	+	+	+	+	0	A	–	–	+
4	"	1952	94	Woman	+	+	+	+	+(CA)	A	–	–	–
5	Lichenstein[3]	1954	54	Man	+	+	+	+	+(CA)	A	+(AS)	–	+
6	"	1954	52	Man	–	+	–	+	0	A	–	+(MR)	+
7	Wagner[4]	1960	54	Man	+	+	+	+	+(CA)	A	+(AS)	–	+
8	Gould[5]	1976	68	Woman	+	+	+	+	+(CA)	A	+(AS)	–	+
9	Butler[6]	1985	57	Woman	0(M)	+(B)	+	0	+(CA)	S	+(AS)	0	+
10	Ptacin[7]	1985	65	Man	+	+	+	0	0	A	+(AS)	–	+
11	Vlay[8]	1986	70	Woman	0	+	–	+	–	S	+(AS)	–	0
12	Gaines[9]	1987	64	Man	+	+	+	+	–	S	+(AS)	–	+
13	Kenny[10]	1990	71	Man	+	+	+	+	+(CA)	A	–	–	+
14	Kragel[11]	1990	72	Man	+	+	+	+	+(CA)	A	+(AS)	–	+
15	Albers[12]	1992	72	Man	+	+	–	–	–	S	+(AS)	–	–
16	Hangaishi[13]	1998	63	Man	+	+	+	+	–	S	+(AS)	–	–
17	Vavuranakis[14]	1998	62	Man	+	+	–	–	–	S	+(AS)	–	+
18	Gonzales[15]	1999	75	Woman	+	+	–	–	–	S	+(AS)	–	+
19	Zünd[16]	1999	67	Woman	+	+	–	+	–	S	+(AS)	+(MR)	+
20	Ambrogio[17]	1999	78	Man	–	+	+	+	+(CA)	A	–	–	+
21	Ghotkar[18]	2003	63	Woman	+	+	–	+	–	S	+(AS)	–	–
22	Yoshikai[19]	2004	65	Man	+	+	+	+	+(CA)	S	+(AS)	–	+
23	Fisher[20]	2004	69	Woman	+	+	–	–	–	S	+(AS)	–	+
24	Erek[21]	2004	67	Woman	+	–	–	+	–	S	+(AS)	+(MR)	0
25	Gerson[22]	2006	76	Woman	0(M)	–	–	+	+(LEA)	A[b]	–	–	–
26	Butany[23]	2006	71	Woman	0	+	–	0	–	S	+(AS)	–	–

No.	Author	Year	Age	Sex									
27	Kovacevic[24]	2006	64	Man	0	+	+	–	–	S	+(AS)	–	+
28	Carman[25]	2006	67	Woman	0(M)	–	–	–	+(LEA)	S	–	–	–
29	Ffolkes[26]	2007	48	Man	+	+	+	+	+(CA)	S	+(AS)	–	+
30	Roser[27]	2008	71	Man	0	+	+	–	–	S	+(AS)	0	–
31	Brueck[28]	2008	69	Man	0	+	+	+	–	S	+(AS)	0	+
32	Laco[29]	2008	75	Woman	+	+	+	+	+(C)	A	+(AS)	+(MS)	–
33	Helliwell[30]	2008	74	Woman	0(M)	+	+	–	–	S	+(AS)	–	–
34	Wauthy[31]	2009	78	Man	0	+	+	–	–	S	+(AS)	–	–
35	Belcher[32]	2009	63	Man	0(M)	+	+	–	–	S	+(AR)[c]	–	–
36	Uchiyama[33]	2010	79	Man	0	+	+	–	–	S	+(AR)[c]	+(MR)	–
37	Wilke[34]	2010	69	Man	+	+	+	–	–	S	+(AR)[c]	+(MR)	+
38	Rios[35]	2010	66	Man	0	+	0	–	+(CA)	S	+(AS)	–	–
39	Steger[36]	2011	65	Woman	+	+	+	–	–	S	+(AS)	–	+
40	Tosya[37]	2012	62	Man	0	+	0	+	–	S	+(AS)	–	+
41	Thakur[38]	2012	65	Man	+	+	0	+	–	S	+(AS)	–	+
42	Hiroyoshi[39]	2013	70	Man	+	+	+	–	0	S	+(AS)	–	+
43	Lok[40]	2013	71	Man	+	+	+	+	+(CA, IMA)	S	+(AS)	–	+
44	"	2013	62	Man	0	+	+	+	–	S	+(AS)	–	+
45	Millucci[41]	2013	65	Woman	+	+	0	+	–	S	+(AS)	–	–
46	Capuano[42]	2014	67	Man	0	+	+	–	+(CA)	S	+(AS)	–	+
47	Tsunekawa[43]	2014	65	Woman	0(M)	+	+	+	+(CA)	S	+(AS)	–	+
48	Pfeffer[44]	2015	64	—	0	+	+	+	–	S	+(AS)	–	+
49	Rizzo[45]	2015	61	Man	0	+	+	+	–	S	+(AS)	–	–
50	Mokashi[46]	2015	64	Woman	0(M)	0	0	–	–	S	+(AS)	–	+
51	Atalay[47]	2015	72	Man	+	+	+	+	–	S	+(AS)	+(MR)	+
52	Roca[48]	2016	78	Man	0	+	+	+	–	S	+(AS)	–	0
53	Cohen[49]	2016	34	Man	0(M)	+	+	+	–	S	+(AR)[c]	–	+
54	Chatzis[50]	2016	63	Man	+	+	+	–	–	S	+(AS)	–	–
55	Schuuring[51]	2016	72	Woman	0	+(B)	0	+	–	S	+(AS)	–	+
56	Parashi[52]	2017	38	Man	+	0	0	0	–	S	+(AS)	–	–
57	Al-Amodi[53]	2017	36	Woman	0(M)	+(U)	0	0	–	S	+(AR)[c]	–	–
58	Tourmousoglou[54]	2017	61	Man	+	+	–	+	–	S	+(AS)	–	–

(Continued)

Table 1: (Continued)

#	First author	Year published	Age (y)	Sex	Ochronosis diagnosed clinically	Black deposits				A/S	Dysfunction		
						AV	MV	Aorta	Other arteries (location)		AV (type)	MV (type)	CAD disease
59	Buckley[55]	2017	56	Man	0(M)	+	0	+	+(CA)	S	-	-	+
60	Karavaggelis[56]	2017	66	Man	+	+	-	+	-	S	+(AS)	-	+
61	Ahmed[57]	2017	61	Woman	+	+	+	+	-	S	+(AS)	-	-
62	Gottschalk[58]	2018	67	Woman	+	-	+	-	+(CA, ITA)	S	-	+(MAC)	+
63	Selvakumar[59]	2018	72	Man	0	+	-	0	-	S	+(AS)	-	+
64	Watanabe[60]	2019	76	Man	+	+	-	0	0	S	+(AS)	-	+
65	Planinc[61]	2019	70	Woman	+	+	-	+	+(CA)	S	+(AS)	-	+
66	"	2019	63	Woman	+	+	-	-	+(CA)	S	+(AS)	-	+

Abbreviations: A=autopsy; AR = aortic regurgitation; AS = aortic stenosis; AV=aortic valve; B = bicuspid aortic valve; C = carotid arteries; CAD = coronary artery disease; CA = coronary arteries; IMA = internal mammary artery; ITA = internal thoracic artery; LEA = lower extremity arteries; M = associated with minocycline; MAC = mitral annular calcification; MR = mitral regurgitation; MS = mitral stenosis; MV = mitral valve; S = surgical; U = unicuspid aortic valve; — = no information available.
a Although published initially in German, Thomas G. Benedek republished Virchow's original article in English in 1966 (62).
b Limited to abdominal and pelvic organs.
c All 4 patients stated to have AR had calcific deposits on the cusps and the black pigment was in the calcific deposits only.

Table 2: Certain clinical and morphologic cardiac findings in the 2 white patients who had Bentall procedures because of aortic valve stenosis and resection of the histologically normal ascending aorta and focally blackened valve and aorta

#	Variable	Case # 1	Case # 2
1	Age at AVR (years)	69	76
2	Gender	Woman	Man
3	Systemic hypertension	+	+
4	Diabetes mellitus	+	0
6	Symptoms	Angina	Fatigue
7	Stroke (by history)	+[a]	0
8	Hypothyroidism	+	+
9	Atrial fibrillation	0	+
10	Body weight in lbs. (in kg)	144[b] (65.3)	203 (92.0)
11	Height (inches)	62	70
12	Body mass index (kg/m^2)	26	29
13	Total cholesterol (mg/dL)	190[c]	152[c]
14	LDL cholesterol (mg/dL)	100[c]	91[c]
15	Total 12-lead QRS voltage (mm)	94	146
16	LV peak systolic pressure (mm Hg)	–	–
17	Aortic peak systolic pressure (mm Hg)	114	136
18	LV-aortic peak systolic gradient (mm Hg)	67	59
19	LV-aorta mean transvalvular gradient (mm Hg)	43	41
20	LV ejection fraction (%)	60	60
21	Ascending aorta diameter (cm)	–	4.4
22	Concomitant cardiac procedures	CABG[d]	0
23	Coronary narrowing	0	0
24	Number of AV cusps	3	2
25	Weight of excised aortic valve (g)	0.79	3.66
26	Weight of excised ascending aorta (g)	1.6	12.8
27	Bovine pericardial valve (size in mm)	+ (23)	+ (29)

Abbreviations: AV=aortic valve; AVR = aortic valve replacement; CABG = coronary artery bypass grafting; LDL = low-density lipoprotein; LV = left ventricular.
[a] Also cerebral artery aneurysm.
[b] Lost 20 lbs. in previous 2 years.
[c] On statin at the time.
[d] Left anterior descending artery narrowed 30% in diameter.

cartilages in various body locations and in plaques in arteries, mainly the aorta. Osler (1849–1919) described this entity clinically in 2 brothers, one of whom had a son with alkaptonuria, an association with ochronosis recognized only 2 years earlier by Albrecht.[65] Osler described the "coal black" and "ebony-black discoloration" in the sclera of the eyes, cartilages of the ears, and on the face.[66] Sir Archibald E. Garrod, who followed Osler as the Regius professor at Oxford, included ochronosis as one of his "Inborn Errors of Metabolism" and he determined ochronosis to be an autosomal recessive disorder.[67]

Although ochronosis was described initially at autopsy, later clinically, and now, at least the cardiovascular features are observed most commonly, as in our 2 cases, at operation when 1 or more cardiac valves are excised. The black deposits, characteristic of ochronosis, appear to be present only in the calcified portions of cardiac valves and atherosclerotic plaques. Thus, ochronosis is common in patients with aortic stenosis and uncommon in patients with aortic regurgitation because the latter usually is devoid of calcific deposit. The black pigment is also common in patients with mitral annular calcium. The characteristic black pigment in these calcific deposits does not appear to either worsen or lessen the function of

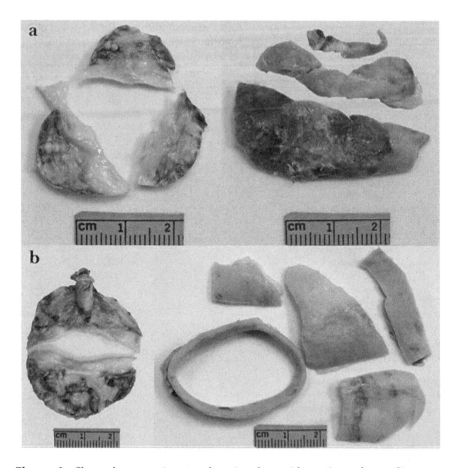

Figure 1 Shown here are pictures of aortic valves with portions of ascending aorta excised surgically: *a*. Case #1, *b*. Case #2. In case #1, the aortic valve is 3-cuspid and in case #2, bicuspid, and the black pigment is present only in the calcific deposits. In case #1, the pigment in the aorta is extensive and in case #2, minimal.

the cardiac valve. Although previously reported, ochronotic pigment in a stenotic congenitally unicuspid[53] or bicuspid[6,52] aortic valve, as in our patient #2, is most unusual. Congenitally bicuspid aortic valves have an estimated frequency of about 1 in 100 adults[68] and clinically manifest ochronosis has an estimated frequency of 1 in 250,000 to 1,000,000,[69] such that the occurrence of both conditions in the same person is indeed unusual. Ochronotic pigment in atherosclerotic plaques, as occurred in our patient #2, was first recognized by Virchow and observed subsequently by many other investigators (Table 1). It appears that cardiovascular ochronosis causes no functional derangement and only exists in previously abnormal cardiac valves or arteries (previous atherosclerosis).

Ochronosis occurs in both primary and secondary forms. The most common secondary form is associated with phenols, a class of chemicals containing a hydroxyl group (-OH) bonded to an aromatic (presence of a benzene ring) hydrocarbon group. Secondary or exogenous ochronosis can be secondary to the topical application of hydroquinone, phenol, resorcinol, or oral administration of antimalarials.[70] Minocycline, one of the tetracyclines, consumed by both patients

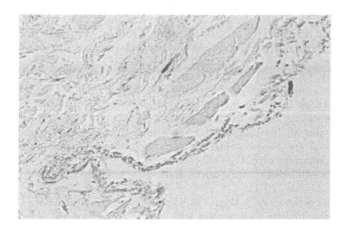

Figure 2 Case # 1. Photomicrograph of a section of aortic valve showing a liner row of dark-staining cells consistent with ochronosis pigment. The pigment stains lightly probably because the tissue was decalcified before processing and staining. Fontana-Masson stain, x25.

described herein, has been recognized, if used chronically, as an exogenous cause of ochronosis.[6,22,25,32,43,46,49,53,55,71] In case #1, this drug was administered for chronic joint pains and in case #2, for neuropathic pain.[71] Whether the minocycline in our 2 patients was the cause of the ochronosis in them is unclear (Figure 2).

DECLARATION OF COMPETING INTEREST
None.

FUNDING
This research did not receive any specific grant from funding agencies in the public, commercial, or not-for-public sectors.

REFERENCES
1. Virchow R. Ein Fall von allgemeiner Ochronose der Knorpel und knorpelaehn-lichen Teile. *Virchows Arch F Path Anat* 1866;37:212–219.
2. Galdston M, Steele JM, Dobriner K. Alcaptonuria and ochronosis: with a report of three patients and metabolic studies in two. *Am J Med* 1952;13(4):432–452.
3. Lichtenstein L, Kaplan L. Hereditary ochronosis: pathologic changes observed in two necropsied cases. *Am J Pathol* 1954;30(1):99–125.
4. Wagner LR, Knott JL, Machaffie RA, Walsh JR. Clinical and pathological find-ings in ochronosis. *J Clin Pathol* 1960;13(1):22–26.
5. Gould L, Reddy CV, DePalma D, De Martino A, Kalish PE. Cardiac manifesta-tions of ochronosis. *J Thorac Cardiovasc Surg* 1976;72(5):788–791.
6. Butler JM, Marks R, Sutherland R. Cutaneous and cardiac valvular pigmentation with minocycline. *Clin Exp Dermatol* 1985;10(5):432–437.
7. Ptacin M, Sebastian J, Bamrah VS. Ochronotic cardiovascular disease. *Clin Cardiol* 1985;8(8):441–445.
8. Vlay SC, Hartman AR, Culliford AT. Alkaptonuria and aortic stenosis. *Ann Intern Med* 1986;104(3):448.
9. Gaines JJ, Pai GM. Cardiovascular ochronosis. *Arch Pathol Lab Med* 1987;111(10): 991–994.

10. Kenny D, Ptacin MJ, Bamrah VS, Almagro U. Cardiovascular ochronosis: a case report and review of the medical literature. *Cardiology* 1990;77(6):477–483.

11. Kragel AH, Lapa JA, Roberts WC. Cardiovascular findings in alkaptonuric ochronosis. *Am Heart J* 1990;120(6 Pt 1):1460–1463.

12. Albers SE, Brozena SJ, Glass LF, Fenske NA. Alkaptonuria and ochronosis: case report and review. *J Am Acad Dermatol* 1992;27(4):609–614.

13. Hangaishi M, Taguchi J, Ikari Y, Ohno M, Kurokawa K, Kotsuka Y, et al. Aortic valve stenosis in alkaptonuria. *Circulation* 1998;98(11):1148–1149.

14. Vavuranakis M, Triantafillidi H, Stefanadis C, Toutouzas P. Aortic stenosis and coronary artery disease caused by alkaptonuria, a rare genetic metabolic syndrome. *Cardiology* 1998;90(4):302–304.

15. Gonzales ME. Alkaptonuric aortic stenosis: a case report. *AANA J* 1999;67(2):145–151.

16. Zünd G, Schmid AC, Vogt PR, Grünenfelder J, Turina MI. Green aortic valve: alcaptonuria (ochronosis) with severe aortic stenosis. *Ann Thorac Surg* 1999;67(6):1805.

17. Sant'Ambrogio S, Connelly J, DiMaio D. Minocycline pigmentation of heart valves. *Cardiovasc Pathol* 1999;8(6):329–332.

18. Ghotkar S, Kuduvalli M, Dihmis W. Ochronosis of the aorta. *Eur J Cardiothorac Surg* 2003;23(3):423.

19. Yoshikai M, Murayama J, Yamada N. Aortic valve regurgitation in alkaptonuria. *J Heart Valve Dis* 2004;13(5):863–865.

20. Fisher AA, Davis MW. Alkaptonuric ochronosis with aortic valve and joint replacements and femoral fracture: a case report and literature review. *Clin Med Res* 2004;2(4):209–215.

21. Erek E, Casselman FR, Vanermen H. Cardiac ochronosis: valvular heart disease with dark green discoloration of the leaflets. *Tex Heart Inst J* 2004;31(4):445–457.

22. Gerson DM, Robinson MJ. Black pigmentation of atherosclerotic plaques associated with chronic minocycline therapy. *Cardiovasc Pathol* 2006;15(3):168–170.

23. Butany JW, Naseemuddin A, Moshkowitz Y, Nair V. Ochronosis and aortic valve stenosis. *J Card Surg* 2006;21(2):182–184.

24. Kovacevic M, Simic O, Medved I, Lucin K, Padovan M. Ochronosis of the aortic valve and aorta. *J Heart Valve Dis* 2006;15(5):730–732.

25. Carman TL, Lyden SP. Images in vascular medicine. Drug-related skin and atherosclerotic plaque pigmentation. *Vasc Med* 2006;11(4):276–277.

26. Ffolkes LV, Brull D, Krywawych S, Hayward M, Hughes SE. Aortic stenosis in cardiovascular ochronosis. *J Clin Pathol* 2007;60:92–93.

27. Roser M, Möller J, Komoda T, Knosalla C, Stawowy P. Alkaptonuric aortic stenosis. *Eur Heart J* 2008;29(4):444.

28. Brueck M, Bandorski D, Kramer W, Schoenburg M, von Gerlach S, Tillmanns H. Aortic valve stenosis due to alkaptonuria. *J Heart Valve Dis* 2008;17(1):127–129.

29. Laco J, Steiner I, Kubicek V, Spacek J. Black aortic valve—ochronosis. *APMIS* 2008;116(11):1011–1012.

30. Helliwell TR, Gallagher JA, Ranganath L. Alkaptonuria—a review of surgical and autopsy pathology. *Histopathology* 2008;53(5):503–512.

31. Wauthy P, Seghers V, Mathonet P, Deuvaert FE. Cardiac ochronosis: not so benign. *Eur J Cardiothorac Surg* 2009;35(4):732–733.

32. Belcher E, Soni M, Azeem F, Sheppard MN, Petrou M. Minocycline-induced pigmentation of the aortic valve and sinuses of Valsalva. *Ann Thorac Surg* 2009;88(5):1704.

33. Uchiyama C, Kondoh H, Shintani H. Acute methemoglobinemia associated with ochronotic valvular heart disease: report of a case. *Thorac Cardiovasc Surg* 2010;58(2):115–117.

34. Wilke A, Dapunt O, Steverding D. Image of the month: Bluish-black pigmentation of the sclera and the aortic valve in a patient with alkaptonuric ochronosis. *Herz* 2010;35(1):41.
35. Caleb Ríos J, Reyes A, Esquivel H, Lescano M. Aortic stenosis and coronary artery disease in alkaptonuria. Case report. *Rev Esp Cardiol* 2010;63(9):1105–1106.
36. Steger CM. Aortic valve ochronosis: a rare manifestation of alkaptonuria. *BMJ Case Rep* 2011. doi:10.1136/bcr.04.2011.4119.
37. Tosya A, Coskun P, Uymaz B, Tarcan O, Aybek T. Black aorta in a patient with alkaptonuric ochronosis. *Anadolu Kardiyoloji Dergisi* 2012;12(5):E27.
38. Thakur S, Markman P, Cullen H. Choice of valve prosthesis in a rare clinical condition: aortic stenosis due to alkaptonuria. *Heart Lung Circ* 2013;22(10):870–872.
39. Hiroyoshi J, Saito A, Panthee N, Imai Y, Kawashima D, Motomura N, et al. Aortic valve replacement for aortic stenosis caused by alkaptonuria. *Ann Thorac Surg* 2013;95(3):1076–1079.
40. Lok ZS, Goldstein J, Smith JA. Alkaptonuria-associated aortic stenosis. *J Card Surg* 2013;28(4):417–420.
41. Millucci L, Ghezzi L, Braconi D, Laschi M, Geminiani M, Amato L, Orlandini M, et al. Secondary amyloidosis in an alkaptonuric aortic valve. *Int J Cardiol* 2014;172(1):e121–e123.
42. Capuano F, Angeloni E, Roscitano A, Bianchini R, Refice S, Lechiancole A, et al. Blackish pigmentation of the aorta in patient with alkaptonuria and Heyde's syndrome. *Aorta (Stamford)* 2014;2(2):74–76.
43. Tsunekawa T, Jones KW, Doty JR. Black pigmented aortic valve and sinus of Valsalva caused by life-long minocycline therapy. *Interact Cardiovasc Thorac Surg* 2014;19(2):339–340.
44. Pfeffer C, Bagaev E, Sotlar K, Hagl C. Aortic valve replacement surgery reveals previously undiagnosed alkaptonuric ochronosis. *Eur J Cardiothorac Surg* 2015;47(1):194.
45. Rizzo S, Basso C, Bottio T. A 61-year-old man with hyperpigmentation: ochronosis. *Heart* 2015;101(17):1412–1421.
46. Mokashi SA, Rajab TK, Burrage PS, Mizuguchi AK, Aranki SF. Mincocycline-induced discoloration of the aorta. *Open Forum Infect Dis* 2015;2(4):1.
47. Atalay A, Gocen U, Basturk Y, Kozanoglu E, Yaliniz H. Ochronotic involvement of the aortic and mitral valves in a 72-year-old man. *Tex Heart Inst J* 2015;42(1):84–86.
48. Roca B, Roca M, Monferrer R. Alkaptonuria presenting with impressive osteoarticular changes and severe aortic stenosis. *Conn Med* 2016;80(3):139–141.
49. Cohen MA, Owens SR, Yang B. Minocycline pigmentation of the cardiac valves and aorta in a 29-year survivor of liver transplant. *J Thorac Cardiovasc Surg* 2016;152(6):1618–1619.
50. Chatzis AC, Kanakis MA, Sofianidou J, Tsoutsinos AJ. Operating the blues. *Clin Case Rep* 2016;4(12):1201–1202.
51. Schuuring MJ, Delemarre B, Keyhan-Falsafi AM, van der Bilt IA. Mending a darkened heart: alkaptonuria discovered during aortic valve replacement. *Circulation* 2016;133(12):e444–e445.
52. Parashi HS, Joshi MM, Jadhao MR. Alkaptonuric ochronosis of congenital bicuspid aortic valve—a case report. *Indian J Thorac Cardiovasc Surg* 2017;33(2):155–158.
53. Al-Amodi HA, Tweedie EJ, Iglesias I, Chu MWA. Black aortic valve: a surprise finding of what clinical relevance? *Can J Cardiol* 2017;33(6):831.e7–831.e8.
54. Tourmousoglou C, Nikoloudakis N, Pitsis A. Aortic valve stenosis in alkaptonuria. *Ann Thorac Surg* 2017;103(6):e557.
55. Buckley T, Lee J, Gipson KE, Earle J. Minocycline-induced hyperpigmentation mimicking aortic dissection. *Ann Thorac Surg* 2017;103(2):e121–e122.

56. Karavaggelis A, Young C, Attia R. Black heart at surgery—primary diagnosis of alkaptonuria at surgery. *J Cardiol Curr Res* 2017;9(5):00335.

57. El-Sayed Ahmed MM, Hussain O, Ott DA, Aftab M. Severe aortic valve stenosis due to alkaptonuric ochronosis. *Semin Cardiothorac Vasc Anesth* 2017;21(4):364–366.

58. Gottschalk BH, Blankenstein J, Guo L. Ochronosis of mitral valve and coronary arteries. *Ann Thorac Surg* 2018;106(1):e19–e20.

59. Selvakumar D, Sian K, Sugito S, Singh T. Ochronosis of the aortic valve. *J Thorac Dis* 2018;10(5):E332–E334.

60. Watanabe T, Harada R, Mikami T, Numaguchi R, Doi H, Kawaharada N. No ochronosis was seen at internal thoracic artery with alkaptonuria. *Asian Cardiovasc Thorac Ann* 2019;27(6):486–488.

61. Planinc M, Unic D, Baric D, Blazekovic R, Sribar A, Sutlic Z, et al. The dark side of the heart: cardiovascular manifestation of ochronosis. *Ann Thorac Surg* 2019;108(4):e257–e259.

62. Virchow RL. Rudolph Virchow on ochronosis: 1866. *Arthritis Rheum* 1966;9(1):66–71.

63. Silver MA, Roberts WC. Detailed anatomy of the normally functioning aortic valve in hearts of normal and increased weight. *Am J Cardiol* 1985;55(4):454–461.

64. Roberts WC, Ko JM. Weights of operatively-excised stenotic unicuspid, bicuspid, and tricuspid aortic valves and their relation to age, sex, body mass index, and presence or absence of concomitant coronary artery bypass grafting. *Am J Cardiol* 2003;92(9):1057–1065.

65. Albrecht H. Über ochronose. *Ztschr Heilk* 1902;23:366.

66. Osler W. Ochronosis: the pigmentation of cartilages, sclerotics, and skin in alkaptonuria. *Lancet* 1904;163(4192):10–11.

67. Garrod AE. The incidence of alkaptonuria: a study in chemical individuality. *Lancet* 1902;160(4137):1616–1620.

68. Roberts WC. The congenitally bicuspid aortic valve. A study of 85 autopsy cases. *Am J Cardiol* 1970;26(1):72–83.

69. Zatkova A. An update on molecular genetics of Alkaptonuria (AKU). *J Inherit Metab Dis* 2011;34(6):1127–1136.

70. Charlín R, Barcaui CB, Kac BK, Soares DB, Rabello-Fonseca R, Azulay-Abulafia L. Hydroquinone-induced exogenous ochronosis: a report of four cases and usefulness of dermoscopy. *Int J Dermatol* 2008;47(1):19–23.

71. Garrido-Mesa N, Zarzuelo A, Gálvez J. Minocycline: far beyond an antibiotic. *Br J Pharmacol* 2013;169(2):337–352.

Case 1760 Virtually All Complications of Active Infective Endocarditis Occurring in a Single Patient

William C. Roberts, MD[a]*, Divya Kapoor, MD[b], and Michael L. Main, MD[b]

Described herein is a 49-year-old black man with advanced polycystic renal disease, on hemodialysis for 6 years, who during his last 12 days of life had his vegetations on the aortic valve extend to the mitral and tricuspid valves, through the aortic wall to produce diffuse pericarditis, to the atrioventricular node to produce complete heart block, and embolize to cerebral arteries producing multiple brain infarcts, to a branch on the left circumflex coronary artery producing acute myocardial infarction, and to mesenteric arteries producing bowel infarction. © 2020 Published by Elsevier Inc.

(Am J Cardiol 2020;137:127–129)

Vegetations dangling on one or more aortic valve cusps (active infective endocarditis) are life threatening because they may extend to adjacent tissues (ring abscess) and/or embolize to arteries causing infarction. It is unusual for aortic valve vegetations to extend to 2 other cardiac valves or to embolize to multiple arteries or to cause septic pericarditis. Such was the case in the patient to be described herein.

CASE DESCRIPTION

A 49-year-old black man with known advanced polycystic renal disease on hemodialysis (for 6 years), diabetes mellitus, systemic hypertension, and obstructive sleep apnea (without obesity—body weight 176 lbs.) had been in his usual health until he developed epigastric, back, and vague chest pain 3 days before hospitalization. Examination in the emergency room disclosed a grade 2/6 systolic murmur along the lower left sternal border. The patient indicated that his chest pain worsened when lying flat. The electrocardiogram was consistent with posterior wall acute myocardial infarction (Figure 1). His troponin level was 1.7 rising to 76 mg/L the next day. From the emergency room he was taken to the cardiac catheterization laboratory where coronary angiogram showed normal right (nondominant), left main, left anterior descending, and left circumflex coronary arteries, and a totally occluded third marginal coronary artery, which could not be opened. The following pressures in mmHg were recorded: pulmonary artery 47/24; pulmonary arterial wedge a 28, v 37, mean 24; aorta 82/54. Blood drawn for culture later disclosed methicillin-sensitive Staphylococcus aureus.

Despite appropriate antibiotic therapy his condition progressively worsened. Because of continued abdominal pain, abdominal imaging was performed which revealed bowel necrosis. Laparoscopic bowel resection was performed the day after admission and a 5 cm portion of necrotic ileum was resected. He became progressively more confused and magnetic resonance imaging of the brain showed several cerebral infarcts. During his 9 days in the hospital he progressed

[a]Baylor Scott & White Heart Institute, Baylor University Medical Center, Dallas, Texas; and [b]Saint Luke's Mid American Heart Institute, Kansas City, Missouri. Manuscript received July 7, 2020; revised manuscript received and accepted September 23, 2020.
* Corresponding author.
E-mail address: William.Roberts1@BSWHealth.org (W.C. Roberts).

DOI: 10.1201/9781003409281-63

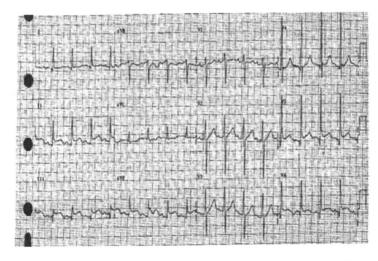

Figure 1 Electrocardiogram shortly after admission with findings of acute myocardial infarction.

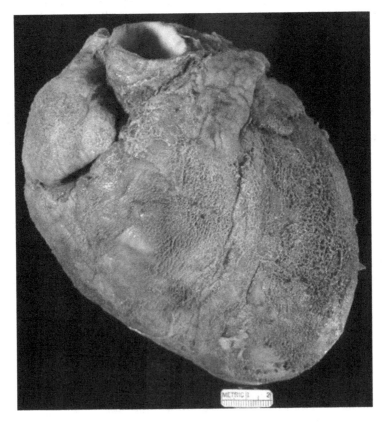

Figure 2 Heart showing acute diffuse pericarditis.

from sinus tachycardia with prolonged PR interval to second degree heart block (Wenckebach), to complete heart block (pacemaker inserted), and finally to fatal ventricular fibrillation.

At necropsy, the pericardial surfaces were diffusely covered by fibrin deposits (fibrinous "pericarditis") (Figure 2). The heart weighed 720g (normal < 350g). The aortic valve was 3 cuspid. Vegetation was present on each of the 3 cusps and calcific deposits were present in the left cusp. The vegetations extended through the wall of aorta to the space between the walls of the aorta and left atrium. The aortic vegetations extended on to the anterior mitral leaflet and into the calcium of the mitral annulus (Figure 3). The infection at the aortic and left atrial wall extended into the atrial septum to destroy the atrioventricular node and infect the adjacent

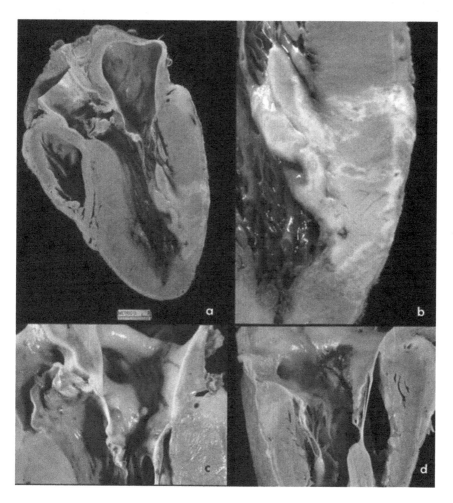

Figure 3 Views of the heart. (*a*) left parasagittal view showing the infection involving the aortic and mitral valves and the posterior wall acute infarct, a close-up of which is shown in (*b*). (*c*). A close-up view of the aortic and mitral valves showing vegetations on each. Ao = aorta; LA = left atrium. (*d*). Right parasagittal view showing vegetation in the area of the atrioventricular node with extension into the septal tricuspid valve leaflet.

tricuspid valve leaflet. All epicardial coronary arteries were wide open except for the third obtuse marginal which was totally occluded by a septic embolus. A large acute myocardial infarct involved the posterior left ventricular free wall and the posteromedial papillary muscle (Figure 3). Septic emboli were found in several small intracerebral arteries and in several mesenteric arteries.

DISCUSSION

Of the various cardiac valves affected by infective endocarditis, the aortic by far is the most common and it also is associated with the most complications.[1] Chronic renal disease, as in the present patient, is a major risk factor for infective endocarditis.[2] These complications include destruction of the aortic valve cusps causing aortic regurgitation, extension of the cuspal infection to adjacent tissues (ring abscess), including the anterior mitral leaflet and its chordae tendinea producing mitral regurgitation; to the atrioventricular node or bundle or both producing heart block; to the atrial septum (or membranous ventricular septum) to infect the tricuspid valve; through the aortic wall to produce pericardial disease, and to embolize to multiple systemic arteries. The patient described herein had all of these complications. The least common is pericardial disease.

REFERENCES

1. Roberts WC, Oluwole O, Fernicola DJ. Comparison of active infective endocarditis involving a previously stenotic versus a previously nonstenotic aortic valve. *Am J Cardiol* 1993;71:1082–1088.
2. Roberts WC, Taylor MA, Shirani J. Cardiac findings at necropsy in patients with chronic kidney disease maintained on chronic hemodialysis. *Medicine (Baltimore)* 2012;91:165–178.

Case 1763 Isolated Mitral Valve Endocarditis with Ring Abscess and Pericarditis in End-Stage Renal Disease

William Ryan Sovic, MD[a], Quynh Ngo, MD[a], Srikant Patlolla, MD[a], Joseph M. Guileyardo, MD[b], and William C. Roberts, MD[a,b,c]

Described herein is a 68-year-old man with end-stage renal disease on hemodialysis who was found to have methicillin-sensitive *Staphylococcus aureus* endocarditis with an associated ring abscess that extended into the left atrioventricular sulcus and ruptured into the pericardial space causing pericardial effusion. In contrast to the frequency of infective endocarditis involving the aortic valve, ring abscess associated with infection of the mitral valve is uncommon.

Infective endocarditis (IE) with ring abscess occurs mainly with infection involving the aortic valve.[1,2] IE with a ring abscess isolated to the mitral valve is uncommon, but such was the case in the patient described herein.

CASE REPORT

A 68-year-old Hispanic man with end-stage renal disease presented to the emergency department with several days of altered mental status, chest pain, dizziness, nausea, and chills. A week earlier he had transitioned from a temporary catheter to an upper extremity fistula for hemodialysis. In the emergency department, he was hypotensive and in atrial fibrillation with a ventricular rate of 134 beats/min. His blood lactate was 6.7 mmol/L, troponin 6.6 ng/mL, D-dimer 14.67 mcg/mL, and C-reactive protein 21.5 mg/dL. He was given fluids, antibiotics, and heparin intravenously. Blood cultures from admission grew methicillin-sensitive *Staphylococcus aureus*. On the third day of hospitalization, the patient had cardiac arrest; resuscitation was successful. An echocardiogram after the cardiac arrest disclosed a pericardial effusion. A subsequent cardiac arrest was fatal. Autopsy revealed mitral valve endocarditis with a ring abscess extending into the left atrioventricular sulcus with rupture into the pericardial space producing hemorrhagic pericardial effusion (*Figure 1*).

DISCUSSION

The patient described herein required hemodialysis for end-stage renal disease, initially with a temporary catheter and recently with an arteriovenous fistula. Patients on chronic hemodialysis have a high incidence of IE. The Danish National Patient Registry reported a frequency of IE in patients undergoing hemodialysis of 1092 per 100,000 person-years.[3] The risk of IE in patients with central venous catheters

[a]Department of Internal Medicine, Baylor University Medical Center, Dallas, Texas; [b]Department of Pathology, Baylor University Medical Center, Dallas, Texas; [c]Baylor Heart and Vascular Institute, Dallas, Texas

Corresponding author: William C. Roberts, MD, Baylor Heart and Vascular Institute, 621 N. Hall Street, Ste. H030, Dallas, TX 75246 (e-mail: William.Roberts1@BSWHealth.org)

The authors report no conflicts of interest. Before his death, the patient gave permission for use of his medical information for educational purposes. Received November 19, 2020; Revised December 30, 2020; Accepted January 19, 2021.

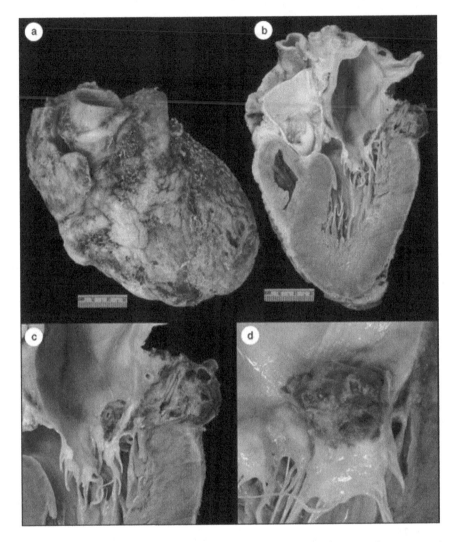

Figure 1 Heart in the patient described. **(a)** Exterior view showing the acute peri-carditis. **(b)** Left parasagittal cut showing the left side of the heart. A vegetation is barely seen on the atrial aspect of the posterior mitral leaflet. As shown better in **(c)**, the mitral vegetation has ruptured into the left atrioventricular sulcus and then out into the pericardial sac, causing a large hemopericardium. **(d)** Shown here is the mitral vegetation "head on." The underlying mitral valve is anatomically normal. Only a minute calcific deposit was present in the mitral annular region.

for hemodialysis was more than double that of those receiving hemodialysis via arteriovenous fistulas.[3]

IE more commonly affects a native aortic valve than a native mitral valve. Analysis of 96 necropsy patients with active left-sided IE studied by Arnett and Roberts[1] disclosed isolated aortic valve involvement in 34 patients (35%), isolated mitral valve involvement in 22 patients (23%), and involvement of both valves in 18 (19%). Of 59 patients with IE involving the aortic valve, 24 (41%) had a ring abscess;

Table 1: Causes of pericarditis in infective endocarditis

I. Extension of inflammation from
A. Mycotic aneurysm of aortic root
B. Valve ring abscess
C. Embolus in extramural coronary artery
II. Rupture of mycotic aneurysm

of 36 patients with IE involving any valve other than the aortic, only 3 (6%) had a ring abscess.[2] At least five patients with IE involving the mitral valve and leading to ring abscess and pericarditis have been reported previously; three had the IE superimposed on a calcified mitral annulus.[3–6]

Pericarditis is a relatively uncommon complication of IE. Arnett and Roberts[2] found pericarditis in 18 (19%) of 95 patients with IE involving the aortic valve, 14 of whom had a ring abscess. The same authors found pericarditis in only 6 (12%) of 48 patients with IE involving the mitral valve, only one of whom had a ring abscess. What makes our patient's pericarditis unusual is that it was in the setting of isolated mitral valve IE. Causes of pericarditis in patients with IE are summarized in Table 1.

REFERENCES

1. Arnett EN, Roberts WC. Active infective endocarditis: a clinicopathologic analysis of 137 necropsy patients. *Curr Prob Cardiol* 1976;1(7):1–76. doi:10.1016/0146-2806(76)90003-7.
2. Arnett EN, Roberts WC. Valve ring abscess in active infective endocarditis. Frequency, location, and clues to clinical diagnosis from the study of 95 necropsy patients. *Circulation* 1976;54(1):140–145. doi:10.1161/01.CIR.54.1.140.
3. Mambo NC, Silver MD, Brunsdon DF. Bacterial endocarditis of the mitral valve associated with annual calcification. *Can Med Assoc J* 1978;119(4):323–326.
4. Sandler MA, Kotler MN, Bloom RD, Jacobson L. Pericardial abscess extending from mitral vegetation: an unusual complication of infective endocarditis. *Am Heart J* 1989;118(4):857–859. doi:10.1016/0002-8703(89)90608-X.
5. Isotalo PA, Mai KT, Stinson WA, Veinot JP. Mitral annular calcification with *Staphylococcus aureus* periannular abscess. *Arch Pathol Lab Med* 2000;124:924.
6. Wentzell S, Nair V. Rare case of infective endocarditis involving mitral annular calcification leading to hemopericardium and sudden cardiac death: a case report. *Cardiovasc Pathol* 2018;33:16–18. doi:10.1016/j.carpath.2017.11.005.

Case 1780 Malignancy-Associated Non-Bacterial Thrombotic Endocarditis Causing Aortic Regurgitation and Leading to Aortic Valve Replacement

Madiha Makhdumi[a], Dan M. Meyer[b,c], and William C. Roberts[a,c],*

Described herein is a 48-year-old woman with metastatic ovarian cancer who developed aortic regurgitation considered clinically to be the result of infective endocarditis but operative resection of the three aortic valve cusps disclosed the valve lesions to be typical of non-bacterial thrombotic endocarditis (NBTE). Aortic regurgitation as a consequence of NBTE is rare but at least 9 cases have been reported previously. © 2021 Published by Elsevier Inc.

(Am J Cardiol 2021;154:120–122)

INTRODUCTION

Recently, we encountered a patient having aortic valve replacement for aortic regurgitation considered clinically to be the result of active infective endocarditis, but examination of an operatively excised aortic valve cusp disclosed the lesion to be typical of non-bacterial thrombotic endocarditis (NBTE), not infective endocarditis. The histological surprise stimulated us to search for previously reported cases of aortic regurgitation secondary to NBTE leading to aortic valve replacement (Table 1).[1-7]

CASE DESCRIPTION

A 48-year-old obese (body mass index of 32 kg/m²) woman with stage IV ovarian cancer, ascites and swollen legs presented to the emergency department at Baylor University Medical Center with dyspnea for two months. She was in no distress and was afebrile. The blood pressure was 140/80mmHg. A precordial murmur (not described further) was heard. No abnormalities were seen on the electrocardiogram. A 2-dimensional transthoracic echocardiogram 3.5 months before aortic valve replacement showed mild aortic regurgitation and cardiac catheterization showed the simultaneous left ventricular and aortic pressures to be 112/2 and 102/63 mmHg, respectively. The left ventricular ejection fraction was about 65%. Computed tomographic imaging disclosed small pleural effusions bilaterally. Transesophageal echocardiography 3 days before aortic valve replacement disclosed moderate aortic regurgitation, a left ventricular ejection fraction of about 35%, and a small mass on the ventricular aspect of the left coronary cusp (Figure 1). The blood cultures were negative. The leukocyte count was 5,600/µL, blood hemoglobin was 12.0 g/dl, and the platelet count was 260,000/µL. At operation, each aortic valve cusp was excised,

[a] From the Baylor Heart and Vascular Institute, Dallas, Texas; [b]The Departments of Cardiac Surgery, Dallas, Texas; and [c]Internal Medicine, Baylor University Medical Center, Dallas, Texas. Manuscript received May 6, 2021; revised manuscript received and accepted May 21, 2021.

* Corresponding author. Telephone 214-820-7911 Fax (214) 820-7533

E-mail address: William.Roberts1@bswhealth.org (W.C. Roberts).

DOI: 10.1201/9781003409281-65

Table 1: Certain observations in previously reported patients with non-bacterial thrombotic endocarditis (NBTE) and valve operation associated with pure regurgitation in one or both left sided valves

Case	First Author (Reference)	Year of Publication	Age at VO (years)	Sex	Valve with NBTE	Severity of Regurgitation	IE Diagnosed in Life	Cancer Location*	Before Valve Operation			
									Antiphospholipid Syndrome	Systemic Emboli	Anticoagulation Therapy†	Antibiotic Therapy
1	Kardaras[1]	1995	48	W	AV	"Significant"	+	0	0	0	0	+
2	Rabinstein[2]	2005	36	M	MV	"New"	+	0	+	+ (B)	+	0
3			42	W	AV	"Moderate"	+	?	0	+ (B,F,K,S)	+	+
4			38	W	MV	"Moderate"	?	0	+	+ (B)	+	0
5	Numnum[3]	2006	38	W	AV	"Severe"	+	Ovary, Uterus	0	+ (B,F,K,S)	0	+
6	Hofstra[4]	2009	34	W	AV, MV	"Severe"	0	Colon	0	+ (B)	0	0
7	Tei[5]	2010	45	W	MV	"Severe"	+	Pancreas	0	+ (B)	0	+
8	Kaneyuki[6]	2017	45	W	AV, MV	"Mild"	+	Uterus	0	+ (B)	+	+
9	Soga[7]	2018	69	M	MV	"Mild"	+	Stomach	0	+ (B, K)	+	+

AV = aortic valve; B = brain; F = finger; IE = infective endocarditis; K = kidney; M = man; MV = mitral valve; NBTE = non-bacterial thrombotic endocarditis; S = spleen; W = woman; VO = valve operation.
* All cancers were adenocarcinomas.
† These patients were treated with anticoagulants for ischemic stroke, not NBTE.

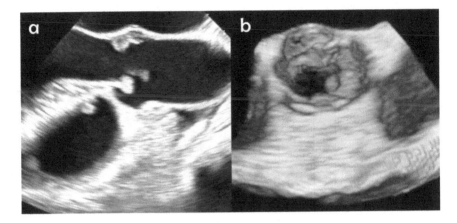

Figure 1 Transesophageal echocardiogram in the patient described showing (A) a mass characteristic of NBTE on the aortic valve; (B) a 3 dimensional image of the mass on one of the aortic valve cusps.

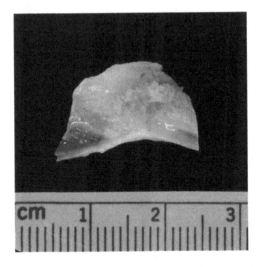

Figure 2 View of one of the three aortic valve cusps showing the mass character- istic of NBTE in the patient described.

and histologically the masses consisted only of fibrin (Figure 2). The underlying cusp was normal.

DISCUSSION

Examination of the operatively excised aortic valve disclosed the presence of NBTE, a lesion consisting entirely of fibrin with a few platelets. Although clinically our patient and 7 of the 9 previously reported patients with NBTE were considered clinically to have infective endocarditis, the latter was not present because the valve lesions consisted only of fibrin without the presence of microorganisms or polymorphonuclear leukocytes, requirements for the diagnosis of infective endocarditis (Figure 3).[6] Also, the underlying cusps were not damaged (no thickening,

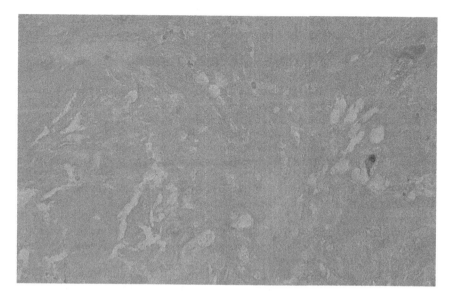

Figure 3 Photomicrograph of the lesion on the excised aortic valve cusp, showing fibrin devoid of microorganisms and polymorphonuclear leukocytes. Hematoxylin and eosin stain, x 400.

no perforations or indentations, or ring abscess). Cultures of the operatively excised aortic valve cusp in our patient were negative for microorganisms and similarly those of the previously reported patients were also negative.[1-7]

The degree of the aortic regurgitation in our patient and in the previously reported ones did not appear to be severe. The left ventricular cavity in our patient was normal in size, the pulse pressure was not widened, and physical examination did not mention the presence of a loud precordial murmur or "pistol-shot" femoral pulses or other signs of severe aortic regurgitation.

Cases have been described with fibrin deposits on previously implanted substitute cardiac valves: on stenotic native cardiac valves, on bioprosthesis and mechanical valve prosthesis, and in patients with systemic lupus erythematosus, and these cases were excluded from this report.[8-15] The patients in whom the aortic valve cusps were quite damaged were also excluded because healing of the active infective endocarditis could not be excluded.[16,17]

DISCLOSURES

The authors declare that they have no known competing financial interests or personal relationships that could have appeared to influence the work reported in this paper.

REFERENCES

1. Kardaras FG, Kardara DF, Rontogiani DP, Sioras EP, Christopoulou-Cokkinou V, Lolas CT, Anthopoulos LP. Acute aortic regurgitation caused by non-bacterial thrombotic endocarditis. *Eur Heart J* 1995;16:1152–1154.
2. Rabinstein AA, Giovanelli C, Ricci M, Romano JG, Koch S, Forteza AM. Surgical treatment of nonbacterial thrombotic endocarditis presenting with stroke. *J Neurol* 2005;252:352–355.

3. Numnum TM, Leath CA, Straughn MJ. Synchronous primary endometrial and ovarian carcinoma in a patient with marantic endocarditis. *Obstet Gynecol* 2006;108:748–750.
4. Hofstra JH, Timmer JR, Breeman A, Havenith MG. Non-bacterial thrombotic endocarditis in metastatic caecal adenocarcinoma. *Neth Heart J* 2009;17:349–350.
5. Tei T, Nomura T, Naito D, Kojima A, Urakabe Y, Enomoto-Uemura S, Nishikawa S, Keira N, Matsubara H, Tatsumi T. Effective surgical treatment for controlling the acute heart failure induced by acutely progressed mitral regurgitation with nonbacterial thrombotic endocarditis. *J Cardiol Cases* 2010;2:59–62.
6. Kaneyuki D, Matsuura K, Ueda H, Kohno H, Kanbe M, Matsumiya G. Surgical management of nonbacterial thrombotic endocarditis in malignancy. *Surg Case Rep* 2017;3:60.
7. Soga Y, Taira K, Sugimoto A, Kurosawa M, Kira H, Su T, Doi K, Nakano A, Himura Y. Mitral valve nonbacterial thrombotic endocarditis: a rare multi-surgery-tolerant survivor of Trousseau's syndrome. *Surg Case Rep* 2018;4:104.
8. Ram D, Armstrong G, Khanijow V, Sibal AK. Nonbacterial thrombotic endocarditis of a bioprosthetic valve: Questions to ponder before replacement of the valve. *J Card Surg* 2020;35:1142–1144.
9. Brock MA, Bleiweis MS, Reid J, Moguillanksy D. Recurrent nonbacterial thrombotic endocarditis: A novel therapeutic approach. *J Cardiol Cases* 2018;17:175–177.
10. Lamba H, Deo S, Altarabsheh S, Elgudin Y, Markowitz A, Park S. Non-bacterial thrombotic endocarditis of aortic valve due to hypereosinophilic syndrome. *J Heart Valve Dis* 2016;25:760–763.
11. Kurdi M, Beanlands DS, Chan KL, Veinot JP. Nonbacterial thrombotic endocarditis presenting as aortic stenosis with suspected infective endocarditis: clinicopathological correlation. *Can J Cardiol* 2004;20:549–552.
12. Moustafa S, Patton DJ, Balon Y, Kidd WT, Alvarez N. Mitral valve surgery for marantic endocarditis and multiple cerebral embolisation. *Heart Lung Circ* 2013;22:545–547.
13. Elikowski W, Jarząbek R, Małek M, Witczak W, Łazowski S, Psuja P. Niebakteryjne zakrzepowe zapalenie wsierdzia na dwupłatkowej zastawce aortalnej u 25-letniego mężczyzny z antykoagulantem toczniowym [Non-bacterial thrombotic endocarditis on the bicuspid aortic valve in a 25-year-old male with lupus anticoagulant]. *Pol Merkur Lekarski* 2016;40:182–185.
14. Basnet S, Stauffer T, Jayswal A, Tharu B. Recurrent nonbacterial thrombotic endocarditis and stroke on anticoagulation. *J Community Hosp Intern Med Perspect* 2020;10:466–469.
15. Yordan-Lopez NM, Hernandez-Suarez DF, Marshall-Perez L, Marrero-Ortiz W, Sánchez-Pérez B, Lopez-Candales A. Nonbacterial thrombotic endocarditis of the tricuspid valve in a male patient with antiphospholipid syndrome. *Cureus* 2018;10:2695.
16. Saito M, Asano N, Ota K, Niimi K, Tanaka K, Gon S, Takano H. Three mitral valve operations in a patient with Trousseau syndrome and nonbacterial thrombotic endocarditis caused by ovarian cancer. *Kyobu Geka* 2016;69:1067–1071.
17. Reid G, Koechlin L, Reuthebuch O, R€uter F, Hopfer H, Eckstein F, Santer D. Noninfective endocarditis: A case report of hereditary coagulation disorders in a 28-year-old male. *Diagnostics (Basel)* 2020;10:384.

Index

Note: Page numbers in *italics* indicate a figure and page numbers in **bold** indicate a table on the corresponding page.

A

abdominal aorta, *189*
active infective endocarditis
    antibiotic therapy, 305
    complications, 308
    diagnostic imaging, 305, *306*
    laparoscopic bowel resection, 305
    patient history, 305
acute myocardial infarction, *109*, 158, *159*
acute rheumatic fever
    Aschoff bodies, 68
    in childhood, 67–69
    incidence of death in, 67
    patient history, 67–68
    with pancarditis, 78–79
Alfieri Stitch
    echocardiographic data before and after
        placement of, **268**
    echocardiographic images, 266, *267*
    operative insertion of, 266–268
    patient history, 266
    surgery, 267
alkaptonuric ochronosis
    complication of, 190
    necropsy, 190, *191*
    patient history, 190
    with pigmentation, 191, *192*
    transverse section of, *192*
ankylosing spondylitis, 88
    diagnostic imaging, 89
    examination, 89
    operation, 93
    patient history, 88–89
antistreptolysin-O, 73
aortic insufficiency, **22–23**
aortic regurgitation, 46, *46*, 47, 88, 274
    and orthotopic heart transplantation,
        272, 274
    fusiform ascending aortic aneurysm,
        119–129
    from systemic hypertension, 152–156
    intermittent, 96–98
aortic stenosis, 158, *159*, 223
    sudden collapse in, 226–228, *227*
aortic valve, *64*
    bulge, *18*
    function, *17*
    operatively excised, 212–214, *213*
    replacement, 223–225, *224*
    ring, 16
aortogram
    ascending aortic aneurysm, 119, *120*
    fatal bioprosthetic regurgitation, 168
aortography, traumatic aortic
        regurgitation, 14
arterial insufficiency, *see* nonobstructive
        mesenteric arterial insufficiency
ascending aortic aneurysm, *125*
    diagnostic imaging, 119, *121*
atrioventricular valves, *61*, *63*
autopsy
    carcinoid heart disease, 31
    mitral valve, 36
    myocardial embolus, 28
    quadrivalvular rheumatoid heart
        disease, 51
    rheumatoid arthritis, 60
    Starr-Edwards prosthetic mitral valve, 81

B

bicuspid aortic valve, 99–103, 179–181, *180*, **181**
    aortic dissection, 292
    aortic valve replacement for, 255
    criteria for, 101
    diagnostic imaging, 99, *100*, 288, *289*
    histologic analysis, 290
    meta-analysis, 291
    in nonagenarian, 223–225, *224*
    occurrence, 254–255
    patient history, 99, 252, 288–289
    posterior mitral valve leaflet, *253*
    surgery, **255**
    surgical intervention, 288
    surgical risk, 292
bioprosthesis
    in aortic valve position, *203*, 203–204
    calcification of, **171**, 171–172, *172*
    massive calcification of, 197–199, *198*
    in mitral valve position, 194–196, *195*,
        205–207, *206*
    in tricuspid and mitral valve positions,
        173, *174*, 175, **175**
bioprosthetic dysfunction, 144–146, *145*,
        145, *146*

bioprosthetic regurgitation, immediately after mitral and tricuspid valve replacements, 168–170, *169, 170*
bioprosthetic valve, massively calcified, 197–199, *198*
bovine pericardial bioprosthetic valve implantation
    after double-valve replacement, 231, **232**, *232, 233,* 233–234
    anatomic studies, 140
    calcification, 136
    cotton fibers, 142
    histologic study, 137, *138*
    host factors and tissue factors, 140
    morphologic observations, 142
    patient history, 136–137
    scanning electron microscopic observations, 139–140, *169*
    transmission electron microscopic observations, 140, *141*
    ultrastructural studies, 140, 142

C

caged-ball prosthetic mitral valve, 85–87
    diagnostic imaging, 85
    patient history, 85–86
Candida organisms, 3, *4*
carcinoid heart disease
    autopsy, 31
    carcinoid plaques location, *260*
    cardiac valve replacement, 246
    clinical features, 262
    computed tomographic image, 262, *262*
    diagnostic imaging, *31,* 243–244, *261*
    electrocardiogram, *31*
    examination, 29–30, 244, *260*
    hemodynamic clues, 263
    histologic section of, 263
    patient history, 29–31, 240–241, 259–260
    pulmonary hypertension, 246
    pulmonic valve, *245,* 246
    QRS voltage on, 264
    surgical options, *241–242*
cardiac catheterization
    bicuspid aortic valve, 252
    bovine pericardial bioprostheses, 231, **232**
    caged-ball prosthetic mitral valve, 85, **87**
    carcinoid heart disease, 29
    combined mitral and aortic stenosis, double-valve replacement, 235
    congenitally bicuspid stenotic aortic valves, 200
    extensive multifocal myocardial infarcts, 182
    fatal bioprosthetic regurgitation, 168
    octogenarian, 221

pulmonary arteriovenous fistula, 35
severe coronary artery disease, 208
severe regurgitation, 205
severe stenosis, **181**
stent-post deformity, 144, **145**
traumatic aortic regurgitation, 14
cardiac valvular bioprosthesis, implantation after removal, *161*
    anatomic findings, 160–163
    cholesterol accumulation, 164
    crystalline material, 163, *163*
    morphologic observations, 164
    patient history, 160
cardiac valvular lesions, in rheumatoid arthritis, 59–66
central cyanosis, 35
chloroquine, disseminated *Petriellidium boydii,* 131
chlorothiazide, nonobstructive mesenteric arterial insufficiency, 40
chordae tendineae, *92*
combined mitral and aortic stenosis, double-valve replacement, 235, *236,* **237**, 237–238
computed tomography, 229, *229*–230
congenitally bicuspid stenotic aortic valves, 200–202, *201,* **201**
congestive heart failure, 158
coronary angiogram
    bicuspid aortic valve, 252
    bicuspid stenotic aortic valves, 200
corticosteroids and gluconeogenesis, 75
cor triatriatum
    concept of, 148
    development of, 151
    M-mode echocardiograms, *148*
    preoperative view, *148*
    ring abscess, 149
    surgical options, 149

D

diastolic murmur, 25
diffuse pericarditis, 76
digitoxin, nonobstructive mesenteric arterial insufficiency, 40
disseminated *Petriellidium boydii*
    diagnostic imaging, 131, *132*
    infections, 133
    with massive vegetations, 133
    patient history, 130–131
    treatment, 134

E

echocardiogram
    Alfieri Stitch, 266, *267*

aortic stenosis, sudden collapse in, 226
ascending aortic aneurysm, *123*
carcinoid heart disease, *261*
disseminated *Petriellidium boydii*, 131
nonbacterial thrombotic endocarditis,
    312, *314*
octogenarian, 221
orthotopic heart transplantation, 270, *271*
severe coronary artery disease, 208, *209*
severe regurgitation, 205
severe stenosis, **181**
Smeloff-Cutter ball-caged mitral valve, *249*
Starr-Edwards model 6120 mechanical
    prosthesis, 215
systemic hypertension, aortic
    regurgitation from, *155*
unicuspid aortic valve, 229
electrocardiogram
    active infective endocarditis, 305, *306*
    ankylosing spondylitis, 89
    aortic stenosis, sudden collapse in, 226
    ascending aortic aneurysm, 119, *121*
    caged-ball prosthetic mitral valve, 85
    carcinoid heart disease, *31, 261*
    congenitally bicuspid aortic valve, 99, *100*
    disseminated *Petriellidium boydii*, 131, *132*
    extensive multifocal myocardial
        infarcts, 182
    fatal bioprosthetic regurgitation, 168
    Marfan cardiovascular disease, 126
    orthotopic heart transplantation, 270, *271*
    prosthetic valve endocarditis, 105, *106*
    quadrivalvular rheumatoid heart
        disease, *51*
    rheumatic heart disease, *100*
    systemic hypertension, aortic
        regurgitation from, *154*
    traumatic aortic regurgitation, 11, *12*, 13
endocardial fibrous lesions, 29
endocarditis, *see* Libman-Sacks (L-S)
    endocarditis

F

fibrinoid necrosis, 3, *5–6*
fibrosis, 3, *5–6*
focal embolic (endocarditic)
    glomerulonephritis, 1, 6, 7, 8
    autopsy, 2–3, *3–6*, 6
    cause of, 7
    examination, 8
    in fungal endocarditis, 1, **8**
    hematuria associated with, 8
    incidence of, 8
    patient report, 1–2
    renal biopsy, 6–7
    uremia, 9

fungal endocarditis, 1, **8**, *see also*
    focal embolic (endocarditic)
    glomerulonephritis
fusiform ascending aortic aneurysm,
    119–129
    aortic root aneurysms of, 125–126
    cardiovascular features, 124
    dilatation of mitral anulus, 128
    hemodynamic and angiographic
        data, **120**
    operative treatment for, 127
    patient history, 119
    postoperative, 120, 122, *122*

G

glomerulonephritis, see *focal embolic
    (endocarditic) glomerulonephritis*
glomerular tufts, 6
glomerulus, *5, 6*
granuloma, cardiac rheumatoid, *56*

H

hyperglycemia, 74
hyperosmolar coma, 74
hypertension, aortic regurgitation from,
    152–156
    diagnostic imaging, *154*
    factors to develop, 156
    frequency and severity of, *153*
    patient history, 152
    systolic and diastolic systemic arterial
        pressures, *153*
hypoglycemia, 43

I

infective endocarditis
    aortic valve, 256
    causes of pericarditis, 310–311, **311**
    development of, 258
    patient history, 256–257, 309
    with ring abscess, 309
    stenotic aortic valve, 258
    surgery, 257, *257*
intestinal infarction, 39–44
Ionescu-Shiley bioprostheses, *170*

L

laparotomy, nonobstructive mesenteric
    arterial insufficiency, 44
left atrial endocardium, inflammatory
    nodule in, 69, *69*
left atrial thrombus, unattached, 186–188,
    187–189

left ventricular apical aneurysm, 158, *159*

left ventricular endocardium, 100
    with multiple typical Aschoff bodies, *102*

left ventricular false aneurysm, *see* cor
    triatriatum

left ventricular fibrous scar, 20, *21*

left ventricular systolic hypertension, 158, *159*

leptospirosis, 74

leukocytes, 8

Libman-Sacks (L-S) endocarditis, 279–282
    bioprosthesis viewed from, 280, *281*
    corticosteroid drug therapy, 282
    diagnosis, 279
    patient history, 279–280

lipid deposits, 160, 164

Listeria monocytogenes, 118

lupus erythematosus, 74

M

Marfan syndrome, 119–129, 274

medial cystic necrosis, 128–129

metabolic acidosis, 44

minocycline, ochronosis, 300

mitral annular calcium, 208–210, *209, 210*

mitral regurgitation, 88
    fusiform ascending aortic aneurysm,
        119–129
    immediately after mitral valve
        replacement, *166,* 166–167

mitral stenosis, 186–188, *187–189*

mitral valve leaflets, *92, 94*

mitral valve prolapse
    echocardiogram, 277
    evidence of, 277, *278*
    occurrence, 254–255
    patient history, 252, 276
    posterior leaflet, *253*
    surgery, **255**

mitral valves, *64*

myocardial contusion, 21

myocardial embolus, 27–28, *27–28*

myocardial infarcts, extensive multifocal,
    182–184, *183, 184*

myocardial rheumatoid granulomas, *64*

myocardium, 76, *78*

N

necropsy
    active infective endocarditis, 307
    alkaptonuric ochronosis, 190, *191*
    aortic stenosis, sudden collapse in, 226
    aortic valve stenosis, 158, *159*
    caged-ball prosthetic mitral valve, 85, 87
    cor triatriatum, 149
    disseminated *Petriellidium boydii*, 133

extensive multifocal myocardial
    infarcts, 183

fatal acute rheumatic fever, in childhood,
    67, 68

fatal bioprosthetic regurgitation, 168

focal embolic (endocarditic)
    glomerulonephritis, 2–3, *3–6*, 6

infective endocarditis, 309

intermittent aortic regurgitation, 96

Marfan cardiovascular disease, 124

mitral stenosis, 187
    prosthetic mitral valve obstruction,
        114, *115*
    prosthetic valve endocarditis,
        106–107, 117

rheumatoid arthritis, 61

severe coronary artery disease, *211*

severe mitral regurgitation, immediately
    after mitral valve replacement, 166

necrosis, 19
    of hepatic lobules, *42*
    fibrinoid, 3, *5–6*
    medial cystic, 128–129

neoantimosan, focal embolic (endocarditic)
    glomerulonephritis, 1

Nocardia asteroides, 47

nonbacterial thrombotic endocarditis
    (NBTE)
    aortic valve replacement, 312, **313**
    diagnostic imaging, 312, *314*
    examination, 314, *315*
    histology, 312
    patient history, 312

nondistensible right atrium, of carcinoid
    disease, 29–34

nonketotic coma, 74

nonobstructive mesenteric arterial
    insufficiency
    abdominal and cardiac
        manifestations, 42
    clinical differentiation, 42
    diagnostic differentiation of, 44
    intestinal ischemia of, 42
    laparotomy, 44
    optimal therapy, 44
    pathologic findings, 40–42
    patient report, 39–40
    physiologic abnormality, 42
    symptoms, 42

O

obstruction, to left ventricular outflow,
    194–196, *195*

ochronosis
    in atherosclerotic plaques, 300
    with black pigment, **296–298**, 299

clinical and cardiovascular findings, 295
morphologic findings, **299**
patient history, 295, 299
secondary form, 300
octogenarian, 200–202, *201*, **201**, 219, *220*, 221,
221, 235–238
orthotopic heart transplantation
aortic regurgitation, 272, 274
diagnostic imaging, 270, *271*
examination, 270
heart and kidney transplant, 272, *273*
laboratory findings, **272**
morphologic findings, 272, *274*
patient history, 270

P

pacemaker endocarditis, 130–134
penicillin
focal embolic (endocarditic)
glomerulonephritis, 1
nonobstructive mesenteric arterial
insufficiency, 40
pericarditis, causes of, 310–311, **311**
pericardium, 76, *76*
peripheral cyanosis, 35
pharyngitis, 73
phonocardiogram, intermittent aortic
regurgitation, *97*
polyarthritis, 73
precordial murmurs, 57
prednisolone, 73
prednisone, in disseminated *Petriellidium
boydii*, 130
prosthetic mitral valve obstruction, 114–115,
115
prosthetic valve endocarditis, 104–113
cause, 108
diagnostic imaging, 105, *106*
with early infection, 110
histologic examination, 118
late, 111
Listeria monocytogenes, 118
patient history, 104, 116
ring abscess, 112, 113
signs of, 111
Staphylococcus, 109, 110
Prussian blue stain, in tubular cells, 6
pullback pressure, from pulmonary
artery, *30*
pulmonary arteriovenous fistula
angiocardiography, 35
cardiac catheterization, 35
in lingular portion, *37*
patient report, 35, 36, *36*, *37*
roentgenograms, 35, *36*
pulmonary nocardiosis, diagnosis of, 47

Q

quadricuspidization, *177*, 177–178
quadrivalvular rheumatoid heart disease, **57**
diagnostic imaging, *51*
electrocardiogram, *51*
patient history, 49–50
roentgenograms, *50*

R

rheumatic heart disease
criterion of, 102
diagnostic imaging, *100*
examination, 99
laboratory study, 100
rheumatic mitral stenosis, 46, *46*, *47*
rheumatoid arthritis, 59, 274, *see also*
quadrivalvular rheumatoid heart
disease
patient summary, 59–60
rheumatoid nodules in, 63
valvular involvement in, 63, 65
rheumatoid granulomas, 55, 57
ring abscess, *109*, 112, 113
roentgenogram
ankylosing spondylitis, 89, *90*
ascending aortic aneurysm, *120*
caged-ball prosthetic mitral valve, 85
congenitally bicuspid aortic valve, 99, *100*
laboratory study, 100
prosthetic valve endocarditis, 104–105, *105*
pulmonary arteriovenous fistula, 35, *36*
quadrivalvular rheumatoid heart
disease, *50*
rheumatic heart disease, *100*
rheumatoid arthritis, 60
systemic hypertension, aortic
regurgitation from, *154*
traumatic aortic regurgitation, 11, *12*, 13, *13*

S

semilunar valves, *62*
severe coronary artery disease, 208–210,
209, *210*
severe regurgitation, 205–207, *206*
silicone rubber poppet, 80
similunar valvular cusp, in cardiac diseases, *66*
Smeloff-Cutter ball-caged mitral valve
ball variance, 248
durability of, 248
dysfunction, 250
implantation, **251**
in mitral position, *250*
patient history, 248
preoperative echocardiogram, *249*

Smeloff-Cutter mechanical prosthesis
    design, 284
    patient history, 284–285
    postmortem, *286, 287*
    radiograph, *285*
    "self-washing" effect, 285
Starr-Edwards prosthesis, *117,* 215, *216,*
        217–218
    lethal ball variance in, 80, 81
    autopsy, 81
    clinical features of, 84
    degeneration of, 80, 81
    patient history, 80–81
    period of implantation, 83–84
stent-post deformity
    left ventricular compression, 146, *146*
    mitral bioprostheses remove, *145*
    obstruction and reoperation, 146
Streptococcus sanguis, 233
streptomycin, in focal embolic (endocarditic)
        glomerulonephritis, 1
sulfonamides, in systemic nocardiosis, 47
syphilis, 93, 274
systemic arterial embolization, 27
systemic lupus erythematosus (SLE), 74
    with corticosteroids, 279
systemic nocardiosis, 47
systolic murmur, 13, 24, 29–30, 50, 59

T

teleoroentgenogram, pulmonary cavity, 47
thrombotic thrombocytopenic purpura, 74

thrombus, 186–188, *187–189*
trauma, nonpenetrating, 11
traumatic aortic regurgitation
    autopsy, 21, 24
    cardiac catheterization, 14
    clinical features, 25
    clinical features of, 24–25
    diagnostic imaging, 11, *12,* 13
    electrocardiograms, 11, *12,* 13
    microscopic findings, 19–20, *19–21*
    pathologic findings, 15–17, *18*
    patient history, 11
    physical examination, 13, 24–25
    retrograde aortography, 14
    roentgenogram, 11, *12,* 13, *13*
    surgical findings, 14, *14–17,* 15
    surgical treatment for, 25
tricuspid regurgitation, 32
tricuspid valve, 55
    vegetation, *132*
tubules, 6

U

unicuspid aortic valve, *229,* 229–230

V

valvular heart disease, **237**
vasculitis, 65
ventricular septum, cephalad
        portion of, *54*
verrucae, 76

Printed in the United States
by Baker & Taylor Publisher Services